INTEGRATIVE MEDICINE AND FUNCTIONAL MEDICINE FOR CHRONIC HYPERTENSION:

AN EVIDENCE-BASED MONOGRAPH ON THE TREATMENT OF HIGH BLOOD PRESSURE

Dietary, Nutritional, Botanical, Surgical, and Manipulative Therapeutics
with Concepts, Perspectives, Algorithms, and Protocols for
the Safe and Effective Management of Chronic High Blood Pressure

DR. ALEX VASQUEZ

- Doctor of Osteopathic Medicine, graduate of University of North Texas Health Science Center, Texas College of Osteopathic Medicine (May 2010)
- Doctor of Naturopathic Medicine, graduate of Bastyr University (September 1999). Licensed Naturopathic Physician with Additional Prescriptive Authority in Washington (2000-2002), Licensed Naturopathic Physician in Oregon (2004-present)
- Doctor of Chiropractic, graduate of Western States Chiropractic College (March 1996). Licensed Doctor of Chiropractic, Washington (1996-2002) and Texas (2002-present)
- Director of the Medical Board of Advisors (2011-present), Researcher and Lecturer (2004-2010), Biotics Research Corporation in Rosenberg, Texas
- Adjunct Faculty (2004-2005, 2010-2011) and Former Forum Consultant (2003-2007), The Institute for Functional Medicine in Gig Harbor, Washington
- Affiliate Faculty, University of Western States in Portland, Oregon
- Former Adjunct Professor of Orthopedics (2000) and Rheumatology (2001), Bastyr University in Kenmore, Washington
- Former Editor (2006-2007), *Naturopathy Digest*
- Private practice of chiropractic and naturopathic medicine in Seattle, Washington (2000-2001) and Houston, Texas (2001-2006) and practice of naturopathic medicine in Oregon (2011-present)
- Author of approximately 80 articles and letters published in *Annals of Pharmacotherapy, The Lancet, Nutritional Perspectives, BMJ (British Medical Journal), Journal of Manipulative and Physiological Therapeutics, JAMA (Journal of the American Medical Association), The Original Internist, Integrative Medicine: A Clinician's Journal, Holistic Primary Care, Nutritional Wellness, Dynamic Chiropractic, Alternative Therapies in Health and Medicine, Journal of the American Osteopathic Association, Evidence-based Complementary and Alternative Medicine, Journal of Clinical Endocrinology and Metabolism*, and *Arthritis & Rheumatism*: Official Journal of the American College of Rheumatology

OPTIMALHEALTHRESEARCH.COM

Vasquez A. <u>Integrative Medicine and Functional Medicine for Chronic Hypertension</u>.
Integrative and Biological Medicine Research and Consulting, LLC
Austin, Texas and Portland, Oregon
10-Digit ISBN: 1451515715
13-Digit EAN: 9781451515718

See website for updated information: www.OptimalHealthResearch.com

The intended audiences for this book are health science students and doctorate-level clinicians. This book has been written with every intention to make it as accurate as possible, and each section has undergone peer-review by an interdisciplinary group of clinicians. In view of the possibility of human error and as well as ongoing discoveries in the biomedical sciences, neither the author nor any party associated in any way with this text warrants that this text is perfect, accurate, or complete in every way, and we disclaim responsibility for harm or loss associated with the application of the material herein. Information and treatments applicable to a specific *condition* may not be appropriate for or applicable to a specific *patient*; this is especially true for patients with multiple comorbidities and those taking pharmaceutical medications with multiple adverse effects and drug/nutrient/herb interactions. Given that this book is available on an open market, lay persons who read this material should discuss the information with a licensed healthcare provider before implementing the treatments and interventions described herein.

Dedications: I dedicate this book to the following people in appreciation for their works, their direct and indirect support of this work, and for their contributions to the advancement of authentic healthcare.

- **To the students and practitioners of chiropractic, naturopathic, and functional medicine**, those who continue to learn so that they can provide the best possible care to their patients.
- **To the researchers** whose works are cited in this text.
- **To Drs Alan Gaby, Jeffrey Bland, Ronald LeFebvre, Robert Richard, and Gilbert Manso,** my most memorable and influential professors and mentors.
- **To Dr Bruce Ames**[1] **and the late Dr Roger Williams**[2], for helping us to view our individuality as biochemically unique.
- **To Dr Chester Wilk**[3,4] **and important others** for documenting and resisting the organized oppression of natural, non-pharmaceutical, non-surgical healthcare.[5,6,7]
- **To my friends, family, supporters, and 'enlightened witnesses', particularly Erika**, Dr Foster, and Carl Robert, who—at a critical time—helped the self-rolling wheel to keep rolling, and who collectively helped solve a most puzzling conundrum.
- **To Jorge Strunz, Ardeshir Farah, Friedrich Nietzsche, Gilberto Gil,** for artistic inspiration.

Acknowledgments for Peer and Editorial Review: Acknowledgement here does not imply that the reviewer fully agrees with or endorses the material in this text but rather that they were willing to review specific sections of the book for clinical applicability and clarity and to make suggestions to their own level of satisfaction. Credit for improvements and refinements to this text are due in part to these reviewers; responsibility for oversights remains that of the author.

- 2011 Edition of *Integrative Medicine and Functional Medicine for Chronic Hypertension*: Erika Mennerick DC, Holly Furlong DC, JoAnn Fawcett DC, Ileana Bourland MSOM LAc, James Bogash DC, Bill Beakey
- 2010 Edition of *Chiropractic Management of Chronic Hypertension*: Joseph Paun MS DC, Joe Brimhall DC, David Candelario OMS4 (TCOM c/o 2010), James Bogash DC, Robert Richard DO, Bill Beakey
- 2009 Edition of *Chiropractic and Naturopathic Mastery of Common Clinical Disorders*: Heather Kahn MD, Robert Richard DO, James Leiber DO, David Candelario (UNT-HSC TCOM DO4)
- 2007 Edition of *Integrative Orthopedics*: Barry Morgan MD, Dennis Harris DC, Richard Brown DC (DACBI candidate), Ron Mariotti ND, Patrick Makarewich MBA, Reena Singh (SCNM ND4), Zachary Watkins DC, Charles Novak MS DC, Marnie Loomis ND, James Bogash DC, Sara Croteau DC, Kris Young DC, Joshua Levitt ND, Jack Powell III MD, Chad Kessler MD, Amy Neuzil ND
- 2006 Edition of *Integrative Rheumatology*: Amy Neuzil ND, Cathryn Harbor MD, Julian Vickers DC, Tamara Sachs MD, Bob Sager BSc MD DABFM (Clinical Instructor in the Department of Family Medicine, University of Kansas), Ron Mariotti ND, Titus Chiu (DC4), Zachary Watkins (DC4), Gilbert Manso MD, Bruce Milliman ND, William Groskopp DC, Robert Silverman DC, Matthew Breske (DC4), Dean Neary ND, Thomas Walton DC, Fraser Smith ND, Ladd Carlston DC, David Jones MD, Joshua Levitt ND
- 2004 Edition of *Integrative Orthopedics*: Peter Knight ND, Kent Littleton ND MS, Barry Morgan MD, Ron Hobbs ND, Joshua Levitt ND, John Neustadt (Bastyr ND4), Allison Gandre BS (Bastyr ND4), Peter Kimble ND, Jack Powell III MD, Chad Kessler MD, Mike Gruber MD, Deirdre O'Neill ND, Mary Webb ND, Leslie Charles ND, Amy Neuzil ND

---

[1] Ames BN, Elson-Schwab I, Silver EA. High-dose vitamin therapy stimulates variant enzymes with decreased coenzyme binding affinity (increased K(m)): relevance to genetic disease and polymorphisms. *Am J Clin Nutr.* 2002 Apr;75(4):616-58 http://www.ajcn.org/cgi/content/full/75/4/616

[2] Williams RJ. *Biochemical Individuality: The Basis for the Genetotrophic Concept.* Austin and London: University of Texas Press; 1956

[3] Wilk CA. *Medicine, Monopolies, and Malice: How the Medical Establishment Tried to Destroy Chiropractic.* Garden City Park: Avery, 1996

[4] Getzendanner S. Permanent injunction order against AMA. *JAMA* 1988 Jan 1;259(1):81-2 http://optimalhealthresearch.com/archives/wilk.html

[5] Carter JP. *Racketeering in Medicine: The Suppression of Alternatives.* Norfolk: Hampton Roads Pub; 1993

[6] Morley J, Rosner AL, Redwood D. A case study of misrepresentation of the scientific literature: recent reviews of chiropractic. *J Altern Complement Med.* 2001 Feb;7(1):65-78

[7] Terrett AG. Misuse of the literature by medical authors in discussing spinal manipulative therapy injury. *J Manipulative Physiol Ther.* 1995 May;18(4):203-10

Format and Layout: The format and layout of this book is designed to efficiently take the reader though the clinically relevant spectrum of considerations for each condition that is detailed. Important topics are given their own section within each chapter, while other less important or less common conditions are only described briefly in terms of the four "clinical essentials" of 1) definition/pathophysiology, 2) clinical presentation, 3) assessment/diagnosis, and 4) treatment/management. Each expanded section which details the more important/common conditions maintains a consistent format, taking the reader through the spectrum of primary clinical considerations: definition/pathophysiology, clinical presentations, differential diagnoses, assessments (physical examination, laboratory, imaging), complications, management, and treatment. As my books have progressed, I am increasingly using an article-by-article review format (especially in the sections on management and treatment) so that readers have more direct access to the information so as to understand and *incorporate* more deeply what the research actually states; the goal and general approach here is to use a *representative sampling* of the research literature.

> **Newsletter & Updates**
> Be alerted to new integrative clinical research and updates to this textbook by signing-up for the free newsletter, sent several times per year as needed. Join at:
> www.OptimalHealthResearch.com/newsletter

References and Citations: Citations to articles, abstracts, texts, and personal communications are footnoted throughout the text to provide supporting information and to provide interested readers the resources to find additional information. Many of the cited articles are available on-line for free, and when possible I have included the website addresses so that readers can access the complete article.

Peer-review and Quality Control: Peer-review is essential to help ensure accuracy and clinical applicability of health-related information. Consistent with the importance of our goals, I have employed several "checks and balances" to increase the accuracy and applicability of the information within my textbooks:

- Reliance upon authoritative references: Nearly all important statements are referenced to peer-reviewed biomedical journals or authoritative texts, such as *The Merck Manual* and *Current Medical Diagnosis and Treatment*. Each citation is provided by a footnote at the bottom of each page so that readers will know quickly and easily exactly from where the information was obtained.
- Extensive cross-referencing: Readers will notice, if not be overwhelmed by, the number of references and citations. Many important statements have several references. Many references (especially textbooks) are referenced several times even on the same page. The purpose of this extensive referencing is three-fold: 1) to guide you to additional information, 2) to help me (as writer) stay organized, and 3) to help you and me (the practicing physicians) employ this information with confidence.
- Periodic revision: All of my books will be updated and revised on an *as-needed* basis. New information is added; superfluous information removed. Inspired by the popular text *Current Medical Diagnosis and Treatment* which is updated every year, I want my books to be accurate, timely, and in pace with the ever-growing literature on natural medicine. Any significant errors that are discovered will be posted at OptimalHealthResearch.com/updates; please

check this page periodically to ensure that you are working with the most accurate information of which I am aware.

- Peer-review: The peer-review process for my books takes several forms. First, colleagues and students are invited to review new and revised sections of the text before publication; every section of the book that you are holding has been independently reviewed by health science students and/or practicing clinicians from various backgrounds: allopathic, chiropractic, osteopathic, naturopathic. Second, you - the reader - are invited to provide feedback about the information in the book, typographical errors, syntax, case reports, new research, etc. If your ideas truly change the nature of the material, I will be glad to acknowledge you in the text (with your permission, of course). If your contribution is hugely significant, such as reviewing three or more chapters or helping in some important way, I will be glad to not only acknowledge you, but to also send you the next edition at a discount or courtesy when your ideas take effect. Third, I keep abreast of new literature by constantly perusing new research and advancements in the health sciences. Having been successful in three separate doctoral programs in the health sciences, I have learned not only to master large amounts of material but to also separate and integrate different viewpoints as appropriate. I also "field test" my protocols with patients in the various clinical arenas in which I work and also with professionals and academicians via presentations and critical dialogue. By implementing these quality control steps, I hope to create a useful text and advance our professions and our practices by improving the quality of care that we deliver to our patients. Readers with suggestions or corrections can email via the website: http://OptimalHealthResearch.com/corrections.

How to Use This Book Safely and Most Effectively: Ideally, these books should be read cover-to-cover within a context of coursework that is supervised by an experienced professor. For post-graduate professionals, they might consider forming a local "book club" and meeting for weekly or monthly discussions to check their understandings and share their clinical experiences to refine the application of clinical knowledge, perceptions, and skills. Virtual groups and internet forums—specifically the forum hosted by the Institute for Functional Medicine at www.FunctionalMedicine.org—can provide access to an assembly of international professional peers wherein sharing of clinical questions and experiences are synergistic. Throughout this book, references are amply provided and are often footnoted with hyperlinks providing full-text access. This book is intended for licensed doctorate-level healthcare professionals with graduate and post-graduate training.

Notice: The intention and scope of this text are to provide doctorate-level clinicians with useful information and a familiarity with available research and resources pertinent to the management of patients in an integrative primary care setting. Specifically, the information in this book is intended to be used by licensed healthcare professionals who have received hands-on clinical training and supervision at accredited health science colleges. Additionally, information in this book should be used in conjunction with other resources, texts, and in combination with the clinician's best judgment and intention to *"first, do no harm"* and second to provide effective healthcare. Information and treatments applicable to a specific *condition* may not be appropriate for or applicable to a specific *patient* in your office; this is especially true for patients with multiple comorbidities and those taking pharmaceutical medications with multiple adverse effects and drug/nutrient/herb interactions. Throughout this text, I describe treatments—manual, dietary, nutritional, botanical, pharmacologic, and occasionally surgical—and their research support for the clinical condition being discussed; each practitioner must determine appropriateness of these treatments for his/her individual patient and with consideration of the doctor's scope of practice, education, training, skill, and the appropriateness of "off label" use of medications and treatments. This book has been carefully written and checked for accuracy by the author and professional colleagues. However, in view of the possibility of human error and new discoveries in the biomedical sciences, neither the author nor any party associated in any way with this text warrants that this text is perfect, accurate, or complete in every way, and we disclaim responsibility for harm or loss associated with the application of the material herein. With all conditions/treatments described herein, each physician must be sure to consider the balance between what is best for the patient and the physician's own level of ability, expertise, and experience. When in doubt, or if the physician is not a specialist in the treatment of a given severe condition, referral is appropriate. These notes are written with the routine "outpatient" in mind and are not tailored to severely injured patients or "playing field" or "emergency response" situations. Consult your First Aid and Emergency Response texts and course materials for appropriate information. These notes represent the author's perspective based on academic education, experience, and post-graduate continuing education and are not inclusive of every fact that a clinician may need to know. This is not an "entry level" book except when used in an academic setting with a knowledgeable professor who can explain the concepts, tests, physical exam procedures, and treatments; this book requires a certain level of knowledge from the reader and familiarity with clinical concepts, laboratory assessments, and physical examination procedures.

Updates, Corrections, and Newsletter: When and if omissions, errata, and the need for important updates become clear, I will post these at the website: OptimalHealthResearch.com/updates. A reader might access this page periodically to ensure staying informed of any corrections that might have clinical relevance. This book consists not only of the text in the printed pages you are holding, but also the footnotes and any updates at the website. Be alerted to new integrative clinical research and updates to this textbook by signing-up for the free newsletter at www.OptimalHealthResearch.com/newsletter.

Preface to the 2009 Edition of *Chiropractic and Naturopathic Mastery of Common Clinical Disorders*: *Chiropractic and Naturopathic Mastery of Common Clinical Disorders* steps beyond the obviously musculoskeletal focus of my first three textbooks *Integrative Orthopedics*, *Integrative Rheumatology*, and *Musculoskeletal Pain: Expanded Clinical Strategies* to provide students and clinicians an evidence-based foundational approach to treating common clinical disorders such as Asthma, Hypertension, Diabetes Mellitus Type-2 and Metabolic Syndrome, and Disorders of Mood and Behavior—a section that emphasizes adult depression and anxiety. Readers of these sections and the works derived from them (e.g., the chapter on hypertension was expanded into the book *Chiropractic Management of Chronic Hypertension* and later *Integrative Medicine and Functional Medicine for Chronic Hypertension*) will note that they differ in format from the other chapters with regard to a stronger emphasis on presenting an article-by-article review in the effort to strengthen the evidence-based nature of the clinical protocols. As with my previous books and all other clinical resources, clinicians should still consult other sources and texts for additional information, updated guidelines, and changes to standards of care. The goal of *Chiropractic and Naturopathic Mastery of Common Clinical Disorders* has been to further bridge the gap that continues to exist between so-called "complementary and alternative medicine" (CAM) and so-called "conventional" medicine.[8]

The Functional Medicine Matrix (version presented in 2003): In *Chiropractic and Naturopathic Mastery of Common Clinical Disorders*, I (re)introduced the Functional Medicine Matrix that I originally diagramed for the Institute for Functional Medicine (IFM) in 2003; the diagram used is updated from the original, and readers should appreciate that IFM has changed the Matrix since this version was made. My perspective is that functional medicine, naturopathic medicine, and *authentic* holistic medicine share much in common in their fundamental models of health and disease. The functional medicine matrix—designed and owned by the Institute for Functional Medicine (FunctionalMedicine.org)—is unique to the discipline functional medicine and provides a conceptual framework for understanding the complexity of health and disease.

2003 Version of the Functional Medicine Matrix: Updated from the original diagram by Vasquez in 2003 for the Institute for Functional Medicine (IFM). See www.FunctionalMedicine.org for updated information and additional training.

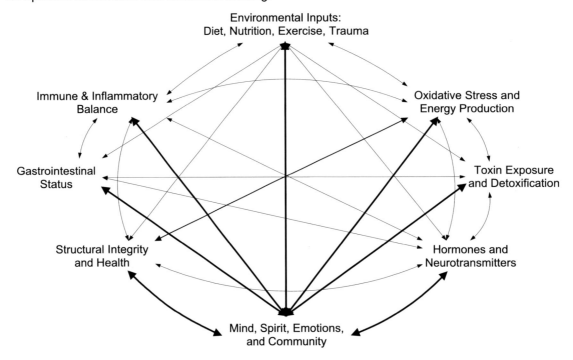

Distinguishing "Integrative Medicine" from "Functional Medicine"—the author's perspective[9]: The distinction of integrative medicine from functional medicine is that of *quantity* from *quality*. Integrative medicine can be understood as a quantitative extension of other already-

---

[8] MacIntosh A. Understanding the Differences between Conventional, Alternative, Complementary, Integrative and Natural Medicine. *Townsend Letter*, July 1999. http://www.tldp.com/medicine.htm Accessed March 2011
[9] Dr Vasquez's perspective: I have trained in functional medicine since 1994, first as a student of Jeffrey Bland PhD *et al* and later as Forum Consultant and Faculty (2003 – present in 2011) for the Institute of Functional Medicine, and I wrote three chapters in *Textbook of Functional Medicine* published by Institute of Functional Medicine. My opinions here are not necessarily currently representative of the Institute of Functional Medicine in this context.

existing healthcare models, to which additional perspectives and treatments are added; in this way, various conceptual models are "integrated" and used together in a more holistic and comprehensive approach. In contrast, functional medicine is a distinct model of health and disease that has developed an identity beyond mere integration of various models and treatments. Functional medicine is qualitatively distinct in its viewpoint of disease causation and treatment by the unique combination of emphases placed on ❶ patient-centered care (in contrast to the disease-centered care of allopathic medicine and most osteopathic medicine), ❷ detailed appreciation of the importance of the web-like interconnected nature of various organ systems[10] and psychological, physiological, and pathological processes (to a greater extent than allopathic, osteopathic, chiropractic and naturopathic medicine), ❸ its rigorous evidence-based standards, and ❹ its willingness to eagerly-yet-appropriately include *all* therapeutic options, ranging from (for example) surgical to meditative, dietary to pharmaceutical, manipulative to botanical, and antidysbiotic to psychological. In short, functional medicine can be described as an ***antiparadigmatic patient-centered discipline***, hence its therapeutic flexibility, broad applicability, and enhanced efficacy; it is antiparadigmatic due to its lack of adherence to a specific and limited set of tools (most professional disciplines are quite limited in their expertise and scope) and due to the emphasis placed on patient-centered healthcare, which first and always foremost seeks to determine the most efficient path for patient empowerment and healing.

Unofficial Functional Medicine Matrix of High Blood Pressure (Hypertension):

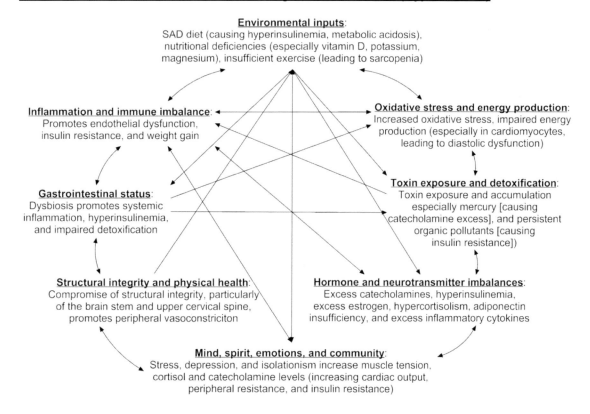

Environmental inputs:
SAD diet (causing hyperinsulinemia, metabolic acidosis), nutritional deficiencies (especially vitamin D, potassium, magnesium), insufficient exercise (leading to sarcopenia)

Oxidative stress and energy production:
Increased oxidative stress, impaired energy production (especially in cardiomyocytes, leading to diastolic dysfunction)

Inflammation and immune imbalance:
Promotes endothelial dysfunction, insulin resistance, and weight gain

Toxin exposure and detoxification:
Toxin exposure and accumulation especially mercury [causing catecholamine excess], and persistent organic pollutants [causing insulin resistance])

Gastrointestinal status:
Dysbiosis promotes systemic inflammation, hyperinsulinemia, and impaired detoxification

Structural integrity and physical health:
Compromise of structural integrity, particularly of the brain stem and upper cervical spine, promotes peripheral vasoconstriciton

Hormone and neurotransmitter imbalances:
Excess catecholamines, hyperinsulinemia, excess estrogen, hypercortisolism, adiponectin insufficiency, and excess inflammatory cytokines

Mind, spirit, emotions, and community:
Stress, depression, and isolationism increase muscle tension, cortisol and catecholamine levels (increasing cardiac output, peripheral resistance, and insulin resistance)

---

[10] **Vasquez A**. Web-like Interconnections of Physiological Factors. *Integrative Medicine: A Clinician's Journal* 2006, April/May, 32-37

Health problems for which patients most often seek CAM treatment are listed in the illustration below from National Center for Complementary and Alternative Medicine, NIH, DHHS (http://nccam.nih.gov/news/camstats/2007/graphics.htm). The table on the following page provides a listing—in order of percentage—of the most common conditions seen in a general family practice of medicine, with hypertension and diabetes mellitus—two conditions highly amenable to integrative therapeutics—clearly dominating the clinical landscape.

Diseases/Conditions for Which CAM Is Most Frequently Used Among Adults - 2007

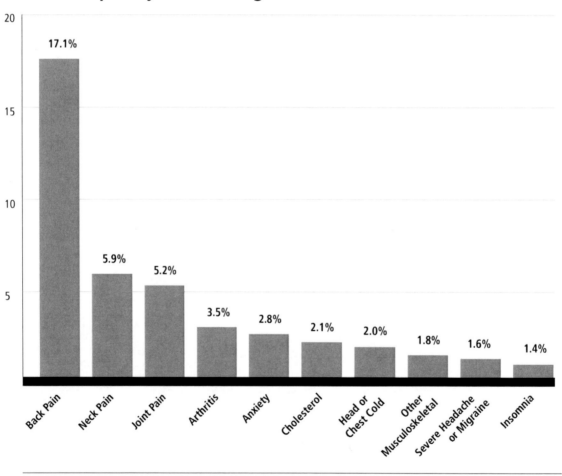

Source: Barnes PM, Bloom B, Nahin R. *CDC National Health Statistics Report #12*. Complementary and Alternative Medicine Use Among Adults and Children: United States, 2007. December 2008.

Top diagnoses	Notes and comments
1. Hypertension	**5.9% of family medicine diagnoses; nearly 11 million patient visits per year.**
2. Diabetes mellitus	4.1% of family medicine diagnoses; more than 7.6 million patient visits per year.
3. Acute upper respiratory infection	3.2% of family medicine diagnoses; more than 10 million patient visits per year. Most of these are caused by viral infections for which there is no direct medical treatment; most patients are treated symptomatically with decongestants and antipyretics. Complications are rare but can be serious.
4. Sinusitis	2.5% of family medicine diagnoses; more than 10 million patient visits per year.
5. Acute pharyngitis	2.3% of family medicine diagnoses; more than 4 million patient visits per year.
6. Otitis media	2.3% of family medicine diagnoses; > 4 million patient visits per year.
7. Bronchitis	1.9% of family medicine diagnoses; > 3 million patient visits per year.
8. Back problems	1.8% of family medicine diagnoses; > 3 million patient visits per year. This is a diverse group of conditions ranging from post-traumatic to benign to developmental problems such as scoliosis. Note that back pain is listed separately below.
9. Hyperlipidemia	1.7% of family medicine diagnoses; > 3 million patient visits per year. This mostly includes the lifestyle-generated dyslipidemia epidemic, with comparably fewer cases of genotropic disorders requiring pharmacotherapy.
10. Urinary tract disorders	1.6% of family medicine diagnoses; almost 3 million patient visits per year. This can include a diverse group of problems ranging from simple and self-limited urinary tract infections to sexually transmitted diseases; these are not covered in this text.
11. Allergic rhinitis	1.2% of family medicine diagnoses; > 2 million patient visits per year. A general approach to allergy treatment is included in this text.
12. Back pain	1.2% of family medicine diagnoses; > 2 million patient visits per year.
13. Abdominal or pelvic symptoms	1.1% of family medicine diagnoses; > 2 million patient visits per year. This can include a wide range of diagnoses ranging from appendicitis to dysmenorrhea. Due to the breadth and complexity, these are not covered in this text.
14. Joint pain	1.1% of family medicine diagnoses; > 2 million patient visits per year.
15. Depression or anxiety	1.1% of family medicine diagnoses; > 2 million patient visits per year. These are mostly mild cases but can also include acute situations that warrant emergency treatment including pharmacotherapy and sedation.
16. Asthma	1.1% of family medicine diagnoses; almost 2 million patient visits per year. An approach to allergy treatment is included in this text, with a section on asthma.
17. Chest pain or shortness of breath	1.1% of family medicine diagnoses; almost 2 million patient visits per year. Some of these are benign musculoskeletal pain or gastroesophageal reflux while others turn out to be life-threatening conditions such as myocardial infarction, pneumothorax, pneumonia, or—rarely—aortic dissection. These are not directly covered in this text.
18. Soft tissue problems	1% of family medicine diagnoses; 1.8 million patient visits per year.
19. Acute bronchitis and bronchiolitis	1% of family medicine diagnoses; 1.8 million patient visits per year. These include bacterial and viral infections, ranging from mild to life-threatening, especially in patients with cardiopulmonary disease.
20. Skin problems	1% of family medicine diagnoses; 1.8 million patient visits per year. Dermatology is not specifically covered in this text except for the chapter on psoriasis. Many patients will benefit from the diet and nutrition protocols described herein.
21. Tendonitis	1% of family medicine diagnoses; 1.7 million patient visits per year.

Data from *Essentials of Family Medicine, 5th edition* edited by Sloane PD, Slatt LM, Ebell MH, Jacques LB, Smith MA published by Lippincott Williams & Wilkins (April 1, 2007)

Introduction to the Hypertension Monograph: In addition to the clinical "front line" information tailored to practicing healthcare providers, this monograph explores a few perspectives which have implications beyond the clinical setting:

1. **The management of chronic hypertension should be *biological*[11] and *integrative* rather than *drug-based*, and clinicians should more frequently utilize natural interventions rather than those sponsored by and leveraged by drug companies**. At present, nondrug care of the chronically hypertensive patient is marginalized to an "alternative and complementary" role, while drug treatment is considered the "standard of care"; this is paradoxical considering that chronic hypertension is generally known to be a Western/industrial lifestyle disease that is avoidable with a lifestyle that pursues wellness and that is amenable to nutritional and physical (i.e., nondrug) interventions. The [allopathic] medical profession has taken *and has been leveraged into* a leadership position for the management of chronic hypertension based on research funded mostly by drug companies and published in journals which reap millions of dollars by selling reprints of drug-endorsing studies.[12,13] A vicious cycle of symbiosis is maintained between drug companies and the medical profession: drug companies publish research extolling the merits of drugs which are available only via medical

> ### Pro-pharmaceutical bias and the molding of antihypertensive prescription practices
>
> "Clinical trials influenced by the corporate bias have been the basis for a massive strategy of promotion of blood pressure drugs that resulted in the shaping of prescription practices departing from the best evidence."
>
> Fuchs FD. The corporate bias and the molding of prescription practices: the case of hypertension. *Braz J Med Biol Res*. 2009 Mar;42(3):224-8

doctors; thus any "therapeutic advancement" (legitimate or not) is an opportunity for sales by the drug company for its product (i.e., the drug) as well as an opportunity for sales by the medical profession for its service (i.e., the office visit, exams, follow-up labs, and return visits). Illegal in nearly every country in the world, direct-to-consumer drug advertising is allowed in the United States and "regulated" by the American Medical Association via a policy that endorses the activity while noting "**direct-to-consumer advertising of pharmaceutical products increases the demand for specific medications**" and "**the major pharmaceutical companies now spend approximately twice as much on 'marketing and administration' as they spend on 'research and development'**"—such expenses on advertising were approximately $25 billion in 2003.[14] Clinicians of all disciplines who have wanted a comprehensive guide to the *natural* nondrug treatment of hypertension have needed a clinical guide founded on evidence, but heretofore no such text existed. This monograph serves to fill that void by providing integrative clinicians with ❶ an overview of the disease, ❷ its differential diagnoses and comprehensive clinical assessments (including: history, physical examination, laboratory and imaging), and ❸ clear evidence-based treatment protocols and interventional options. Many nondrug treatments from nutritional supplementation to physical medicine and spinal manipulation can safely reduce elevated blood pressure with cost-effectiveness and safety profiles superior to drug treatment.

---

[11] "Bio-logical" (i.e., the logic of life, or wisdom in accord with life) in this context implies working with the logic of physiology and life by optimizing function rather than using symptom-blocking chemicals to mask the expression of disordered physiology that has become errant largely due to discord between Western/industrialized lifestyles and inherent physiologic needs and expectations.

[12] Fuchs FD. The corporate bias and the molding of prescription practices: the case of hypertension. *Braz J Med Biol Res*. 2009 Mar;42(3):224-8

[13] Smith R. Medical journals are an extension of the marketing arm of pharmaceutical companies. *PLoS Med*. 2005 May;2(5):e138

[14] American Academy of Child and Adolescent Psychiatry American Psychiatric Association. Direct-to-consumer Advertising of Pharmaceutical Products. http://www.aacap.org/galleries/LegislativeAction/Direct-to-Consumer_Advertising.pdf Accessed September 4, 2010

2. **Medical (drug-based) management of hypertension is by no means a panacea, leaving significant numbers of patients untreated, undertreated, or mistreated**. According to recent peer-reviewed research, shortcomings in the medical management of hypertension place patients at high risk of adverse effects, inefficacy, and unnecessary expense. By generally failing to address the underlying causes of high blood pressure and by failing to treat the constellation of comorbid conditions (e.g., insulin resistance, obesity, hyperuricemia, and nutritional deficiencies), medical management of hypertension that focuses with near exclusivity on the numeric reduction of elevated blood pressure cannot be viewed as optimal therapy.

Evidence sample from *New England Journal of Medicine* in 2003: The data from this study show that the medical profession leaves many hypertensive patients untreated and undertreated. Specifically, profession-wide deficiencies were noted in the following areas:
❶ Lifestyle modification for patients with mild hypertension: ***underused***
❷ Change in treatment when blood pressure is persistently uncontrolled: ***underused***
❸ Pharmacotherapy for uncontrolled mild hypertension: ***underused***
The authors wrote, "METHODS: We telephoned a random sample of adults living in 12 metropolitan areas [initial sample: n=20,028] in the United States and asked them about selected health care experiences. We also received written consent to copy their medical records for the most recent two-year period and used this information to evaluate performance on 439 indicators of quality of care for 30 acute and chronic conditions as well as preventive care. We then constructed aggregate scores. RESULTS: **Participants received 54.9 percent (95 percent confidence interval, 54.3 to 55.5) of recommended care**. … CONCLUSIONS: **The deficits we have identified in adherence to recommended processes for basic care pose serious threats to the health of the American public**. Strategies to reduce these deficits in care are warranted."[15]

Evidence sample from *Milbank Quarterly—A Multidisciplinary Journal of Population Health and Health Policy* in 1998: The authors review pertinent literature on healthcare quality and note that among Americans only "41%–54% of patients had their hypertension controlled (mean blood pressure (150/90)." By weak criteria of HTN control, 55% of people with hypertension had blood pressure "under control" with pressures of 160/95 treated with at least one antihypertensive medication; when using more strict medical criteria (achievement medicated blood pressure of 140/90) only 21% of Americans were properly treated. **On average, medical care provided only 41%–54% of the appropriate treatment for HTN**—note that these criteria do *not* include evidence-based nutritional interventions such as fish oil supplementation which has been shown to reduce cardiovascular mortality more effectively and cost-effectively than the "approved" drugs and medical treatments. The authors conclude, "Studies over the past decade show that some people are receiving more care than they need, and some are receiving less. Simple averages from a number of studies indicate that 50 percent of people received recommended preventive care; 70 percent, recommended acute care; 30 percent, contraindicated acute care; 60 percent, recommended chronic care; and 20 percent, contraindicated chronic care. **These studies strongly suggest that the [medical] care delivered in the United States often does not meet professional standards**."[16]

---

[15] McGlynn EA, Asch SM, Adams J, Keesey J, Hicks J, DeCristofaro A, Kerr EA. The quality of health care delivered to adults in the United States. *N Engl J Med*. 2003 Jun 26;348(26):2635-45
[16] Schuster MA, McGlynn EA, Brook RH. How good is the quality of health care in the United States? *Milbank Q*. 1998;76(4):517-63

> Evidence sample regarding "The corporate bias and the molding of prescription practices: the case of hypertension" published in 2009: In this review article, the author provides several examples of glaring divergences between the raw data from antihypertensive research and the frequently misguided policies and practices that result. "**Drug management of hypertension has been a noticeable example of the influence of the pharmaceutical industry on prescription practices**. … Commercial strategies have been based on the results of clinical trials sponsored by drug companies. Most of them presented distortions in their planning, presentation or interpretation that favored the drugs from the sponsor, i.e., corporate bias. Atenolol, an ineffective blood pressure agent in elderly individuals, was the comparator drug in several trials. In a re-analysis of the INSIGHT trial, deaths appeared to have been counted twice. The LIFE trial appears in the title of more than 120 reproductions of **the main and flawed trial, as a massive strategy of scientific marketing. Most guidelines have incorporated the corporate bias from the original studies,** and the evidence from better designed studies, such as the ALLHAT trial, have been largely ignored. In trials published recently corporate influences have touched on ethical limits. In the ADVANCE trial, elderly patients with type 2 diabetes and cardiovascular disease or risk factors, allocated to placebo, were not allowed to use diuretic and full doses of an ACE inhibitor, despite the sound evidence of benefit demonstrated in previous trials. As a consequence, they had a 14% higher mortality rate than the participants allocated to the active treatment arm. This reality should be modified immediately, and a greater independence of the academy from the pharmaceutical industry is necessary."[17]

3. **Because hypertension is a major patient-centered and public health concern, healthcare providers must have an evidence-based treatment protocol that includes instruction on how to use diet, nutritional supplements, and other nondrug interventions**. Chronic hypertension is a "disease" of epidemic and indeed pandemic proportions in America and increasingly in other nations. The lifetime incidence of high blood pressure among Americans is 90%, while on any given day, approximately one-in-three to one-in-four Americans has high blood pressure. These patients and potential patients would benefit more from integrative care and the nutrition-based protocols in this text than they can hope to benefit from drug-only treatment. **The evidence supporting the lifestyle and nutritional prevention and treatment of chronic primary hypertension is irrefutable, particularly when used as described this text—that is, when used as a comprehensive multicomponent synergistic intervention.** Many of the biological and physiology-based (rather than pharmacology-based) treatments in this book are superior to drug treatment with regard to safety, the provision of collateral benefits, and the correction of the primary underlying pathophysiology that is the true cause of hypertension. Clinicians should and must realize and recall that elevated blood pressure is a superficial manifestation of underlying dysfunction; in routine non-emergent situations, identification and correction of this dysfunction should be the clinician's main goal.

Language, Semantics, and Perspective: As a diligent student who previously aspired to be an English professor, I have written this text with great (though inevitably imperfect) attention to detail. Individual words were chosen with care. I confess to knowing, pushing, and creatively breaking several rules of grammar and punctuation. With regard to the he/she and him/her

---

[17] Fuchs FD. The corporate bias and the molding of prescription practices: the case of hypertension. *Braz J Med Biol Res*. 2009 Mar;42(3):224-8

debacle of the English language, I've mixed singular and plural pronouns for the sake of being efficient and so that the images remain gender-neutral to the extent reasonable. The subtitle *The art of creating wellness while effectively managing acute and chronic musculoskeletal/health disorders* was chosen to emphasize the intentional creation of wellness rather than a limited focus on disease treatment and symptom suppression. For the 2009 printing of *Chiropractic and Naturopathic Mastery of Common Clinical Disorders*, this subtitle was slightly modified from "creating" to "co-creating" to emphasize the **team effort** required between physician and patient. *Managing* was chosen to emphasize the importance of treating-monitoring-referring-reassessing, rather than merely *treating*. *Disorders* was chosen to reflect the fact that a distinguishing characteristic of *life* is the ability to habitually create *organized structure* and *higher order* from chaos and *disorder*. For example, plants organize the randomly moving molecules of air and water into the organized structure of biomolecules which eventually take shape as plant structure—fiber, leaves, flowers, petals. Similarly, the human body creates organized structure of increased complexity from consumed plants and other foods; molecules ingested and inhaled from the environment are organized into specific biochemicals and tissue structures with distinct characteristics and definite functions. Injury and disease *result in* or *result from* a lack of order, hence my use of the word "disorders" to characterize human illness and disease. A motor vehicle accident that results in bodily injury, for example, is an example of an external chaotic force, which, when imparted upon human body tissues, results in a disruption (disorder) of the normal structure and organization that previously defined and characterized the now-damaged tissues of the body. Likewise, an autoimmune disease process that results in tissue destruction is an *anti-evolutionary* process that takes molecules of higher complexity and reverts them to simpler, fragmented, and non-functional forms. From the perspective of "health" as *organized structure and meaningful function* and "disease" as *the reversion to chaos, destruction of structure, and the loss of function*, the task of healthcare providers is essentially to restore order, and to acutely reduce and proactively prevent/eliminate clinical-biochemical-biomechanical-emotional chaos insofar as it adversely affects the patient's life experience as an individual and our collective experience as an interdependent society. What is required of clinicians then is the ability first to create conceptual order from what appears to be chaotic phenomena, and then second to materialize that conceptual order into our physical world; this is our task, and no small task it is.

Integrity and Creativity: I have endeavored to accurately represent the facts as they have been presented in texts and research, and to specifically resist any temptation to embellish or misrepresent data as others have done.[18,19] Conversely, I have not endeavored to make this book appeal to the "average" student or reader; my goal is to write and teach to the students at the top of the class, thereby affirming them and pulling the other students forward and upward. While I offer *explanations*, I intentionally resist *simplifications*, except when one simplification might facilitate the comprehension of a more complex phenomenon, or when such a simplification might facilitation the conveyance of information from clinician to patient. I have allowed this text to be unique in format, content, and style, so that the personality of this text can be contrasted with that of the instructor and reader, thus enabling the learner to at least benefit from an intentionally different – and intentionally honest – perspective and approach. Students using this

---

[18] **Vasquez A**. Zinc treatment for reduction of hyperplasia of prostate. *Townsend Letter for Doctors and Patients* 1996; January: 100
[19] Broad W, Wade N. *Betrayers of the Truth: Fraud and Deceit in the Halls of Science*. New York: Simon and Schuster; 1982

text with the guidance of a qualified professor will benefit from the experience of "two teachers" rather than just one.

Linearity, Nonlinearity, Redundancy, Asynchronicity: Although the overall flow of the text is highly linear and sequential, occasionally I place a conclusion before its introduction for the sake of foreshadowing and therefore for preparing the reader for what is to come. The purpose of this is not simply one of preparation for the sake of allowing the reader to know what is already lying ahead on the path, but more to begin creating new "shelf space" in the reader's intellectual-neuronal "library" so that when the new—particularly if *neoparadigmatic*—information is encountered, a space will already exist for it; it other words: the intent is to make learning easier. Likewise, for the sake of *information retention*—or what is better understood as synaptogenesis—important points are presented more than once, either identically or variantly. Given that "*No one ever reads the same book twice*"[20] (because the "person who starts" the reading of a meaningful book is changed into the "person who finishes" the reading of that book (assuming proper intentionality and application of one's "self"), the person reading these words might consider a second glace after the first.

> ### Authentic learning is life integration
> "Ultimately, no one can extract from things—*books included*—more than he already knows. What one has no access to through experience, one has no ear for."
>
> Friedrich Nietzsche [translated by RJ Hollingdale]. *Ecce Homo: How One Becomes What One Is*. New York & London: Penguin Books; 1979, page 70

Bon Voyage: All artists and scientists—regardless of genre—grapple with the divergent goals of perfecting their work and presenting their work; the former is impossible, while the latter is the only means by which the effort can create the desired effect in the world, whether that is pleasure, progress, or both. At some point, we must all agree that it is "good enough" and that it contains the essence of what needs to be communicated. While neither this nor any future edition of this book is likely to be "perfect", I am content with the literature reviewed, presented, and the new conclusions and implications which are described—many for the first time ever—in this text. Particularly for *Integrative Rheumatology* and *Chiropractic and Naturopathic Mastery*, each chapter aims to achieve a paradigm shift which distances us further from the simplistic pharmacocentric model and toward one which authentically empowers both practitioners and patients. With time, I will make future editions more complete and perhaps less polemical—but not less passionate. I hope you are able to implement these conclusions and research findings *into your own life* and into the treatment plans for your patients. In short time, I believe that we will see many of these concepts more broadly implemented. Hopefully this work's value and veracity will promote patients' vitality via the vigilant and virtuous clinicians viewing this volume. To the more attentive and thoroughgoing reader, more is revealed.

Thank you, and I wish you and your patients the best of success and health.

[signature]

Alex Vasquez, D.C., N.D., D.O.
March 2, 2011

---

[20] Davies R. *Reading and Writing*. Salt Lake City: University of Utah Press; 1992, page 23

Foreword to *Functional Medicine and Integrative Medicine for Chronic Hypertension*

In his newly updated publication, Dr. Vasquez's expanded volume encourages and challenges clinicians to further re-imagine their roles in the delivery of health care services. His particular focus on the care of patients with chronic hypertension emphasizes that high blood pressure is both an indicator of underlying functional disorders and a contributor to other serious health problems.

As Dr. Vasquez notes, heart disease and vascular disorders cause tremendous losses in quality of life for a large segment of the population and are the primary causes of death in our society. Chronic high blood pressure is both *a cause of* and *an indicator of* vascular dysfunction and disease. For the most part, these health problems are self-inflicted, meaning that they are the result of how we live, what we eat, and how we view health (and healthcare) in general. Consequently, Dr. Vasquez submits that patients with vascular problems as indicated by chronic hypertension are best managed through dietary changes, nutritional interventions, exercise and other lifestyle modifications. These natural approaches are almost always more safe and effective than conventional drug-based therapies.

Throughout his series of patient-management reference texts for functional integrative clinicians, Dr. Vasquez promotes a simple yet profound principle; "*The art of co-creating wellness while effectively managing common health disorders.*" Chiropractic physicians, as with other functional integrative clinicians, are uniquely positioned to implement this advice. The methods he recommends are specifically designed to optimize function and facilitate health. As healthcare professionals, we can provide no higher service than that of addressing the needs of those patients who seek our care by treating them as *individuals*, and by seeing them as *whole people* and not just as hosts of disease.

Clinical evaluation and management of patients with chronic hypertension should and can be done by all functional integrative clinicians, and Dr. Vasquez's text shows how this can be accomplished. The benefits of this protocol extend beyond reduced hypertensive morbidity and mortality to include the alleviation of comorbid conditions such as depression, migraines, and back pain and the enhancement of vitality and sense of well-being.

Dramatic change in health care delivery is in the air; it is the clinician's responsibility to ensure that the conversation centers on the *care of the patient.* In placing as first priority the needs and preferences of the patient, functional integrative clinicians demonstrate capacity to improve health care choices for individuals while also positively impacting the entire healthcare delivery system by reorienting it toward *health optimization* rather than *symptom suppression* and *disease treatment.*

The quest for a better way to achieve and maintain a healthy life compels us to adapt, to modify, and to transform. Such is the path of advancement and growth. I commend Dr. Vasquez's excellent work and encourage functional integrative clinicians to embrace and apply his recommendations.

Joseph Brimhall, D.C.
President, University of Western States
http://uws.edu/
September 2010

Foreword to *Functional Medicine and Integrative Medicine for Chronic Hypertension*

Dr. Alex Vasquez comes to the question of the *origins of hypertension* with a perspective and set of tools that presage 21st century functional systems medicine. We currently have in place in the industrialized world a method of healthcare developed and based on the 20th century acute-care medical model. Such a model is characterized by rapid differential diagnosis—with an organ-system focus—aimed at prescribing a drug (or procedure) that will ameliorate the patient's presenting symptoms and signs, averting the immediate threat.[1] It is a model that evolved in response to the primary causes of morbidity and mortality in the last century, namely acute infections and trauma. The experts within this organ-system model are the various specialists within conventional medicine, such as cardiologists, pulmonologists, endocrinologists, neurologists, and orthopaedic surgeons.

Inherently, this methodology minimises the involvement of the patient, who functions mostly as a passive recipient of the procedure or prescription. It is not a model that reimburses the practitioner for looking into *why* the patient became ill, the origins of illnesses. Instead, it prioritises immediate solutions to the most pressing problems. It is, of course, absolutely essential in emergency and hospital-based care of many kinds, but difficulties arise when this model is applied to ongoing, community-based care for the non-acute, chronic, complex conditions that represent 80% of the daily work of present day clinicians.[2]

This new book, *Integrative Medicine and Functional Medicine for Chronic Hypertension,* discusses the principles of functional integrative medicine and shows how they can be usefully applied to the frequently encountered clinical condition of chronic hypertension. In so doing, it illustrates the shift that will be required to enfold into 21st century medical practice the innovative clinical practises of patient-centred, personalised, systems-based medicine. A core principle of functional integrative medicine maintains that diagnosis is the *starting point* for the clinician's primary set of responsibilities, not the last step before prescriptive interventions. The most complex of skills, *clinical decision making* and *medical judgment,* in the medical context of chronic, complex co-morbid illnesses such as chronic hypertension, require:
- A persistent exploration of the accretion of the relevant scientific evidence, tempered by...
- the wealth of knowledge and judgment inherent in clinical experience, along with...
- the creation of a real partnership with the patient in educing a lifestyle-based personalized, therapeutic plan.

Clinical decision making, when exercised at the most efficacious level, drills deeply into the "why" of every diagnosis. Pursuit of the elusive network of causality in the deeper intersections of genetic individuality, within each client's unique context of living, is an essential responsibility of the clinician. This clinical guide focused on chronic hypertension illustrates, using step-by-step illustration, how to achieve more satisfying outcomes through an integrated clinical assessment and treatment program.

Stepping out of the shadow of conventional poly-pharmacology and procedure-based interventions, into the bright sunlight afforded by 21st century breakthroughs in personalised medicine, systems biology, and systems medicine re-enchants and illuminates the practice of clinical medicine. The blending of the foundational sciences of genomics (unique genes embedded in a unique environment) with the intellectual architecture of functional, integrative, systems-thinking enables the creation of a more comprehensive portfolio of clinical service for the patient. The author's careful explanations in this volume illustrate how clinical practice, coupled with skills learned through rigorous training in both conventional medicine and functional, integrative systems medicine can successfully bring to the therapeutic relationship real patient-centred answers for chronic, complex illnesses.

The most powerful motivator for changes in our behaviour as physicians is listening attentively to compelling stories brought to the clinic by our patients. The intense satisfaction of successfully resolving their hitherto unanswered questions about the root causes of chronic hypertension, by applying a different lens for evaluation and assessment, is transformative. Functional, integrative, systems medicine provides such a lens. Hence, *Integrative Medicine and Functional Medicine for Chronic Hypertension* will prove to be an important publication about functional and integrative medicine in clinical practice.

David S Jones, M.D.
President, Institute for Functional Medicine
http://www.functionalmedicine.org/
August, 2010

[1] Ely JW, Osheroff JA, Gorman PN, et al. A taxonomy of generic clinical questions: classification study. *BMJ* 2000;321:429-32
[2] Holman H. Chronic disease—The need for a new clinical education. *JAMA* 2004;292(9):1057-1059

Work as love

"You work that you may keep pace with the earth and the soul of the earth.
For to be idle is to become a stranger unto the seasons, and to step out of life's procession. ...
Work is love made visible."

Kahlil Gibran (1883-1930). The Prophet. Publisher Alfred A. Knopf, 1973

Newsletter & Updates

Be alerted to new integrative clinical research and updates to this textbook by registering for the free newsletter, sent 4-6 times per year. Subscribe via
www.OptimalHealthResearch.com/newsletter

Pro-pharmaceutical bias and the molding of antihypertensive prescription practices

"Clinical trials influenced by the corporate bias have been the basis for a massive strategy of promotion of blood pressure drugs that resulted in the shaping of prescription practices departing from the best evidence."

Fuchs FD. The corporate bias and the molding of prescription practices: the case of hypertension. *Braz J Med Biol Res*. 2009 Mar;42(3):224-8

Section 2:
Integrative & Functional Medicine for High Blood Pressure & Chronic Hypertension

---

Integrative & Functional Medicine for Chronic Hypertension:

This section reviews clinically relevant information related to chronic hypertension—its cause(s), its social and economic impacts, selected aspects of its pathophysiology and complications, differential diagnosis, assessments, overall management and specific treatments. Throughout, emphasis is placed on clinical accuracy, therapeutic efficacy, and patient safety.

Treatment options reviewed include drugs, diet, lifestyle, metabolic modifications such as weight loss and improvement in insulin sensitivity, nutritional supplementation, manipulative therapeutics and surgical treatment for the alleviation of medullary neurovascular compression.

Clearly, most of the non-drug non-surgery treatments reviewed here are natural, nonpatentable, and widely available; they work with the body's physiology to improve metabolic function and to thereby improve overall health and cardiovascular dynamics. Side effects are minimal, and collateral benefits are many; therefore, as overall health improves, various complaints and disorders are alleviated, vitality is enhanced, and patient compliance increases while the need for medical management of other issues decreases.

A *quantitative* compilation can effect a *qualitative* transformation in the reader's perception of the nature of the disease and its place in clinical care and healthcare policy; such is the goal of this section on chronic hypertension.

Topics:

- **Description, Pathophysiology, and Key Concepts**
  - The silent disease and tremendous opportunity
  - Overview and perspective
  - Blood pressure and mortality
  - Hypertension and vascular disease
  - Medical physiology-pharmacology of hypertension
  - Acceleration of atherogenesis and atherosclerosis
  - Obesity, type-2 diabetes mellitus, and hypertension—unnecessary epidemics
  - Hypertension control—an international health priority
  - Hypertension—multifaceted entity with clinical, political, social, and economic components and implications
  - Hypertension—primarily a "disease of Western civilization"
  - The clinician's responsibilities
- **Clinical Presentations**
- **Major Differential Diagnoses**
  - Aortic coarctation
  - Cocaine use
  - Cushing's disease/syndrome
  - Drug side-effect
  - Estrogen, oral contraceptives
  - Ethanol overconsumption
  - Gestational hypertension and preeclampsia
  - Hypercalcemia
  - Insulin resistance and hyperinsulinemia
  - Licorice (*Glycyrrhiza glabra*) over-consumption
  - Mercury toxicity
  - Neurogenic hypertension (central and peripheral)
  - Nonsteroidal anti-inflammatory drugs (NSAIDs)
  - Pheochromocytoma
  - Primary hyperaldosteronism (Conn's syndrome)
  - Renal artery (renovascular) stenosis
  - Renal parenchymal disease
  - Sleep apnea
  - Systemic sclerosis
  - Thyroid disease, including both hyperthyroidism and hypothyroidism
  - Tobacco use
  - Upper cervical spine dysfunction/subluxation
  - Vitamin D deficiency
- **Clinical Assessments**
- **Laboratory Assessments**
- **Imaging, Biopsy/Procedure**
- **Establishing the Diagnosis**
- **Disease Complications**
- **Clinical Management**
- **Treatment Considerations for "Primary" Hypertension**
- **Selected Essays, Perspectives, and Previously Published Articles**

Commonly Used Abbreviations:

- **25-OH-D** = serum 25-hydroxy-vitamin D(3)
- **ACEi** = angiotensin-2 converting enzyme inhibitor
- **Alpha-blocker** = alpha-adrenergic antagonist
- **ARB** = angiotensin-2 receptor blocker/antagonist
- **ARF** = acute renal failure
- **BB** = beta blocker or beta-adrenergic antagonist
- **BMP** = basic metabolic panel, includes serum Na, K, Cl, CO2, BUN, creatinine, and glucose
- **BP** = blood pressure, **HBP** = high blood pressure
- **BUN** = blood urea nitrogen
- **CAD** = coronary artery disease
- **CBC** = complete blood count
- **CCB** = calcium channel blocker/antagonist
- **CE** = cardiac enzymes, generally including creatine kinase (CK), creatine kinase myocardial band (CKMB), and troponin-1, with the latter being the most specific serologic marker for acute myocardial injury; for the evaluation of acute MI, these are generally tested 2-3 times at 6-hour intervals with ECG performed at least as often.
- **CHF** = congestive heart failure
- **CK** = creatine kinase, historically named creatine phosphokinase (CPK)
- **CKD** = chronic kidney disease, generally stratified into five stages based on GFR of roughly <90, 90-60, 60-30, 30-15, and >15, respectively
- **CMP** = comprehensive metabolic panel, also called a chemistry panel, includes the BMP along with markers of hepatic status albumin, protein, ALT, AST, may also include alkaline phosphatase and rarely GGT; panels vary per laboratory and hospital
- **COPD** = chronic obstructive pulmonary disease
- **CRF**, **CRI** = chronic renal failure/insufficiency
- **CRP** = c-reactive protein, **hsCRP** = high-sensitivity c-reactive protein
- **CT** = computed tomography
- **CVD** = cardiovascular disease
- **DM** = diabetes mellitus
- **ECG** or **EKG** = electrocardiograph
- **Echo** = echocardiography
- **GFR** = glomerular filtration rate
- **HDL** = high density lipoprotein cholesterol
- **HTN** = hypertension
- **IHD** = ischemic heart disease
- **IV** = intravenous
- **MI** = myocardial infarction
- **MRI** = magnetic resonance imaging, **MRI** = magnetic resonance angiography
- **PRN** = from the Latin "pro re nata" meaning "on occasion" or "when necessary"
- **PTH** = parathyroid hormone, **iPTH** = intact parathyroid hormone
- **PVD** = peripheral vascular disease
- **RAD** = reactive airway disease
- **TRIG(s)** = serum triglycerides
- **UA** = urinalysis
- **US** = ultrasound

[handwritten annotation: CAM Complementary and alternative medicine]

Dosing shorthand (mostly Latin abbreviations): q = each; qd = each day; bid = twice daily; tid = thrice daily; qid = four times per day; po = per os = by mouth; prn = as needed.

Hypertension (HTN)
High Blood Pressure (HBP)

Description, Pathophysiology, and Key Concepts:

- <u>Chronic high blood pressure: The silent disease and tremendous opportunity</u>: High blood pressure (chronic hypertension) is the most common disease diagnosis encountered in clinical practice worldwide. As such, the diagnosis and successful integrative management of chronic hypertension represents an opportunity for clinicians to achieve higher levels of practice success and for patients to receive the healthcare that they need. In America, 30% of adults have hypertension. For those of us specializing in adult healthcare, these hypertensive adults in the population can be thought of as

> **Recent review: 1 in 3 US adults has hypertension; the vast majority of these cases have no clear "medical" cause**
>
> "In the United States, one in three adults has hypertension. Most of these patients have no clear etiology and are classified as having essential hypertension."
>
> Viera AJ, Neutze DM. Diagnosis of secondary hypertension: an age-based approach. *Am Fam Physician*. 2010 Dec 15;82(12):1471-8

belonging to two categories: ❶ patients receiving comprehensive integrative functional medicine care (very small minority), and ❷ patients who are either undiagnosed, untreated, or treated only with drugs and therefore in need of comprehensive integrative functional medicine care for optimal hypertension management, disease prevention, and wellness promotion (the vast majority of hypertensive patients).

   Most hypertensive patients have no symptoms of their disorder and are therefore reliant upon a competent clinician to reveal the problem and to provide the appropriate education and the motivation to initiate and maintain compliance with treatment. Clinicians have the responsibility to detect and effectively manage high blood pressure. High blood pressure accelerates the development of cardiovascular disease and additional complications including stroke, heart attack (myocardial infarction), heart failure, renal failure, blindness, peripheral vascular disease and endothelial dysfunction which can contribute to (for example) lower leg amputation and sexual dysfunction[1] in both men and women.

   Clinicians have three core responsibilities related to hypertension management. First, the condition must be diagnosed by the clinician; this is a simple physical exam procedure. Second, the patient must be assessed for underlying causes and disease complications. Third, the patient must be enrolled in a treatment program to ensure proper lowering of elevated pressures; this is best accomplished with diet optimization, nutritional supplementation, therapeutic lifestyle changes, spinal manipulation, and—rarely—use of medications.

- <u>Overview and perspective</u>: The emphasis of this section will be the integrative management of so-called "primary" or "essential" hypertension (HTN), which is generally considered "idiopathic" from an outdated medical perspective that has failed to appreciate and integrate the research that has clarified the numerous causes of and contributors to HTN. From the allopathic medical perspective, >90-95% of HTN is considered idiopathic and thus by

---

[1] "Available data indicate that essential hypertension is a risk factor for sexual dysfunction, as male and female sexual dysfunction is more prevalent in hypertensive patients than normotensive individuals. Several mechanisms have been implicated in the pathogenesis of sexual dysfunction in hypertensive patients, and major determinants include severity and duration of hypertension, age, and antihypertensive therapy. Female sexual dysfunction, although more frequent than its male counterpart, remains largely under-recognized." Manolis A, Doumas M. Sexual dysfunction: the 'prima ballerina' of hypertension-related quality-of-life complications. *J Hypertens*. 2008 Nov;26(11):2074-84

definition "of no known cause" and therefore appropriate for treatment with drugs. Most (more than 70%) medically managed patients with HTN take two or more antihypertensive drugs from the time of diagnosis until the end of their lives; these drugs commonly cause adverse effects, are relatively devoid of collateral benefits, and do not address the underlying causative physiologic imbalances. Patients managed with nutritional and lifestyle modifications must likewise remain compliant with the prescribed health-promoting treatment-diet-lifestyle, but they generally experience clinically and statistically meaningful *collateral benefits*; for example, ❶ **correction of vitamin D deficiency can alleviate hypertension**[2] and musculoskeletal pain[3] while improving mood[4,5]; ❷ **fish oil supplementation slightly lowers blood pressure** but tremendously and safely lowers cardiovascular mortality and all-cause mortality[6] while also improving mental health[7] and alleviating pain and inflammation[8,9]; ❸ **CoQ-10 is very effective for the treatment of HTN**[10] while also restoring lost renal function[11,12], alleviating migraine headaches[13], and helping to control asthma.[14] The exemplary nutritional interventions listed in the previous sentence are virtually devoid of adverse effects when employed with a modicum of competence, and each of these natural and nonpatentable interventions is widely available. Furthermore, **their clinical benefit (in this case, the reduction of elevated blood pressure) is derived from their ability to restore proper physiologic function** rather than—as with most pharmaceutical drugs—the blockade of normal physiology. If the routine outpatient medical treatment of HTN were to shift away from synthetic chemical drugs that function by interfering with normal physiology (e.g., beta-adrenergic *blockers*, calcium channel *blockers*, ACE *inhibitors*, angiotensin-2 receptor *blockers*, etc) and toward the favor of natural treatments—diet optimization, body weight reduction/optimization, and evidence-based nutritional supplementation—that promote normalization of blood pressure by helping restore balance to the body's physiology (i.e., by facilitating the restoration of homeostasis),

---

[2] "A short-term supplementation with vitamin D(3) and calcium is more effective in reducing SBP than calcium alone. Inadequate vitamin D(3) and calcium intake could play a contributory role in the pathogenesis and progression of hypertension and cardiovascular disease in elderly women." Pfeifer M, Begerow B, Minne HW, Nachtigall D, Hansen C. Effects of a short-term vitamin D(3) and calcium supplementation on blood pressure and parathyroid hormone levels in elderly women. *J Clin Endocrinol Metab*. 2001 Apr;86(4):1633-7

[3] "Findings showed that 83% of the study patients (n = 299) had an abnormally low level of vitamin D before treatment with vitamin D supplements. After treatment, clinical improvement in symptoms was seen in all the groups that had a low level of vitamin D, and in 95% of all the patients (n = 341). CONCLUSIONS: Vitamin D deficiency is a major contributor to chronic low back pain in areas where vitamin D deficiency is endemic." Al Faraj S, Al Mutairi K. Vitamin D deficiency and chronic low back pain in Saudi Arabia. *Spine*. 2003;28:177-9

[4] Vieth R, Kimball S, Hu A, Walfish PG. Randomized comparison of the effects of the vitamin D3 adequate intake versus 100 mcg (4000 IU) per day on biochemical responses and the wellbeing of patients. *Nutrition Journal* 2004, 3:8 http://www.nutritionj.com/content/3/1/8

[5] Lansdowne AT, Provost SC: Vitamin D3 enhances mood in healthy subjects during winter. *Psychopharmacology* (Berl) 1998, 135:319-323

[6] GISSI-Prevenzione Investigators. Dietary supplementation with n-3 polyunsaturated fatty acids and vitamin E after myocardial infarction: results of the GISSI-Prevenzione trial. Gruppo Italiano per lo Studio della Sopravvivenza nell'Infarto miocardico. *Lancet*. 1999 Aug 7;354(9177):447-55

[7] Peet M, Stokes C. Omega-3 fatty acids in the treatment of psychiatric disorders. *Drugs*. 2005;65(8):1051-9

[8] Maroon JC, Bost JW. Omega-3 fatty acids (fish oil) as an anti-inflammatory: an alternative to nonsteroidal anti-inflammatory drugs for discogenic pain. *Surg Neurol*. 2006 Apr;65(4):326-31

[9] "Many of the placebo-controlled trials of fish oil in chronic inflammatory diseases reveal significant benefit, including decreased disease activity and a lowered use of anti-inflammatory drugs." Simopoulos AP. Omega-3 fatty acids in inflammation and autoimmune diseases. *J Am Coll Nutr*. 2002 Dec;21(6):495-505

[10] Singh RB, Niaz MA, Rastogi SS, Shukla PK, Thakur AS. Effect of hydrosoluble coenzyme Q10 on blood pressures and insulin resistance in hypertensive patients with coronary artery disease. *J Hum Hypertens*. 1999 Mar;13(3):203-8

[11] Singh RB, Khanna HK, Niaz MA. Randomized, double-blind placebo-controlled trial of coenzyme Q10 in chronic renal failure: discovery of a new role. *J Nutr Environ Med* 2000;10:281-8

[12] Singh RB, Kumar A, Naiz MA, Singh RG, Gujrati S, Singh VP, Singh M, Singh UP, Taneja C, AND Rastogi SS. Randomized, Double-blind, Placebo-controlled Trial of Coenzyme Q10 in Patients with Endstage Renal Failure. *J Nutr Environ Med* 2003; 13 (1): 13–22

[13] Rozen TD, Oshinsky ML, Gebeline CA, Bradley KC, Young WB, Shechter AL, Silberstein SD. Open label trial of coenzyme Q10 as a migraine preventive. *Cephalalgia* 2002;22(2):137-41

[14] Gvozdjáková A, Kucharská J, Bartkovjaková M, Gazdíková K, Gazdík FE. Coenzyme Q10 supplementation reduces corticosteroids dosage in patients with bronchial asthma. *Biofactors*. 2005;25(1-4):235-40

then meaningful and authentic progress in the otherwise never-ending "fight against hypertension" would be made. (For more discussion, see "Thinking Outside the (Pill) Box" at the end of this chapter.)

- Blood pressure and mortality: Increased risk for cardiovascular mortality begins with blood pressures that are still well within the accepted normal range; therefore blood pressure that is consistent with an official diagnosis of hypertension—blood pressure consistently greater than 140 mm Hg systolic and/or greater than 90 mm Hg diastolic—is clearly worthy of treatment if part of the clinical goal is—*as it should be*—to reduce unnecessary morbidity and early mortality. Benowitz[15] wrote, "Starting at 115/75 mm Hg, cardiovascular risk doubles with each

---

Antihypertensive drugs function by blocking *normal* physiology (rather than by *correcting* dysfunctional physiology)

"All antihypertensive [drugs]… produce their effects by interfering with normal mechanisms of blood pressure regulation."

Benowitz NL. "Antihypertensive Agents." In Katzung BG (editor). Basic and Clinical Pharmacology. Tenth Edition. New York: McGraw Hill Medical; 2007, p159

"In Western medicine, because of the prevailing mechanistic view, we treat our bodies as dumb machines. We move in with surgery and drugs to make them do what we want [a reflection of the *power-over model*, or the *control paradigm*], bypassing strategies that support the body's capacity to solve its own problems, learn, and regenerate itself."

Breton D, Largent C. The paradigm conspiracy: why our social systems violate human potential and how we can change them. Center City, Minnesota: Hazelden Publishing; 1998, pages 147-148

---

increment of 20/10 mm Hg throughout the blood pressure range." Thus, from both *wellness-centered* as well as *disease-prevention* perspectives, pro-active integrative clinicians can define mild HTN as > 115/75 mm Hg. Data from the Framingham study showed that sustained BP > 140/90 induces left ventricular hypertrophy.[16] A reduction of systolic BP (sBP) of -5 mm Hg correlates with a -7% reduction in cardiovascular mortality[17]; thus, patients must be encouraged to take HTN and its effective treatment seriously, since even small numerical decrements in BP can have impressive ameliorating effects on the risk for cardiovascular complications. Except in younger age groups, sBP is more predictive of adverse cardiovascular outcomes than is diastolic BP. Systolic hypertension indicates the presence of vascular abnormalities including reductions in elasticity/compliance of large and medium arteries; thus, the finding of systolic HTN simultaneously indicates *current* vascular abnormalities and *future* cardiovascular disease (CV) risk elevation.

"Prehypertension" is deadly: mortality increases starting at 115/75 mm Hg

"Hypertension-related diseases are the leading causes of morbidity and mortality in industrially developed societies. Surprisingly, **68% of all mortality attributed to high blood pressure (BP) occurs with systolic BP between 120 and 140 mm Hg and diastolic BP below 90 mm Hg**. Dietary and lifestyle modifications are effective in the treatment of borderline hypertension."

Goldhamer AC, Lisle DJ, Sultana P, Anderson SV, Parpia B, Hughes B, Campbell TC. Medically supervised water-only fasting in the treatment of borderline hypertension. *J Altern Complement Med*. 2002 Oct;8(5):643-50

---

[15] Benowitz NL. "Antihypertensive Agents." In Katzung BG (editor). Basic and Clinical Pharmacology. Tenth Edition. New York: McGraw Hill Medical; 2007, 159
[16] Kumar V, Abbas AK, Fausto N (Editors). Robbins and Cotran Pathologic Basis of Disease. Seventh Edition. Philadelphia: Elsevier; 2005, 587
[17] Nahas R. Complementary and alternative medicine approaches to blood pressure reduction: An evidence-based review. *Can Fam Physician*. 2008 Nov;54(11):1529-33 http://www.cfp.ca/cgi/content/full/54/11/1529

- <u>Hypertension and vascular disease</u>: Sustained HTN accelerates the development of CVD and end-organ damage by several mechanisms including promotion of endothelial damage resulting in accelerated atherosclerosis (e.g., stroke, myocardial infarction, peripheral vascular disease), direct pressure (e.g., retinal hemorrhages, aortic aneurysm), hyperplastic arteriolosclerosis and occlusive vasculopathy due to smooth muscle proliferation, fibrosis, and hyaline deposition (e.g., hypertensive nephrosclerosis), interstitial edema (e.g., cerebral edema, peripheral edema), and pathologic myocardial adaptation (e.g., hypertrophic cardiomyopathy, hypertensive heart disease, congestive heart failure). Hyperplastic arteriolosclerosis causes hypertensive nephrosclerosis, characterized by renal ischemia which triggers release of renin and increased formation of angiotensin-2 which exacerbates renal ischemia and systemic hypertension.[18]

- <u>Medical physiology-pharmacology of hypertension</u>: Drug treatment of hypertension must have some physiologic basis, even if this basis is simplistic, limited, and outdated by current research and emerging paradigms that might surpass and supplant previous and well entrenched models. In the medical/allopathic paradigm, "physiology" must be tailored to support pharmacology, since the latter is the profession's primary intervention. Thus, the study of physiology must be made to fit pharmacology by limiting the variables considered to those which are amenable to drug intervention. Thus, per medical pharmacology textbooks[19], the primary variables considered for the support of antihypertensive pharmacotherapy are ❶ cardiac output ("to be controlled with beta-blockers"), ❷ peripheral resistance ("to be treated with vasodilators such as ACEi and CCB"), and ❸ blood volume ("to be reduced by the first-line use of diuretics"). While this perspective is necessarily limited in the service of the medical paradigm, it is also useful for provisionally grasping a view of some of the key factors involved in blood pressure regulation, including those that are relevant for drug intervention in the acute care setting as well as the long-term nondrug treatment of HTN. Given that this text details the "functional" and "integrative" management of HTN and must therefore provide a variety of perspectives, a concise review of medical physiology is appropriate. The medical paradigm views most HTN as idiopathic and "somehow" resulting from a complex dysregulation of normal physiology; thereby, the "appropriate" intervention is to interfere with the normal physiologic mechanisms that have gone astray. One interconnecting theme in this paradigm is that of activation of the sympathetic nervous system by some unknown insult or combination thereof. Whether due to "stress", faulty disinhibition of baroreceptors in the aortic arch, carotid sinuses, or renal juxtaglomerular cells, sympathetic activation increases cardiac output via increased rate and contractility, increases peripheral resistance via

> **Affective interpretations: emotional needs influence intellectual perspectives**
>
> "…to see differently in this way for once, to *want* to see differently, is no small discipline and preparation of the intellect for its future "objectivity"—the latter understood not as "contemplation without interest" (which is a nonsensical absurdity), but as the ability *to control* one's Pro and Con and to dispose of them, so that one knows how to employ a *variety* of perspectives and *affective interpretations* in the service of knowledge."
>
> Nietzsche FW. <u>Genealogy of Morals [1887]</u>. Essay #3, section #12.

---

[18] Kumar V, Abbas AK, Fausto N (Editors). <u>Robbins and Cotran Pathologic Basis of Disease. Seventh Edition</u>. Philadelphia: Elsevier; 2005, 1007-8
[19] Harvey RA, Champe PC (eds). <u>Lippincott's Illustrated Reviews: Pharmacology, Third Edition</u>. Philadelphia, Lippincott Williams and Wilkins; 1997

vasoconstriction, and increases blood volume via aldosterone-enhanced sodium retention. The enzyme renin converts angiotensinogen into angiotensin-1, which is converted via angiotensin converting enzyme (ACE) into angiotensin-2, which is a powerful vasoconstrictor and trigger for the release of aldosterone, which promotes sodium reabsorption and thus sodium-water retention. With this simple and simplistic model, one can grasp the rationale employed for antihypertensive pharmacotherapeutics as well as some of the natural and *eu*physiologic[20] interventions detailed in this text; drug treatments for HTN are detailed toward the end of this chapter.

- Acceleration of atherogenesis and atherosclerosis: HTN is the single most important risk factor for the development of CVD. On a population-wide basis, achieving the target of ≤ 140 mmHg systolic would result in a 28-44% reduction in stroke and a 20-35% reduction in ischemic heart disease (IHD). In describing these benefits for the United Kingdom (population ~60 million in 2005), Tomson and Lip[21] noted in 2005 that control of HTN would prevent approximately 42,800 strokes and 82,800 IHD events per year.

- Basic pathology: Reviewed here are several of the more direct and salient effects of high blood pressure on important organs, the most relevant of which are brain, eye, heart, and kidney.

  o Brain—intracerebral hemorrhage, lacunar infarcts, slit hemorrhages, hypertensive encephalopathy: HTN can cause intracerebral hemorrhage and cerebellar hemorrhage. Arteriolar sclerosis of small vessels can lead to ischemia of the basal ganglia, cerebral white matter, and brainstem. Cavitary lacunar ("lake-like") infarcts classically affect the lenticular nucleus, thalamus, internal capsule, caudate nucleus, and pons. Rupture of small vessels can leave a slit-like cavity of discoloration, cell destruction, and gliosis termed a *slit hemorrhage*. Hypertensive encephalopathy presents with headache, confusion, vomiting, seizure, and/or coma; cerebral edema, petechiae, and transtentorial or tonsillar herniation may be noted at autopsy.[22]

  o Eye—ocular vascular disease and hypertensive retinopathy: Hypertensive sclerosis of arteries and arterioles serving the eye results in the "copper wire" then "silver wire" fundoscopic changes that occur as the arteriole wall thickens and obscures visualization of luminal blood. Within the nerve fiber layer of the retina, "cotton-wool spots" are infarcts, and "flame hemorrhages" are due to vascular rupture. Retinal exudates secondary to vascular leak due to severe hypertension may induce retinal detachment and acute vision loss. Occlusion of retinal arterioles causes retinal infarction.[23]

  o Heart—hypertensive cardiomyopathy and cardiac hypertrophy: HTN increases the work demands placed on the heart and leads to myocyte hypertrophy followed by altered proportions of cardiac anatomy as well as functional abnormalities: left atrial enlargement leads to conduction defects such as atrial fibrillation; ventricular walls thicken and encroach upon intraventricular volume leading to reduced ejection volume. Adaptations to chronically increased blood pressure lead to alterations in cardiac

---

[20] The prefix "eu" means good or beneficial. The term "euphysiologic" was used more commonly in medical literature of the early 1900's than it is today. Here, euphysiologic means "properly-working physiology" or "beneficial to physiology" in contrast to interventions that are contrary to normal physiology ("antiphysiologic" or—per Greenblatt [*Obstet Gynecol Clin North Am*. 1987;14:251-68]—"contraphysiologic") such as enzyme-blocking drugs which have their therapeutic and adverse effects by working against normal physiology and enzyme function.

[21] Tomson J, Lip GY. Blood pressure demographics: nature or nurture…genes or environment? *BMC Med*. 2005;3:3 biomedcentral.com/1741-7015/3/3

[22] Frosch MP, Anthony DC, DeGirolami U. "Chapter 28: The central nervous system." in Kumar V, Abbas AK, Fausto N (eds). Robins and Cotran Pathologic Basis of Disease. Seventh Edition. Elsevier: Philadelphia; 2005, 1368-1369

[23] Folberg R. "Chapter 29: The eye." in Kumar V, Abbas AK, Fausto N (eds). Robins and Cotran Pathologic Basis of Disease. Seventh Edition. Elsevier: Philadelphia; 2005, 1436-1437

anatomy, histology, physiology, and gene expression that—if persistent and progressive—eventually culminate in cardiac failure.[24] Acute-onset hypertension can induce oxygen/nutrient delivery-demand mismatch resulting in myocardial infarction.

o Kidney—malignant hypertension and accelerated nephrosclerosis: Malignant hypertension—the full syndrome of which includes diastolic pressure > 130 mm Hg, papilledema/retinopathy, encephalopathy, renal failure, and cardiovascular complications—occurs in 1-5% of hypertensive patients; it is more common in patients who are male, young, and of African descent. Risk factors include pre-existing chronic hypertension (whether primary or secondary), scleroderma, and preexisting renal disease such as reflux nephropathy or glomerulonephritis. The main pathophysiologic sequence appears to include intrarenal vascular damage followed by vascular occlusion secondary to intimal smooth muscle hypertrophy and hyperplastic arteriolosclerosis; eventually this leads to renal hypoperfusion and ischemia. Renal hypoperfusion, besides leading to azotemia and oliguria in acute severe hypertension, leads to activation of the renin-angiotensin-aldosterone system (RAAS) which leads to additional vasoconstriction and the cascade of events (including sodium and water retention) which leads to further elevations in blood pressure. Histologic changes in the kidney include fibrinoid necrosis of the arterioles, hyperplastic arteriolitis, intrarenal arterial thrombosis, and glomerular necrosis.[25]

- Treatment-resistant hypertension: "Resistant hypertension" was defined in a December 2010 review as "elevated blood pressure despite patient adherence to optimal dosages of three antihypertensive agents, including a diuretic."[26]

- Obesity, type-2 diabetes mellitus, and hypertension—*unnecessary* epidemics: **In the United States (population ~300 million in 2005), 65% of adults are overweight or obese,** generally as a direct result of *overconsumption malnutrition* and physical inactivity). In the US, the number of deaths attributable to obesity is greater than 280,200 yearly. At least 11 million Americans have type-2 diabetes mellitus, while **50 million Americans have hypertension.**[27]

- Hypertension diagnosis and control—an international health priority: Control of HTN is a worldwide healthcare priority. According to a 2001 editorial by Chobanian[28] in *New England Journal of Medicine*, "…more than one-fourth of the estimated 42 million people with hypertension in the United States remain unaware that they have the disorder, and approximately three-fourths of those with known hypertension have blood pressure that exceeds recommended levels." Dr Chobanian goes

Prevalence of HTN
• 50 million people in the U.S.
• 1 billion worldwide
• European Americans:
o 15% of women,
o 25% of men > age 45 years
• African Americans:
o 35% of women,
o 40% of men > age 45 years
Villela T. Hypertension: Diagnosis and Management. University of California, San Francisco-San Francisco General Hospital. Family and Community Medicine Residency Program. July 2010

---

[24] Schoen FJ. "Chapter 12: The heart" in Kumar V, Abbas AK, Fausto N (eds). Robins and Cotran Pathologic Basis of Disease. Seventh Edition. Elsevier: Philadelphia; 2005, 560-562

[25] Alpers CE. "Chapter 20: The kidney" in Kumar V, Abbas AK, Fausto N (eds). Robins and Cotran Pathologic Basis of Disease. Seventh Edition. Elsevier: Philadelphia; 2005, 1007-1008

[26] Viera AJ, Neutze DM. Diagnosis of secondary hypertension: an age-based approach. *Am Fam Physician*. 2010 Dec 15;82(12):1471-8

[27] Cordain L, Eaton SB, Sebastian A, Mann N, Lindeberg S, Watkins BA, O'Keefe JH, Brand-Miller J. Origins and evolution of the Western diet: health implications for the 21st century. *Am J Clin Nutr*. 2005 Feb;81(2):341-54 http://www.ajcn.org/cgi/content/full/81/2/341

[28] Chobanian AV. Control of hypertension--an important national priority. *N Engl J Med*. 2001 Aug 16;345(7):534-5

on to note that the prevalence and severity of the problem is comparable in the rest of the world, where approximately 20% of the adult population (more than 800 million people) are hypertensive, and rates of control are even worse than in the United States. According to an extensive review of international data published in *The Lancet* in 2005, the global prevalence of HTN was 26.4% (972 million people) in 2000 and is projected to increase to 29.2% (1.56 billion people) by the year 2025; the authors concluded, "Hypertension is an important public-health challenge worldwide."[29]

- Hypertension—a multifaceted entity with clinical, political, social, and economic components and implications: First, as previously noted, HTN is a treatable and therefore avoidable contributor to CVD and other forms of end-organ damage—stroke, myocardial infarction, congestive heart failure, peripheral vascular disease, renal failure, and hypertensive retinopathy. Second, HTN as a clinical manifestation is *always* a sign of underlying dysfunction or disease; HTN does not cause itself (at least initially) and therefore the "treatment of hypertension" should focus on the identification and "treatment of underlying dysfunction" rather than simply suppressing the visible manifestation of this dysfunction— the elevated blood pressure. **The finding of HTN is a sign to the clinician that one or more underlying physiologic imbalances are present and in need of detection and/or corrective intervention**. The environmental-social factors that predispose toward the development of HTN—including overconsumption malnutrition, lack of exercise, and psychoemotional stress—tend to disproportionately affect people of lower socioeconomic status. Third, HTN is not merely a disease; it is a *business* (leading diagnosis in Family Medicine practices[30]), and an industry (direct costs approach $200 billion per year in the United States). Among allopathic and osteopathic physicians, HTN is the most common clinical diagnosis in Family Medicine practice. For the medical profession and pharmaceutical industry, antihypertensive medications and services are a major source of revenue. Direct annual medical expenses related to HTN exceed $185 billion per year in the United States. Most patients treated exclusively with drugs require *multiple drugs* for adequate BP control[31], and— from the day of diagnosis—they are prescribed to take these drugs for the rest of their lives. **Thus, the term "hypertension" describes much more than one individual patient's elevated blood pressure; the term refers to an entity that spans and interconnects clinical, political, social, and economic phenomena and institutions.** To change the management of hypertension is to change—or at least begin changing in an important way—the practice of medicine as previously known. By perceiving high blood pressure as a barometer of poor health rather than as an isolated clinical entity, clinicians have license to intervene in numerous ways to improve each patient's overall health, thereby reducing suffering and death *beyond that attributable to hypertension-related illness* because most of the natural interventions described in

> **Hypertension costs more than 12% of total US healthcare expenditures: more than $185 billion per year**
>
> "In 1998, the direct costs of hypertension in the USA were calculated to be 12.6% of health care expenditures ($185 billion)... A similar figure was found based on analysis of the 1996 Medical Expenditure Panel Survey (i.e., $177 billion)."
>
> Tarride JE, Lim M, DesMeules M, Luo W, Burke N, O'Reilly D, Bowen J, Goeree R. A review of the cost of cardiovascular disease. *Can J Cardiol*. 2009 Jun;25(6):e195-202

---

[29] Kearney PM, Whelton M, Reynolds K, Muntner P, Whelton PK, He J. Global burden of hypertension: analysis of worldwide data. *Lancet*. 2005 Jan 15-21;365(9455):217-23

[30] Sloane PD, Slatt LM, Ebell MH, Jacques LB, Smith MA (Eds). Essentials of Family Medicine, 5th Edition. Lippincott Williams & Wilkins, 2007

[31] Domino FJ (editor in chief). The 5-Minute Clinical Consult. 2010. 18th Edition. Philadelphia; Wolters Kluwer: 2009, 656-7

this chapter provide clinically meaningful collateral benefits and reduce blood pressure *en passant*.[32]

- Hypertension—primarily a "disease of Western civilization": The prevalence of HTN among hunter-gatherer societies is virtually zero.[33] Contrasting the absence of CVD noted in *physically active* societies that consume *natural diets* against the pandemics of HTN and CVD seen in Westernized/industrialized nations, O'Keefe and Cordain[34] wrote, **"The lifetime incidence of hypertension [among Americans] is an astounding 90%**, and the metabolic syndrome is present in up to 40% of middle-aged American adults. **Cardiovascular disease remains the number 1 cause of death**, accounting for 41% of all fatalities, and the prevalence of heart disease in the United States is projected to double during the next 50 years." In industrialized nations, the prevalence of HTN in adults is approximately 1 per 4-5 (20-25%) with the vast majority of these considered idiopathic, chronic, and unresponsive to diet and lifestyle improvements from the dominant allopathic medical perspective. Integrative clinicians who appreciate the broad range of causes of and *synergistic contributors to hypertension* do not generally view this disorder as *idiopathic*, nor as necessarily *chronic*, nor as *unresponsive*, but rather find it *understandable* and *highly amenable* to numerous interventions—necessarily specific for each patient (e.g., food allergies and/or hypothyroidism and/or nutrient deficiencies)—supported by publications in

---

"Diseases of Western civilization"

- Primary hypertension
- Diabetes mellitus, type-2
- Metabolic syndrome
- Dental carries and malocclusion
- Common neuropsychiatric problems
- Dermatopathies such as eczema, psoriasis, and acne
- Obesity

"Diseases of Western civilization" can be understood by appreciation of the physiologic effects caused by the lifestyle and dietary changes historically imposed upon indigenous hunter-gather societies from incoming Westerners/Europeans. These changes include what was *added* (white flour, grains, table salt, white sugar, alcohol, and other so-called "refined" foods, which were poor in substance and vitality compared to their more "natural" and "primitive" counterparts) and what was *removed* (exercise, whole fruits, vegetables, nuts, seeds, berries, roots [i.e., fiber and phytonutrients], multigenerational community, natural living, full-body exposure to sunshine and therefore ensured adequacy of vitamin D). Important to appreciate is that these diseases were once exceedingly rare but are now commonplace. The fact that most of these conditions are common these days in children dispels the shibboleth espoused by pharmacosurgical proponents that these diseases have become more common simply because people are living longer due to "advances in medicine." Quite to the contrary, medicine as generally practiced has reinforced and abetted the conditions which generate many of these illnesses; thankfully, we are seeing positive changes in medicine, but only recently, and mainly due to outside pressures and the popularity of and market demand for open-mindedness toward healthy living.

The classic text on this subject is Price W A. Nutrition and Physical Degeneration: A Comparison of Primitive and Modern Diets and Their Effects. Santa Monica; Price-Pottinger Nutrition Foundation: 1945

---

[32] French: *in passing* or *in passage*. Capturing "en passant" is a strategy used in the game of chess wherein a player is allowed to capture an opponent's pawn in an adjacent row after the opponent has moved the pawn forward by two spaces. In this context, I use the phrase *en passant* to denote that most of the natural treatments detailed in the following pages do not directly and intentionally target hypertension *per se* but rather reduce hypertension *in passing* as overall health is improved.

[33] Eaton SB, Shostak M, Konner M. The Paleolithic Prescription. New York: Harper and Row Publishers; 1988, 49

[34] O'Keefe JH Jr, Cordain L. Cardiovascular disease resulting from a diet and lifestyle at odds with our Paleolithic genome. *Mayo ClinProc* 2004;79:101-8

peer-reviewed biomedical journals. **The high prevalence of primary hypertension seen in industrial "Westernized" societies does not necessarily imply that the people in these societies are as a group genetically defective and therefore "in need of medical intervention" but perhaps rather that the industrialized/Westernized lifestyle is inherently adverse to the preservation of human health, well-being, and longevity.**[35] In early biomedical and socioanthropologic literature such as Dr Weston Price's *Nutrition and Physical Degeneration: A Comparison of Primitive and Modern Diets and Their Effects*[36] published in 1945, hypertension—just like diabetes mellitus, dental carries, malocclusion, chronic dermatopathies such as acne, eczema, and psoriasis, and a myriad of clinical and subclinical neuropsychiatric problems—was often described as one of the "diseases of Western civilization", i.e., a disease that did not generally exist within primitive hunter-gatherer societies until such societies were infiltrated with white flour, white sugar, alcohol, salt [sodium chloride], and other aspects of the Western/industrialized way of existing and surviving.

- The clinician's responsibilities: The obligations imposed upon clinicians in the management of hypertension include:

    1. Comprehensive clinical assessment: Assess for urgent situations (BP > 210/120 mm Hg) and end-organ damage, particularly of the **eyes** (fundoscopic examination), **kidneys** (measure serum BUN and creatinine; determine GFR; obtain UA, perhaps also look for albumin:creatinine ratio to detect early proteinuria), and **cardiovascular system** (cardiopulmonary auscultation and blood pressure measurement with every visit; consider bruit screening, ECG, echocardiography, ankle-brachial index, and assessment for other cardiovascular risk factors such as hyperglycemia, dyslipidemia, and inflammation with hsCRP. Assessing for other risk factors such as n-3 fatty acid insufficiency (generally dietary history is sufficient for assessment; laboratory analysis is expensive and generally not required), vitamin D3 insufficiency, serum cystatin C, serum ferritin, lipoprotein a (Lp-a), aldosterone, renin, and fibrinogen can also be performed.

    2. Differential diagnosis: Competently assess for and exclude genuine causes of HTN before ascribing HTN to a "genetic" or familial cause requiring perpetual medicalization; detailed information on assessment (e.g., physical exam, lab tests, and diagnostic/therapeutic interventions) is reviewed later in this chapter.

    3. Effective treatment: Effective intervention must be prescribed by the physician and implemented by the patient; results must be documented in the patient's chart. The clinician has the responsibility to effect improved outcome, document patient noncompliance, and/or initiate a *complete referral* to a specialist for recalcitrant cases, for additional testing, advanced treatment, and/or liability defense.

    4. Patient education: Because hypertension—like diabetes and hemochromatosis—is generally asymptomatic in its early stages and in milder cases, doctors (derived from the Latin *docere,* which means "to teach"[37]) have the responsibility to instruct patients on the nature of their disorder, its effects and treatment options, and the consequences of nontreatment. Patients have the responsibility to comply with the

---

[35] O'Keefe JH Jr, Cordain L. Cardiovascular disease resulting from a diet and lifestyle at odds with our Paleolithic genome. *Mayo ClinProc* 2004;79:101-8
[36] Price WA. Nutrition and Physical Degeneration: A Comparison of Primitive and Modern Diets and Their Effects. Price-Pottinger Nutr Foundtn: 1945
[37] Prakash R, Misra R, Misra R. Doctors as Teachers. *Psychiatric News* 2002; 37: 37 http://www.pn.psychiatryonline.org/content/37/9/37.1.full

treatment plan, implement an effective alternate plan, or absorb the consequences of noncompliance and disease progression.

5. <u>Implement a follow-up plan</u>: Doctors must (pre)schedule patients for follow-up in-office visits to monitor treatment adherence and therapeutic effectiveness.

6. <u>Complete referral for nonresponsive or noncompliant patients</u>: "Complete referral" includes a professional letter of referral including the patient's history, examination findings, lab results, and any imaging and other assessments that are within the referring clinician's scope of competence/practice. Generally, the referring clinician's office should call the specialist's office to make the appointment for the patient, then provide the appointment time and address to the patient; the components of this complete referral are then documented in the patient's chart. Simply telling a patient, "You need to see a specialist" is often insufficient because doing so places the burden of responsibility onto the patient, and many of our patients lack the sophistication and knowledge to successfully navigate various overlapping healthcare systems. By ensuring that the patient's appointment is made with the specialist, the physician facilitates patient care and protects herself/himself from undue liability.

Consequences of failing to adequately manage hypertension
• Accelerated atherosclerosis, CVD
• Hemorrhagic and ischemic stroke,
• Peripheral arterial disease,
• Mesenteric ischemia,
• Erectile dysfunction in men,
• Myocardial infarction,
• Heart failure,
• Cerebral and aortic aneurysm,
• Nephropathy, dialysis, transplant,
• Retinopathy, intra ocular hemorrhage, vision loss,
• Patient dissatisfaction
• Physician dissatisfaction, malpractice litigation

<u>**Clinical Presentations**</u>:

- Clearly the vast majority of clinical presentations of HTN are silent, discovered only when the clinician finds elevated blood pressure on routine examination. This underscores the importance of hypertension screening among asymptomatic patients. The second and remaining group of clinical presentations of HTN includes those of end-organ damage: nephropathy, retinopathy, cardiomyopathy, and the consequences of HTN-accelerated CVD including stroke, myocardial infarction, aortic dissection, and rupture of an enlarged (generally >5.5 cm) abdominal aortic aneurysm.

- Typical clinical presentations of the hypertensive patient can range from incidental to catastrophic and include the following:
  - Asymptomatic: incidental finding during presentation and evaluation for another concern such as routine examination, injury, or infection
  - Headache, altered mental status
  - Congestive heart failure presenting with fatigue, lower extremity edema, or dyspnea
  - Retinopathy, vision impairment
  - Myocardial infarction or sudden death due to accelerated CVD complicated by cardiac hypertrophy (i.e., supply-demand mismatch)
  - Hypertensive nephropathy presenting with renal insufficiency: azotemia, edema, malignant hypertension, anuria/oliguria

Major Differential Diagnoses: Characteristics of secondary hypertension include therapeutic recalcitrance (defined as inefficacy or subefficacy of simultaneous use of three or more drugs[38]), onset at an early age (< 30y) or at a more advanced age (>50y), and the typical associated features of the causative disorder, such as hypokalemia with hyperaldosteronism, depression or musculoskeletal pain with hypovitaminosis D, and cold intolerance, bradycardia, and delayed Achilles reflex return with hypothyroidism. Listed below are most of the primary causes of hypertension with a brief sketch of their classic clinical characteristics, including physical examination and laboratory findings. Additionally, the December 2010 review by Vierra and Neutze[39] recommends an age-based approach which will also be included in the following descriptions of differential diagnoses; of note, 70-85% of hypertension in children is secondary to an identifiable primary disorder. While the purpose of this text is to focus on *adult* hypertension, many of the diagnostic and treatment considerations are appropriately applicable to children. Normal and abnormal values for blood pressure in infants and children differ from those of adults and are stratified based on age, gender, and height in a chart from the International Pediatric Hypertension Association available at http://PediatricHypertension.org.

- Aortic coarctation: Coarctation of the aorta is the second most common cause of HTN in children. (Kidney disease is the most common cause of HTN in children, as reviewed later.) Aortic coarctation is 2-5x more common in males, and typical age of diagnosis is 5 years. Classic presentation includes upper extremity hypertension with lower extremity hypotension/hypoperfusion/claudication, with or without discrepancies in bilateral brachial pressure, in a child or young adult; secondary activation of the renin-angiotensin system due to renal hypoperfusion exacerbates the HTN and complicates this *focal* anatomic disorder by adding a *systemic* neurohormonal component. Physical examination findings may include leg blood pressure at least 20 mm Hg less than arm blood pressure, delayed or absent femoral pulses, and an audible murmur or bruit. Imaging modalities of choice are transthoracic ultrasonography for children and MRI for adults; computed tomography (CT), magnetic resonance angiography/aortography (MRA) may also be used. Treatment includes antihypertensive interventions (reviewed in the section on *Therapeutic Considerations*) to manage the hypertension until surgery corrects the coarctation.

- Cocaine use: Cocaine use can cause acute and chronic elevations in blood pressure. Drug cessation is the key to treatment; urine drug testing is appropriate for patients suspected of undisclosed drug use or noncompliance with cessation. In hospital practice, patients presenting with hypertensive disorders, chest pain, and other cardiovascular syndromes are routinely tested for acute (serum drug screen) and chronic (urine drug screen) drug exposure; an impressive number of these tests come back positive even among patients who swear to have never used or not recently used recreational drugs.

- Cushing's disease/syndrome, hypercortisolism: Excess glucocorticoids whether endogenous or exogenous promote sodium retention directly via their mineralocorticoid effect and by causing hyperinsulinemia via induction of peripheral insulin resistance; both of these pathophysiologic processes contribute to HTN. Determination of iatrogenic hypercortisolism can be determined by reviewing the patient's medication intake. Endogenous hypercortisolism (2-5 diagnoses per million patients per year) can be assessed with measurements of serum adrenocorticotropic hormone (ACTH), 24-hour urinary free cortisol,

---

[38] Viera AJ, Neutze DM. Diagnosis of secondary hypertension: an age-based approach. *Am Fam Physician*. 2010 Dec 15;82(12):1471-8
[39] Viera AJ, Neutze DM. Diagnosis of secondary hypertension: an age-based approach. *Am Fam Physician*. 2010 Dec 15;82(12):1471-8

nighttime salivary cortisol, and the low-dose dexamethasone suppression test in addition to looking for the clinical characteristics of moon facies, striae, sarcopenia, and abdominal obesity. Treatment is withdrawal of exogenous steroids (if possible) for iatrogenic Cushing's syndrome, or surgical removal of the ACTH-producing pituitary corticotroph adenoma (classically) in cases of endogenous Cushing's disease. An additional type of Cushing's syndrome can result from ectopic ACTH production from tumors such as small cell carcinoma of the lung or a carcinoid tumor.

- Drug side-effect: Many pharmaceutical drugs can cause an elevation in blood pressure. Reviewing the adverse effects of each drug that a patient is taking may be sufficient to identify the offending agent; a clinical trial of discontinuation may be appropriate to determine if a drug causes or contributes to elevated blood pressure in a particular patient. Many options to the use of pharmaceutical drugs exist, allowing the prevention and alleviation of many diseases and disorders commonly encountered in clinical practice.[40] Several common hypertension-inducing drugs are listed in separate paragraphs within this section on differential diagnosis; drugs worthy of specific mention include amphetamines, buspirone, carbamazapine, clozapine, fluoxetine, lithium, tricyclic antidepressants, prednisone and methylprednisolone, and sympathomimetic decongestants.[41]

- Estrogen, oral contraceptives: As a group of various hormones with divergent effects, estrogens generally tend to promote sodium and water retention, which promotes volume overload and the development of HTN. For women with "estrogen dominance" due to excess endogenous production or exogenous administration of estrogens, supplementation with pyridoxine 50-250 mg/d (nearly always co-administered with magnesium 600-1,200 mg/d or to bowel tolerance; pyridoxal-5-phosphate [p5p] might also be used) and/or natural progesterone (rather than a synthetic progestin, since many of these preparations have inherent glucocorticoid/mineralocorticoid activity) can frequently offset the HTN-inducing effects of estrogens. Clinicians desiring a more comprehensive anti-estrogen protocol within a context of practical hormone optimization ("orthoendocrinology") may find helpful the review in chapter 4 of *Integrative Rheumatology*.[42]

- Ethanol overconsumption: Excess ethanol consumption raises blood pressure and makes HTN more difficult to treat. Many patients fail to accurately disclose the extent and duration of their alcohol consumption. In acute care and hospital settings, plasma ethanol (blood alcohol concentration, BAC) can be measured, along with either serum toxicology screening for acute/recent intoxication or urinary toxicology screening for chronic/past drug use. Many patients who claim to have not used drugs ever or recently will be found to have positive drug tests with replicable results. Clues to occult alcoholism may include socioeconomic problems and elevations of serum AST (aspartate transaminase) greater than ALT (alanine transaminase), along with elevations of GGT (gamma glutamyl transpeptidase) and triglycerides; hepatic cirrhosis, splenomegally, and pancytopenia may also be noted among patients with chronic alcoholism, even among patients who deny alcohol use. Differential diagnosis of occult alcoholism includes chronic viral hepatitis B or C, hemochromatosis and

---

[40] **Vasquez A**. Chiropractic and Naturopathic Mastery of Common Clinical Disorders. IBMRC 2009. http://optimalhealthresearch.com/

[41] Viera AJ, Neutze DM. Diagnosis of secondary hypertension: an age-based approach. *Am Fam Physician*. 2010 Dec 15;82(12):1471-8

[42] **Vasquez A**. Integrative Rheumatology. IBMRC 2006, 2007 and all future editions. http://optimalhealthresearch.com/rheumatology.html

other forms of iron overload, overuse of other drugs or medications, and psychiatric disorders.

- Gestational hypertension and preeclampsia: Pregnancy-induced (after week 20 of gestation) hypertension without proteinuria is termed *gestational hypertension*; gestational hypertension with concomitant proteinuria is termed *preeclampsia*, while the addition of seizures advances the diagnosis to *eclampsia*—all of these pregnancy-related hypertenive syndromes can present with acute HTN. Preeclampsia can accelerate rapidly and cause life-threatening complications for the mother and/or fetus; treatment requires parenteral therapy (intravenous magnesium sulfate for seizure prophylaxis; hydralazine and/or labetolol for HTN control) and/or emergency interventions— namely, delivery.[43] Some evidence suggests that the incidence of preeclampsia can be reduced via increased intake of aspirin, ascorbate, calcium, tocopherol(s), and magnesium[44], and by pre-pregnancy treatment/cure of obesity, diabetes mellitus, and HTN.

- Hypercalcemia: Easily diagnosed by routine laboratory testing, hypercalcemia may be caused by hyperparathyroidism, malignancy, Paget's disease of bone, sarcoidosis, or rarely by

> **Rapid-onset HTN must be managed early and assertively**
>
> Rapid-onset HTN of 160 mm Hg systolic or 110 mm Hg diastolic requires urgent treatment. *Rapid-onset* HTN can cause stroke at pressures generally tolerated in *chronic* HTN because, in the latter, the vasculature has time to adapt to the higher pressures, while in the former, the cardiovascular system has not had time to adapt, thus leaving the patient particularly vulnerable to hemorrhagic stroke. Acute-onset HTN *from any cause* should be treated urgently when pressures approximate or exceed 160-180 mm Hg systolic or 110 mm Hg diastolic, especially *but not exclusively* if accompanied by complications such as angina (test serum cardiac enzymes), shortness of breath (consider pulmonary edema and auscultate for crackles), vision changes, papilledema, headache/ confusion/ seizures (which suggest cerebral edema or cerebral vasospasm), proteinuria, or edema of the face, peripheral extremities, or of the general body (anasarca, check for sacral edema and weight gain).

nutritional excesses of calcium and/or vitamin D. Most hypercalcemia (80-90%) is due to hyperparathyroidism or malignancy; the most common cause of hypercalcemia in the outpatient setting is hyperparathyroidism, while in the hospital setting the most common cause is malignancy, particularly multiple myeloma, lymphoma, lymphosarcomas, and metastatic disease.[45] While other differential diagnoses also need to be considered, some endocrinologist particularly advocate testing 24-h urinary calcium levels as a test for familial hypocalciuric hypercalcemia. When primary hyperparathyroidism is suspected, the serum level of intact parathyroid hormone (iPTH) is tested. When malignancy is suspected (particularly from the finding of an unexplained serum calcium > 13 mg/dL [> 3.25 mmol/L]), patient-centered evaluation is performed, which often includes initial chest radiograph followed by *pan-scanning* with CT for occult malignancies in the thorax (e.g., lung cancers), abdomen and pelvis (e.g., gastrointestinal tumors).

- Insulin resistance and hyperinsulinemia: Insulin promotes renal retention of sodium which leads to water retention and the subsequent volume overload and systemic hypertension which logically follow in sequence. This explains the well proven and replicable benefit of

---

[43] Wagner LK. Diagnosis and management of preeclampsia. *Am Fam Physician*. 2004 Dec 15;70(12):2317-24

[44] Domino FJ (editor in chief). The 5-Minute Clinical Consult. 2010. 18th Edition. Philadelphia; Wolters Kluwer: 2009, 1062

[45] Bent S, Gensler LS, Frances C. Saint-Frances Guide: Clinical Clerkship in Outpatient Medicine. 2nd Edition. Philadelphia; Wolters Kluwer: 2008, 490

low-carbohydrate diets in treating "idiopathic" HTN in the general population. Elevated or high-normal serum insulin along with chronic hyperglycemia is most suggestive of insulin resistance; the most effective treatments for insulin resistance are integrative nutritional interventions as detailed in *Chiropractic and Naturopathic Mastery of Common Clinical Disorders*.[46]

- Licorice (*Glycyrrhiza glabra*) over-consumption: Used medicinally for thousands of years with excellent safety and effectiveness, *Glycyrrhiza glabra* is particularly useful against several common human viral infections. The active constituent glycyrrhizin (also known as glycyrrhizic acid, the hydrolysis product of which is glycyrrhetinic acid) can cause clinically severe hypertension with hypokalemia via potentiation of endogenous mineralocorticoids leading to clinical syndrome called "pseudo-hyperaldosteronism." More specifically, glycyrrhizin inhibits 11-beta hydroxysteroid dehydrogenase thus preventing cortisol's inactivation to cortisone in the kidney; this potentiates the mineralocorticoid effect of endogenous cortisol leading to sodium retention and potassium excretion. The hypertension resolves following discontinuation of the excess licorice.

- Mercury toxicity: Mercury is an established neurotoxin, immunotoxin, and nephrotoxin. Because pathophysiologic effects are noted even with very small doses of exposure, one could reasonably argue that no safe amount exists and therefore that any detected mercury is an indication for therapeutic intervention to remove this toxicant. According to an article by Schober et al[47] published in *JAMA—Journal of the American Medical Association* in 2003, "Approximately 8% of [1,709 American] women had [blood mercury] concentrations higher than the US Environmental Protection Agency's recommended reference dose (5.8 µg/L), below which exposures are considered to be without adverse effects." Sources of exposure include dental amalgams, vaccinations, airborne pollution, and fish; recently, high-fructose corn syrup was shown to contain mercury.[48] Mercury impairs catecholamine degradation and can thereby cause a clinical syndrome that can include hypertension, tremor, tachycardia, diaphoresis, and neurocognitive changes.[49] Per Shih and Gartner[50], "Mercury combines with the sulfhydryl group of S-adenosylmethionine, which is a cofactor for catecholamine-O-methyltransferase (COMT), and this inhibition of COMT allows accumulation of norepinephrine, epinephrine, and dopamine." The clinical presentation of mercury toxicity can include any of the following: diffuse erythematosus rash, dermatitis (acrodynia), anorexia, malaise, fatigue, muscle pain, proximal and/or distal muscle weakness, tremor, weight loss, insomnia, night sweats, burning peripheral neuropathy (axonal neuropathy), renal insufficiency/failure, inattention, neurocognitive compromise, personality

[46] **Vasquez A**. Chiropractic and Naturopathic Mastery of Common Clinical Disorders. IBMRC 2009. http://optimalhealthresearch.com/textbooks/clinical_mastery.html
[47] Schober SE, Sinks TH, Jones RL, Bolger PM, McDowell M, Osterloh J, Garrett ES, Canady RA, Dillon CF, Sun Y, Joseph CB, Mahaffey KR. Blood mercury levels in US children and women of childbearing age, 1999-2000. *JAMA*. 2003 Apr 2;289(13):1667-74 http://jama.ama-assn.org/content/289/13/1667.long
[48] "Average daily consumption of high fructose corn syrup is about 50 grams per person in the United States. With respect to total mercury exposure, it may be necessary to account for this source of mercury in the diet of children and sensitive populations." Dufault R, LeBlanc B, Schnoll R, Cornett C, Schweitzer L, Wallinga D, Hightower J, Patrick L, Lukiw WJ. Mercury from chlor-alkali plants: measured concentrations in food product sugar. *Environ Health*. 2009 Jan 26;8:2. See also: "High fructose corn syrup has been shown to contain trace amounts of mercury as a result of some manufacturing processes, and its consumption can also lead to zinc loss." Dufault R, Schnoll R, Lukiw WJ, Leblanc B, Cornett C, Patrick L, Wallinga D, Gilbert SG, Crider R. Mercury exposure, nutritional deficiencies and metabolic disruptions may affect learning in children. *Behav Brain Funct*. 2009 Oct 27;5:44.
[49] Wössmann W, Kohl M, Grüning G, Bucsky P. Mercury intoxication presenting with hypertension and tachycardia. *Arch Dis Child*. 1999 Jun;80(6):556-7 http://www.ncbi.nlm.nih.gov/pmc/articles/PMC1717944/pdf/v080p00556.pdf
[50] Shih H, Gartner JC Jr. Weight loss, hypertension, weakness, and limb pain in an 11-year-old boy. *J Pediatr*. 2001 Apr;138(4):566-9

changes, depression, diaphoresis, tachycardia, and hypertension. Differential diagnoses for mercury toxicity are numerous, including pheochromocytoma, hyperthyroidism, conversion disorder, viral infection, toxic shock syndrome, and Kawasaki disease. Laboratory assessment can include 24-hour urinary catecholamines, random urine mercury, and whole blood mercury; these tests are particularly appropriate for acute and subacute intoxications. For distant and chronic mercury intoxications, many clinicians including this author prefer to use dimercaptosuccinic acid (DMSA) dosed orally at 10 mg per kilogram of body weight to enhance the sensitivity of urine toxic metal testing. The use of DMSA for children and adults is supported by peer-reviewed literature[51,52,53,54,55] and has been reviewed in more detail by this author in *Integrative Rheumatology*[56] and to a lesser extent in *Musculoskeletal Pain: Expanded Clinical Strategies.*[57] DMSA chelation is approved by the US Food and Drug Administration (FDA) for the treatment of lead toxicity in children.[58]

- Neurogenic hypertension: In the context of discussing HTN, "neurogenic" was historically interchangeable with "essential", "primary", and "idiopathic." Since *neurogenic* is no longer generally used for this purpose, and because new research advocates the term's reinstitution, *neurogenic hypertension* should be exonerated from its previous identification with *idiopathicity* and given revised meaning. For the purposes of this discussion and as detailed later in this chapter, **the term "neurogenic hypertension" will mean what its name implies,** namely **chronic HTN induced principally by the nervous system due to** *irritation* **or** *functional disturbance* **rather than overt pathology**. Given its basis in physiology rather than pathology per se, the term

> **Physiologic irritation of the nucleus tract solitarius (NTS) and other nearby structures in the brainstem appears to contribute to some cases of hypertension**
>
> "Impaired NTS (CNS) function can produce an amplification of the action of the environmental stresses on blood pressure. Thus environmental stimuli or the expression of behaviors which normally result in trivial elevations of blood pressure will, after the NTS is perturbed, result in marked elevations (of blood pressure)."
>
> Reis DJ. The nucleus tractus solitarius and experimental neurogenic hypertension: evidence for a central neural imbalance hypothesis of hypertensive disease. *Adv Biochem Psychopharmacol*. 1981;28:409-20

"functional neurogenic hypertension" would serve to further emphasize the functional and therefore largely reversible mechanism of the disorder. Foci of neurogenic hypertension can reside in the central nervous system (CNS) or peripheral nervous system (PNS). In this text, "**central neurogenic hypertension**" describes hypertensive states induced by irritation of the central nervous system, in particular at the level of the brainstem (i.e., medulla oblongata in general and the root entry zones [REZ] of cranial nerves 9 and 10 as well as the nucleus tract

[51] Bradstreet J, Geier DA, Kartzinel JJ, Adams JB, Geier MR. A case-control study of mercury burden in children with autistic spectrum disorders. *Journal of American Physicians and Surgeons* 2003; 8: 76-79   http://www.jpands.org/vol8no3/geier.pdf
[52] Crinnion WJ. Environmental medicine, part three: long-term effects of chronic low-dose mercury exposure. *Altern Med Rev*. 2000 Jun;5(3):209-23
[53] Forman J, Moline J, Cernichiari E, Sayegh S, Torres JC, Landrigan MM, Hudson J, Adel HN, Landrigan PJ. A cluster of pediatric metallic mercury exposure cases treated with meso-2,3-dimercaptosuccinic acid (DMSA). *Environ Health Perspect*. 2000 Jun;108(6):575-7 http://ehp.niehs.nih.gov/docs/2000/108p575-577forman/abstract.html
[54] Miller AL. Dimercaptosuccinic acid (DMSA), a non-toxic, water-soluble treatment for heavy metal toxicity. *Altern Med Rev*. 1998 Jun;3(3):199-207 http://www.thorne.com/altmedrev/.fulltext/3/3/199.pdf
[55] DMSA. *Altern Med Rev*. 2000 Jun;5(3):264-7 http://thorne.com/altmedrev/.fulltext/5/3/264.pdf
[56] **Vasquez A**. Integrative Rheumatology. IBMRC 2006, 2007 and all future editions. http://optimalhealthresearch.com/rheumatology.html
[57] **Vasquez A**. Musculoskeletal Pain: Expanded Clinical Strategies. Institute for Functional Medicine. 2008
[58] "The Food and Drug Administration has recently licensed the drug DMSA (succimer) for reduction of blood lead levels >/= 45 micrograms/dl. This decision was based on the demonstrated ability of DMSA to reduce blood lead levels. An advantage of this drug is that it can be given orally." Goyer RA, Cherian MG, Jones MM, Reigart JR. Role of chelating agents for prevention, intervention, and treatment of exposures to toxic metals. *Environ Health Perspect*. 1995 Nov;103(11):1048-52 Http://ehp.niehs.nih.gov/docs/1995/103-11/meetingreport.html

solitarius [NTS] in particular) as will be reviewed in a following section on surgical interventions for the treatment of medullary neurovascular compression. The first use of the term "central neurogenic hypertension" of which this author is aware was published by Reis[59] in a 1981 review, mostly of animal research. In this review, Reis included the hypothesis that irritation of the CNS by either mechanical or neurochemical means could serve as a predisposition or antecedent to the manifest development of clinical HTN. The diagnosis of central neurogenic hypertension is generally based upon ❶ MRI/MRA or CT findings of neurovascular compression of the left medulla oblongata in conjunction with ❷ reduction in blood pressure following decompressive intervention.

"**Peripheral neurogenic hypertension**" as an entity is more theoretical, less studied, and might be exemplified by irritation of spinal nerve roots and sympathetic ganglia as discussed primarily in the chiropractic[60,61,62,63,64] and osteopathic literature.[65,66] Functional compromise in general and **facilitation**[67] in particular of the nerve roots and sympathetic ganglia as a potential *cause of* or *contributor to* chronic HTN supports the rationale for the use of spinal manipulation and manual medicine for the treatment of HTN and other nonmusculoskeletal disorders. Peripheral neurogenic hypertension may be diagnosed based on clinical/electrographic/vasodynamic evidence of functional PNS compromise/ facilitation/ irritation and alleviation of HTN following appropriate regional intervention such as manual manipulative treatment of the spine and adjacent neuromusculoskeletal structures applied to effect restoration of proper nervous system function and balance. Central and peripheral types of neurogenic HTN will be discussed in more detail later in this chapter within the context of their surgical and manipulative treatments, respectively.

> ### Facilitation: chronic low-threshold nerve discharge
>
> "Previous studies have indicated the existence, in man, of pools of spinal extensor motoneurons which are in a state of enduring excitation, as reflected in low reflex thresholds. ... The data indicate that differences in pressure thresholds reflect differences in central facilitation, and that the facilitation is due to a bombardment of the motoneurons by impulses originating, in part at least, from points other than the spinous process which was the site of stimulation."
>
> Denslow JS, Korr IM, Krems AD. Quantitative studies of chronic facilitation in human motoneuron pools. *Am J Physiology* 1947: 150; 229-238

---

[59] "The abnormalities of pressure control resulting from abnormal transmission in NTS met most of the criteria of an animal model of central neurogenic hypertension. ... Impaired NTS function can produce an amplification of the action of the environmental stresses on blood pressure." Reis DJ. The nucleus tractus solitarius and experimental neurogenic hypertension: evidence for a central neural imbalance hypothesis of hypertensive disease. *Adv Biochem Psychopharmacol*. 1981;28:409-20

[60] Bakris G, Dickholtz M Sr, Meyer PM, Kravitz G, Avery E, Miller M, Brown J, Woodfield C, Bell B. Atlas vertebra realignment and achievement of arterial pressure goal in hypertensive patients: a pilot study. *J Hum Hypertens*. 2007 May;21(5):347-52

[61] Plaugher G, Bachman TR. Chiropractic management of a hypertensive patient. *J Manipulative Physiol Ther*. 1993 Oct;16(8):544-9

[62] Yates RG, Lamping DL, Abram NL, Wright C. Effects of chiropractic treatment on blood pressure and anxiety: a randomized, controlled trial. *J Manipulative Physiol Ther*. 1988 Dec;11(6):484-8

[63] Plaugher G, Long CR, Alcantara J, Silveus AD, Wood H, Lotun K, Menke JM, Meeker WC, Rowe SH. Practice-based randomized controlled-comparison clinical trial of chiropractic adjustments and brief massage treatment at sites of subluxation in subjects with essential hypertension: pilot study. *J Manipulative Physiol Ther*. 2002 May;25(4):221-39

[64] Crawford JP, Hickson GS, Wiles MR. The management of hypertensive disease: a review of spinal manipulation and the efficacy of conservative therapeusis. *J Manipulative Physiol Ther* 1986 Mar ;9(1):27-32

[65] Celander E, Koenig AJ, Celander DR. Effect of osteopathic manipulative therapy on autonomic tone as evidenced by blood pressure changes and activity of the fibrinolytic system. *J Am Osteopath Assoc*. 1968 May;67(9):1037-8

[66] Fichera AP, Celander DR. Effect of osteopathic manipulative therapy on autonomic tone as evidenced by blood pressure changes and activity of the fibrinolytic system. *J Am Osteopath Assoc*. 1969 Jun;68(10):1036-8

[67] Denslow JS, Korr IM, Krems AD. Quantitative studies of chronic facilitation in human motoneuron pools. *Am J Physiol*. 1947 Aug;150(2):229-38

- Nonsteroidal anti-inflammatory drugs (NSAIDs): NSAIDs in general such as ibuprofen and naproxen and COX-2 inhibitors (coxibs) in particular reduce endogenous production of vasodilating prostacyclin and thus cause pharmacologic/iatrogenic renal artery constriction, which leads to varying degrees of HTN via activation of the renin-angiotensin system. This explains, in part, the increased cardiovascular mortality due to overutilization of coxibs such as rofecoxib/Vioxx, withdrawn from the US market in 2005 by the US FDA due to its causal role in increasing cardiovascular deaths.[68] Evidence of increased cardiovascular morbidity and mortality secondary to coxib use was widely publicized for several years before rofecoxib/Vioxx and a similar drug valdecoxib/Bextra were belatedly withdrawn from the consumer market.[69,70] The multiple failures involved in this politicopharmaceutical phenomenon include ❶ failure of Merck to act on data showing that its popular

> **Fraudulent marketing of valdecoxib/Bextra contributed to the largest healthcare fraud settlement in the history of the US Department of Justice—US $2.3 billion**
>
> Pharmacia and Upjohn Company, a subsidiary of Pfizer Inc, pled guilty to a felony violation of the Food, Drug & Cosmetic Act for misbranding the drug Bextra with the intent to defraud or mislead. Pharmacia and Upjohn Company admitted to its criminal conduct in the promotion of Bextra and agreed to pay a criminal fine of $1.195 billion, the largest criminal fine ever imposed in the United States for any matter. Pharmacia and Upjohn Company also agreed to forfeit $105 million, for a total criminal resolution of $1.3 billion. In addition Pfizer agreed to pay an additional $1 billion plus interest to settle civil allegations that it fraudulently promoted and marketed Bextra, as well as three other drugs in its portfolio, Geodon, an anti-psychotic drug, Zyvox, an antibiotic, and Lyrica, an anti-epileptic drug, as well as claims that it paid kickbacks for these, as well as other drugs, to induce physician prescribing.
>
> http://www.justice.gov/usao/ma/Press Office Press Release Files/Sept2009/PharmaciaPlea.html. Posted September 15, 2009. Accessed November 23, 2010. See also http://news.bbc.co.uk/2/hi/business/8234533.stm

and profitable new drug was harming and killing an unacceptable proportion of patients who took it, ❷ failure of the US FDA to regulate the pharmaceutical industry, ❸ failure of the medical profession as a whole to police itself and call for a ban on the use of this drug before either Merck or the FDA took action. See Eric Topol's "Failing the public health—rofecoxib, Merck, and the FDA" published in the October 21, 2004 issue of *New England Journal of Medicine* for authoritative discussion.

- Pheochromocytoma: An exceedingly rare cause of secondary HTN (0.5%) in contrast to the high frequency with which it is covered in textbooks and licensing board exams, pheochromocytoma's classic presentation includes episodic HTN, headache, tremor, and diaphoresis. Pheochromocytoma is diagnosed with increased 24-hour urinary catecholamines, metanephrines, and vanillylmandelic acid with or without plasma free metanephrines followed by CT/MRI to localize the secreting neuroendocrine tumor. Mercury

---

[68] Topol EJ. Failing the public health—rofecoxib, Merck, and the FDA. *N Engl J Med*. 2004 Oct 21;351(17):1707-9

[69] "The results from VIGOR showed that the relative risk of developing a confirmed adjudicated thrombotic cardiovascular event (myocardial infarction, unstable angina, cardiac thrombus, resuscitated cardiac arrest, sudden or unexplained death, ischemic stroke, and transient ischemic attacks) with rofecoxib treatment compared with naproxen was 2.38 (95% confidence interval, 1.39-4.00; P =.002)." Mukherjee D, Nissen SE, Topol EJ. Risk of cardiovascular events associated with selective COX-2 inhibitors. *JAMA* 2001 Aug 22-29;286(8):954-9

[70] "Systolic blood pressure increased significantly in 17% of rofecoxib- compared with 11% of celecoxib-treated patients (P = 0.032) at any study time point. Diastolic blood pressure increased in 2.3% of rofecoxib- compared with 1.5% of celecoxib-treated patients (P = 0.44)." Whelton A, Fort JG, Puma JA, Normandin D, Bello AE, Verburg KM; SUCCESS VI Study Group. Cyclooxygenase-2--specific inhibitors and cardiorenal function: a randomized, controlled trial of celecoxib and rofecoxib in older hypertensive osteoarthritis patients. *Am J Ther* 2001 Mar-Apr;8(2):85-95

intoxication whether acute or chronic must be considered in the differential diagnosis of pheochromocytoma and similar clinical presentations.[71,72] Treatment is surgical excision of the adrenal/extra-adrenal catecholamine-producing tumor.

- <u>Primary hyperaldosteronism (Conn's syndrome)</u>: Primary hyperaldosteronism is caused by a unilateral adrenal adenoma or bilateral adrenal hyperplasia; this condition accounts for approximately 6% of adult HTN and 10-20% of cases of treatment-resistant HTN.[73] The classic finding is HTN with hypokalemia (30%), occasionally with slight hypernatremia, and the diagnosis is established by documentation of an elevated serum aldosterone:renin ratio. Importantly, aldosterone must be tested with renin (i.e., plasma renin activity) since measurement of serum aldosterone alone is insensitive; 25% of patients with hyperaldosteronism will have a normal serum aldosterone level.[74] Per *The Merck Manual*:

  "Initial laboratory testing consists of plasma aldosterone levels and plasma renin activity (PRA). Ideally, tests are done with the patient off of drugs that affect the renin-angiotensin system (e.g., thiazide diuretics, ACE inhibitors, angiotensin antagonists, β-blockers) for 4 to 6 wk. PRA is usually measured in the morning with the patient recumbent [or upright[75]]. Patients with primary aldosteronism typically have plasma aldosterone > 15 ng/dL (> 0.42 nmol/L, [or > 416.10 pmol/L[76]]) and low levels of PRA, with a ratio of plasma aldosterone (in nanograms/dL) to PRA (in nanograms/mL/h) > 20."[77]

  Diagnosis is confirmed by an endocrinologist performing a salt-suppression test. CT imaging is insensitive for detecting microadenomas and milder degrees of glandular hyperplasia. Curative treatment is laparoscopic removal/resection of the hypersecreting adrenal tumor; for patients who are not surgical candidates, drug treatment with an aldosterone-blocking drug (e.g., spironolactone or eplerenone) is used. Pseudohyperaldosteronism can be caused by overconsumption of *Glycyrrhiza glabra* (licorice) and by Liddle's syndrome, a genotropic disorder causing increased sodium reabsorption, characterized by early onset (<35y) HTN with hypokalemia, low urinary sodium levels, and normal serum aldosterone levels.

- <u>Renal artery (renovascular) stenosis</u>: Partial obstruction of the renal arteries whether by thrombus (rare), atherosclerosis, or fibromuscular dysplasia causes renal hypoperfusion and activation of the renin-angiotensin system. Accounting for approximately 10% of renal artery stenosis (RAS), fibromuscular dysplasia is the most common cause of renovascular stenosis in young adults (19-39 years of age); women are affected much more commonly than are men. The other 90% of renovascular stenosis is caused by atherosclerosis and is therefore mostly seen in older adults (>50y), particularly those with clinically significant CVD risk factors such as smoking and dyslipidemia and/or already established vascular disease. Renovascular stenosis is suggested by elevation of serum potassium, BUN, and/or creatinine following administration of an ACEi or an ARB; a high-pitched holosystolic renal artery bruit may be heard upon careful physical examination. The diagnosis of renal artery stenosis, per

---

[71] Wössmann W, Kohl M, Grüning G, Bucsky P. Mercury intoxication presenting with hypertension and tachycardia. *Arch Dis Child*. 1999 Jun;80(6):556-7 http://www.ncbi.nlm.nih.gov/pmc/articles/PMC1717944/pdf/v080p00556.pdf

[72] Shih H, Gartner JC Jr. Weight loss, hypertension, weakness, and limb pain in an 11-year-old boy. *J Pediatr*. 2001 Apr;138(4):566-9

[73] Viera AJ, Neutze DM. Diagnosis of secondary hypertension: an age-based approach. *Am Fam Physician*. 2010 Dec 15;82(12):1471-8

[74] Viera AJ, Neutze DM. Diagnosis of secondary hypertension: an age-based approach. *Am Fam Physician*. 2010 Dec 15;82(12):1471-8

[75] Viera AJ, Neutze DM. Diagnosis of secondary hypertension: an age-based approach. *Am Fam Physician*. 2010 Dec 15;82(12):1471-8

[76] Viera AJ, Neutze DM. Diagnosis of secondary hypertension: an age-based approach. *Am Fam Physician*. 2010 Dec 15;82(12):1471-8

[77] http://www.unboundmedicine.com/merckmanual/ub/view/Merck-Manual-Pro/503850/all/Primary_Aldosteronism Accessed October 2, 2010

review by Zhang et al[78] in December 2009, can be made via imaging or invasive procedures, each with distinct advantages, disadvantages, safety profiles and costs. Catheter angiography with pressure gradient measurements is the definitive gold standard but is invasive, expensive, and thus reserved for surgical revascularization candidates. Ultrasonography is safe and inexpensive but the least accurate. Contrast-enhanced computed tomographic angiography and magnetic resonance angiography are intermediate in safety and accuracy. Magnetic resonance angiography *without any contrast* has become progressively more accurate and

> **Clinical pearl: Increase in serum K, BUN, or creatinine following ACEi or ARB treatment suggests RAS**
>
> An increase in serum creatinine (0.5-1.0 mg/dL [44.2-88.4 micromol/L]) following initiation of ACEi or ARB treatment suggests renal artery stenosis (RAS). Additional considerations include heart failure, renal insufficiency, dehydration, and drug intolerance with secondary acute renal injury. The drug does not necessarily have to be stopped until the creatinine has increased >30% over baseline or unless another compelling reason exists; monitor serum K and recheck GFR within 10 days.

can rival contrast-enhanced techniques in its clinical utility, thereby making it the preferred imaging assessment for patients with renal insufficiency. Captopril-augmented renography lacks sensitivity and specificity and is no longer recommended. Treatment options are generally surgical (e.g., stent placement, angioplasty, or other revascularization technique) and/or pharmaceutical, with surgical approaches generally preferred for fibromuscular dysplasia and pharmaceutical treatment preferred for atherosclerotic renovascular stenosis.

- Renal parenchymal disease (nephrogenic hypertension): Renal disease can both lead to and result from HTN. Kidney diseases are the most common cause of hypertension in childhood; the leading primary etiologies are glomerulonephritis, congenital abnormalities, and reflux nephropathy. Over time and especially in adults, chronic HTN causes renal parenchymal damage, and parenchymal damage (whether due to HTN or another cause such as glomerulonephritis, pyelonephritis, polycystic kidneys, etc) leads to water retention and activation of the renin-angiotensin-aldosterone system, thus promoting a vicious cycle of progressive HTN and renal failure. The clinical picture commonly includes edema, elevated BUN and creatinine, proteinuria, anemia due to insufficient production of erythropoietin, and osteomalacia and osteodystrophy due to hyperphosphatemia, hypocalcemia, and insufficient renal formation of 1,25-dihydroxyvitamin D3. The diagnosis of renal disease is suggested by the finding of elevated BUN and creatinine on routine chemistry/metabolic panel blood tests; the diagnosis is further verified and refined by the use of CT, MRI, or US imaging, followed if necessary by renal biopsy. The Cockcroft-Gault formula has commonly been used for bedside

> **Clinical pearls for managing the patient with declining renal function**
>
> - When the GFR < 60 (CKD stage 3), modify dosages or withdraw certain drugs. Treat the causative problem and/or begin specialist co-management. Avoid intravenous contrast agents and other nephrotoxic drugs when feasible. Blood pressure and glucose control are important; initiation of ACEi or ARB should be considered.
> - When the GFR < 30 (CKD stage 4), the patient needs to consult a nephrologist.
> - When the GFR < 15 (CKD stage 5), the patient needs transplant or dialysis.

---

[78] Zhang HL, Sos TA, Winchester PA, Gao J, Prince MR. Renal artery stenosis: imaging options, pitfalls, and concerns. *Prog Cardiovasc Dis.* 2009 Nov-Dec;52(3):209-19

estimation of renal function based on the patient's age, weight, gender, and serum creatinine (sCr); the formula is provided below in two versions, one using American-favored mg/dL as the unit for sCr, and the other using the international units of micromol/L—note that the latter formula employs a different constant value per gender in the numerator of the equation. The Cockcroft-Gault formula estimates creatinine clearance, which in turn is an estimate of the glomerular filtration rate (GFR), a measure of kidney function; thus creatinine clearance and GFR are somewhat interchangeable from a practical clinical perspective. Clinicians should appreciate the importance of the patient's age in determining GFR; sCr in the upper end of the normal range may indicate renal insufficiency in a patient of advanced age.

$$\text{Estimated Creatinine Clearance} = \frac{(140 - \text{age in years}) \times \text{Weight in kilograms} \times (0.85 \text{ if female})}{72 \times \text{serum } \mathbf{creatinine\ in\ mg/dL}}$$

$$\text{Estimated Creatinine Clearance} = \frac{(140 - \text{age in years}) \times \text{Weight in kilograms} \times (1.23 \text{ for men or } 1.04 \text{ for women})}{72 \times \text{serum } \mathbf{creatinine\ in\ micromol/L}}$$

Although the Cockcroft-Gault formula is the best-known and longest-used formula for the estimation of GFR, currently the best equation for more accurately estimating GFR from serum creatinine is the Modification of Diet in Renal Disease (MDRD) Study equation, available on-line: http://nkdep.nih.gov/professionals/gfr_calculators/.[79]

Finally on this topic of renal disease, clinicians should be aware of measuring serum cystatin C to assess renal function. Cystatin C is a cysteine protease inhibitor produced by all nucleated cells, and its serum level is not affected by diet or muscle mass (unlike serum creatinine). The normal range for cystatin C when measured by particle-enhanced nephelometric immunoassay (PENIA) is <0.28 mg/L or <0.95 mg/L when measured by other immunologic methods. Cystatin C is a more sensitive indicator of declining renal function than is serum creatinine, and—like elevating serum creatinine or declining GFR (or elevated CRP for that matter)—cystatin C predicts risk and severity of CVD, CHF, and CKD; furthermore, cystatin C is directly involved in the pathogenesis of atherosclerosis.[80]

- Sleep apnea: Obstructive sleep apnea (OSA) is a risk factor for HTN, and treatment for OSA with continuous positive airway pressure (C-PAP) can produce modest reductions in BP that are proportionate to the severity of the HTN and compliance with treatment. Diagnosis is suggested by history of unrestful sleep, fatigue, depression, and/or a spouse's report of interrupted nighttime breathing. Physical exam may show obesity and impairment of upper airway airflow. An overnight sleep study (polysomnography) provides data on sleep, respiratory effort, and blood oxygenation and has been considered the standard for the diagnosis of sleep apnea; however, nocturnal pulse oximetry may be sufficient for the diagnosis in selected high-index patients and is less cumbersome and less expensive.
- Systemic sclerosis: HTN in general and treatment-resistant HTN in particular are seen in systemic sclerosis, a disease in which cardiopulmonary disease (e.g., pulmonary

---

[79] National Kidney Disease Education Program, National Institutes of Health (NIH). http://www.nkdep.nih.gov/professionals/gfr_calculators/

[80] "Prospective studies have shown, in various clinical scenarios, that patients with increased cystatin C are at a higher risk of developing both CVD and CKD. Importantly, cystatin C appears to be a useful marker for identifying individuals at a higher risk for cardiovascular events among patients belonging to a relatively low-risk category as assessed by both creatinine and estimated glomerular filtration rate values." Taglieri N, Koenig W, Kaski JC. Cystatin C and cardiovascular risk. *Clin Chem.* 2009 Nov;55(11):1932-43

hypertension, congestive heart failure) and renal compromise (e.g., acute renal crisis heralded by nephrogenic hypertension) are the most common causes of death. Abnormalities disclosed on history and physical exam may include Raynaud's phenomenon, sclerodactyly, mask-like face, telangiectasia, and esophageal dysfunction. Laboratory findings typically include some combination of positive antinuclear antibodies (ANA), anticentromere antibodies, anti-SCL-70 antibodies, and (more rarely) anti-fibrillarin antibodies. Treatment for scleroderma and other common autoimmune disorders is reviewed in *Integrative Rheumatology*.[81]

- <u>Thyroid disease, including both hyperthyroidism and hypothyroidism</u>: Hypothyroidism generally causes diastolic HTN, whereas hyperthyroidism generally causes systolic HTN and widened pulse pressure. Assess clinically (e.g., pulse rate, physical exam, weight loss/gain, Achilles reflex return speed, body temperature), and with laboratory testing. A low TSH and elevated free T4 is sufficient to diagnose hyperthyroidism. The diagnosis of hypothyroidism is indicated by any one or more of the following: elevated TSH, low free T4, low free T3 and/or total T3. Elevated titers of antithyroid antibodies (e.g., either anti-thyroid peroxidase or anti-thyroglobulin) can provide sufficient indication for treatment with thyroid hormone to prevent overt hypothyroidism from developing. Elevated reverse T3 and/or a ratio of total T3 to reverse T3 less than 10:1 indicates impaired peripheral metabolism of thyroid hormones; many integrative clinicians—including this author—hold that the ratio of total T3 to reverse T3 should be > 10:1 to ensure proper peripheral thyroid metabolism.[82]

- <u>Tobacco use</u>: Tobacco smoke constituents cause arterioconstriction which promotes HTN. Constituents and free radicals in tobacco smoke are more pathogenic than nicotine, while the latter in isolation indeed causes adverse cardiovascular effects.

- <u>Upper cervical spine dysfunction/subluxation</u>: A remarkable clinical trial published in *Journal of Human Hypertension* in 2007 by Bakris et al[83] showed that **correction of upper cervical spine subluxation/dysfunction by chiropractic spinal manipulation causes "marked and sustained reductions in BP [blood pressure] similar to the use of two-drug combination therapy."** These results suggest and perhaps indicate that subtle biomechanical dysfunction of the upper cervical spine can cause hypertension, perhaps via neuronal reflex mechanisms or possibly—as suggested by Bakris et al—by alleviating neurovascular compression and/or by alleviating circulatory compromise of the vertebral artery.

- <u>Vitamin D deficiency</u>: Vitamin D deficiency is common in the general population—often up to 90-100% of subjects in large population-based studies—and causes intracellular hypercalcinosis[84] via elevated PTH levels and contributes to chronic HTN[85] via endothelial dysfunction, systemic inflammation, insulin resistance, and activation of the renin-angiotensin-aldosterone system.[86] **Correction of vitamin D deficiency can cause a reduction**

---

[81] **Vasquez A**. Integrative Rheumatology. IBMRC 2006, 2007 and all future editions. http://optimalhealthresearch.com/rheumatology.html
[82] McDaniel AB. Thyroid Assessment: Controversies and Conundrums. Institute for Functional Medicine Fourteenth International Symposium. Tuscon, Arizona. May 23-26, 2007. Reviewed in more detail in: **Vasquez A**. Musculoskeletal Pain: Expanded Clinical Strategies. Institute for Functional Medicine. 2008
[83] Bakris G, Dickholtz M Sr, Meyer PM, Kravitz G, Avery E, Miller M, Brown J, Woodfield C, Bell B. Atlas vertebra realignment and achievement of arterial pressure goal in hypertensive patients: a pilot study. *J Hum Hypertens*. 2007 May;21(5):347-52
[84] **Vasquez A**. Intracellular Hypercalcinosis: A Functional Nutritional Disorder with Implications Ranging from Myofascial Trigger Points to Affective Disorders, Hypertension, and Cancer. *Naturopathy Digest* 2006 Previously published in-print and on-line at http://www.naturopathydigest.com/archives/2006/sep/vasquez.php and included at the end of this chapter.
[85] **Vasquez A**. Nutritional Treatments for Hypertension. *Naturopathy Digest* 2006. Previously published in-print and on-line at http://www.naturopathydigest.com/archives/2006/nov/vasquez.php and included at the end of this chapter.
[86] Pilz S, Tomaschitz A, Ritz E, Pieber TR; Medscape. Vitamin D status and arterial hypertension: a systematic review. *Nat Rev Cardiol*. 2009 Oct;6(10):621-30

in elevated blood pressure comparable to that which can be achieved by single-drug oral antihypertensive medication[87] while also providing numerous collateral benefits (including reductions in depression, pain, and risks for autoimmune and malignant diseases) at lower cost and greater safety than can be achieved with pharmaceutical drugs.[88,89]

<u>Clinical Assessments</u>:

- <u>**History/subjective**</u>: As stated previously, **most patients with HTN are asymptomatic** and only become symptomatic as a result of severe HTN which results in end-organ compromise, such as renal insufficiency, cerebral edema, or transient myocardial ischemia. The clinical history should include inquiry about chest pain, shortness of breath, family history of CVD or diabetes mellitus (DM), morning occipital headaches, new stressors, tobacco/caffeine use, and current medications/drugs including antihypertensives, nonsteroidal anti-inflammatory drugs (NSAIDs), estrogens, ethanol, cocaine, sympathomimetics and decongestants. During this standard *history of the present illness* (HPI) which all clinicians are taught to master before graduation from their respective colleges, astute clinicians have already begun the psychographic assessment (described hereafter as "BVG-LOC profiling") which will enable them to couch the treatment objectives and details in a manner tailored for that particular patient. In this context, the patient's BVG-LOC profile (i.e., personal profile of beliefs, values, goals, and locus of control) must be appreciated by the clinician since each aspect is essential to the understanding needed by the clinician in order to address or "speak to" the patient in such a way as to improve treatment compliance—these concepts are discussed more under the section *Clinical Management* below.

- <u>**Physical Examination/Objective**</u>:
  - <u>Physical examination and vital signs</u>: A screening physical examination is necessary (with details emphasized below) along with documentation of findings and vital signs, including blood pressure, pulse rate, breathing rate, temperature, pain level; weight and body mass index should be noted. Auscultation of the heart, lungs, carotid and renal arteries is performed, and cranial nerves are screened.

  - <u>Blood pressure measurement</u>: Screening for HTN should be performed at least once every two years starting at 18 years of age. The blood pressure cuff must be at heart level and properly fitted to the patient; the patient should be seated and relaxed for 5-10 minutes prior to blood

---

How to measure waist circumference

"To measure your waist circumference, place a tape measure around your bare abdomen just above your hip bone. [Waist circumference is the distance around your natural waist (just above the navel).*] Be sure that the tape is snug (but does not compress your skin) and that it is parallel to the floor. Relax, exhale, and measure your waist."

Weight and Waist Measurement: Tools for Adults. http://win.niddk.nih.gov/Publications/tools.htm Accessed February 12, 2009
* Body Composition Tests. Accessed February 12, 2009 http://americanheart.org/presenter.jhtml?identifier=4489

---

[87] "Inadequate vitamin D(3) and calcium intake could play a contributory role in the pathogenesis and progression of hypertension and cardiovascular disease in elderly women." Pfeifer M, Begerow B, Minne HW, Nachtigall D, Hansen C. Effects of a short-term vitamin D(3) and calcium supplementation on blood pressure and parathyroid hormone levels in elderly women. *J Clin Endocrinol Metab*. 2001 Apr;86(4):1633-7

[88] **Vasquez A**, Manso G, Cannell J. The clinical importance of vitamin D (cholecalciferol): a paradigm shift with implications for all healthcare providers. *Altern Ther Health Med*. 2004 Sep-Oct;10(5):28-36 http://optimalhealthresearch.com/cholecalciferol.html

[89] Faloon B. Millions of Needless Deaths. *Life Extension Magazine*. 2009 January http://lef.org/magazine/mag2009/jan2009_Millions-of-Needless-Deaths_01.htm

pressure measurement. At initial evaluation and periodically thereafter, blood pressure should be assessed in both the right and left arms; a significant side-to-side discrepancy > 20/10 mm Hg suggests a partial unilateral occlusion and is worthy of further evaluation. The two measurements upon which the diagnosis of HTN is being considered should occur on different visits at least 3 days apart; alternatively, if the blood pressure is >160/100 mm Hg on any one visit, then a presumptive diagnosis of HTN can be made and treatment initiated—in the pharmaceutical paradigm, treatment for BP >160/100 mm Hg is often initiated with two drugs. Blood pressure 120/80-139/89 mm Hg is considered "prehypertension" and is observed for progression without drug treatment in standard allopathic medicine[90] but is obviously a prime opportunity to intervene with nutritional and lifestyle improvements for those clinicians more progressively inclined. Blood pressure ≥140/90-160/100 is considered "stage 1 hypertension" and in the medical model is initially treated with one drug—generally a thiazide—while blood pressure ≥160/100-210/120 ("stage 2 hypertension") is often treated initially with a two-drug combination, with one of those drugs generally being a thiazide and the other drug selected based on patient characteristics. (Antihypertensive drug treatments are summarized at the end of this chapter). Blood pressures ≥210/120 are worthy of urgent or emergency treatment, based on the absence or presence of symptoms or organ damage, respectively, in an emergency hospital setting—additional details are provided in a following section on *Clinical Management*.

o **Cardiopulmonary examination:** Auscultation for rate, rhythm, rales/crackles; localize the cardiac point of maximal impulse (PMI) for evidence of lateral displacement or increased intensity which could indicate cardiomegaly or left ventricular hypertrophy.

o **Eye and fundoscopic examination:** Look for cotton-wool spots, retinal/flame hemorrhages, arteriovenous nicking, and papilledema; manifestations of diabetic retinopathy may also be seen if DM is concomitant. Patients with DM are referred for ophthalmologic evaluation at the time of diagnosis and annually/biannually thereafter depending on severity and compliance with and effectiveness of treatment.

o **Inspection for diagonal ear lobe crease:** Numerous studies have shown that the diagonal ear lobe crease is one of the easiest and most sensitive (~75%) and specific (~80%) physical examination findings to correlate with advanced atherosclerosis and cardiovascular disease.[91,92]

o **Examination of the extremities:** Assess pulse strength, arm:leg blood pressure differences[93] (ankle:brachial index should be > 1), lower extremity edema, capillary refill/perfusion and trophic changes consistent with peripheral vascular disease.

o **Renal disease survey:** Renal diseases are the most common causes of secondary hypertension. No physical examination finding correlates specifically with renal disease; peripheral edema is correlative but not indicative. Laboratory assessments include serum BUN, serum creatinine, serum cystatin C, and urine albumin:creatinine ratio (microalbuminuria) and/or urine albumin (proteinuria).

---

[90] Le T, Dehlendorf C, Mendoza M, Ohata C. First Aid for the Family Medicine Boards. New York: McGraw-Hill Medical; 2008, 50
[91] Edston E. The earlobe crease, coronary artery disease, and sudden cardiac death: an autopsy study of 520 individuals. *Am J Forensic Med Pathol.* 2006 Jun;27(2):129-33
[92] Motamed M, Pelekoudas N. The predictive value of diagonal ear-lobe crease sign. *Int J Clin Pract.* 1998 Jul-Aug;52(5):305-6
[93] Ankle-brachial index test. http://www.webmd.com/heart-disease/ankle-brachial-index-test Referenced January 2010

o <u>Auscultation for bruits</u>: Use the stethoscope bell over the carotid arteries (atherosclerosis) and renal arteries (renovascular hypertension due to atherosclerosis or fibromuscular dysplasia). Occasionally, an aortic bruit may be heard, particularly in cases of malformation or dissection. Higher degrees of arterial occlusion may reduce blood flow to such an extent that no bruit is heard.

o <u>Neurologic examination</u>: Observation for facial symmetry, inquiry about headache and mental status, and quick screening for symmetric and normal extremity muscle strength and reflexes may be sufficient for "low index" cases of mild hypertension in middle-aged patients without concomitant disease, such dyslipidemia or diabetes mellitus. However, as the number and severity of risk factors accumulate, the case becomes progressively worthy of a "high index" examination to establish a comprehensive assessment of baseline status and to screen for underlying causes or contributors to the HTN, as well as for other risk factors for CVD and complications from HTN. Situations indicating the appropriateness of a more thorough examination include younger or older patients in whom the HTN is more likely to be secondary to an underlying cause, patients with comorbidities or increased risk for complications, patients with more severe hypertension, and in patients with possible or impending complications from chronic HTN. Deep tendon reflexes are checked for hyperreflexia (particularly with preeclampsia), and the Achilles reflex return is assessed for noteworthy delay that can indicate hypothyroidism[94], a well-documented cause of HTN and dyslipidemia. All patients deserve a thorough exam, whether for the assessment of baseline status, complications, contributions, or for the reassurance (for both doctor and patient) that is attained after a competent professional evaluation reveals no abnormalities.

o <u>Body mass index (BMI) for assessing current BMI and predicting amount and duration of weight loss</u>: Given that the average citizen of industrialized nations is overweight, nearly all patients can benefit from developing a specific goal-oriented and time-oriented plan for the achievement of weight optimization. **Contrasting current BMI with optimal BMI** clarifies the **amount of weight** that needs to be lost and provides an estimate of the **duration of the weight loss program**, given that adherent patients can lose an average of 4-8 lbs (~9-15 kg) per month. Although some patients can achieve highly significant improvements in various parameters such as glycemic control and blood pressure *without* significant weight loss, the fact remains that obesity (more specifically, abdominal obesity) is a **risk factor** and often the **primary determinant** for CVD-HTN-dyslipidemia-hyperglycemia-inflammation as well as osteoarthritis, many types of cancer, and significant but immeasurable (and generally unspoken) suffering associated with diminished self-esteem, inefficacy, social isolation, and depression. Patients have a myriad of reasons and rationalizations for maintaining their

> **Clinical wisdom**
>
> Patients with lifestyle-generated diseases should be coached in the reversal of the patterns that have caused their disease rather than being enabled to pursue their disease-promoting lifestyles while surrogate markers of metabolic-physiologic dysfunction (e.g., hypertension) are pharmacologically suppressed.

---

[94] Degowin RL. *DeGowin and DeGowin's Diagnostic Evaluation. Sixth Edition*. New York: McGraw Hill: 1994, 900. See also Khurana AK, Sinha RS, Ghorai BK, Bihari N. Ankle reflex photomotogram in thyroid dysfunctions. *J Assoc Physicians India*. 1990 Mar;38(3):201-3

overweight status quo—every excuse from being "big boned" to "big framed" to "I've always been big" to "Everyone in my family is big" to "I don't have time to take care of myself" to "I don't know how to cook" to "I simply cannot [eat right, exercise, say no to candy, give up wheat, give up ice cream, drink coffee without sugar and cream]." Clinicians need to anticipate this resistance and have a diverse array of techniques—ranging from patient to insistent, from gentle to confrontational, from emotional to intellectual—to use *as appropriate to the individual patient's needs* to coax, inspire, lead, or push the patient who will benefit from weight loss. Elevated BMI correlates with numerous biochemical risk factors for CVD—progressively elevated levels of blood glucose, insulin, triglycerides, increasing severity of insulin resistance, and progressively lower levels of beneficial high-density lipoprotein (HDL) cholesterol—and an increased risk for cardiovascular death, various cancers, psychosocial problems including low self-esteem, reduced academic performance, and impaired interpersonal relationships, e.g., being a target for prejudice.[95] Elevated BMI is a preventable and treatable condition; physicians should not ignore this problem simply because it is common or difficult for some patients to acknowledge and effectively address.

Body mass index (BMI) interpretation

- ❑ Severely underweight: < 16.5
- ❑ Underweight: 16.5 - 18.4
- ❑ **Normal: 18.5 - 24.9**
- ❑ Overweight: 25 - 29.9
- ❑ Obese Class 1: 30 - 34.9
- ❑ Obese Class 2 (severe obesity): 35 - 39.9
- ❑ Obese Class 3 (morbid obesity): 40 - 47.9
- ❑ Obese Class 4 (supermorbid obesity): ≥ 48

WEIGHT in pounds

HEIGHT	100	110	120	130	140	150	160	170	180	190	200	210	220	230	240	250
5'0"	20	21	23	25	27	29	31	33	35	37	39	41	43	45	47	49
5'1"	19	21	23	25	26	28	30	32	34	36	38	40	42	43	45	47
5'2"	18	20	22	24	26	27	29	31	33	35	37	38	40	42	44	46
5'3"	18	19	21	23	25	27	28	30	32	34	35	37	39	41	43	44
5'4"	17	19	21	22	24	26	27	29	31	33	34	36	38	39	41	43
5'5"	17	18	20	22	23	25	27	28	30	32	33	35	37	38	40	42
5'6"	16	18	19	21	23	24	26	27	29	31	32	34	36	37	39	40
5'7"	16	17	19	20	22	23	25	27	28	30	31	33	34	36	38	39
5'8"	15	17	18	20	21	23	24	26	27	29	30	32	33	35	36	38
5'9"	15	16	18	19	21	22	24	25	27	28	30	31	32	34	35	37
5'10"	14	16	17	19	20	22	23	24	26	27	29	30	32	33	34	36
5'11"	14	15	17	18	20	21	22	24	25	26	27	28	30	32	33	35
6'0"	14	15	16	18	19	20	22	23	24	26	27	28	30	31	33	34
6'1"	13	15	16	17	18	20	21	22	24	25	26	28	29	30	32	33
6'2"	13	14	15	17	18	19	21	22	23	24	26	27	28	30	31	32
6'3"	12	14	15	16	17	19	20	21	22	24	25	26	27	29	30	31
6'4"	12	13	15	16	17	18	19	21	22	23	24	26	27	28	29	30

[95] Costa GB, Horta N, Resende ZF, et al. Body mass index has a good correlation with proatherosclerotic profile in children and adolescents. *Arq Bras Cardiol*. 2009 Sep;93(3):261-7 http://www.scielo.br/pdf/abc/v93n3/en_a10v93n3.pdf

- **Laboratory Assessments**:
  - <u>Chemistry/metabolic panel</u>: Heightened attention is given to glucose, BUN, creatinine, calcium, and potassium. To screen for a renal cause of HTN, test serum BUN and creatinine and check urine albumin:creatinine ratio on a random urine sample; these tests are generally sufficient to confirm or refute a renal etiology of HTN. Renal US or CT imaging can be used for further renal evaluation. Glomerular filtration rate (GFR) can be estimated by the Cockcroft-Gault equation and should be used by clinicians to monitor renal function in patients at risk for renal insufficiency, namely patients with HTN, diabetes mellitus, advanced age, and known renal disease. **Estimated GFR = (140 - age) x weight (kg) / (72 x serum creatinine); in women, multiply this result by .85.** GFR values consistently less than 60 for 3 months are consistent with chronic kidney disease and approximately 50% loss of renal function; at this level of impaired renal function, drug doses need to be modified. Hypercalcemia is a rare cause of HTN and requires evaluation for underlying cause, such as hyperparathyroidism, hyperthyroidism, malignancy (especially multiple myeloma, lymphoma, or cancer of the breast, lung, or kidney), granulomatous diseases such as sarcoidosis, vitamin D or vitamin A excess, adverse drug effect (especially lithium or thiazide diuretics), Paget disease of bone, adrenal insufficiency, or genotropic metabolic disorder such as familial hypocalciuric hypercalcemia.
  - <u>Routine urinalysis (UA)</u>: Test for hematuria, proteinuria, and glucosuria; random albumin:creatinine ratio is indicated in diabetic patients to assess for microalbuminuria.
  - <u>Thyroid assessment—glandular function, peripheral metabolism, and autoimmunity</u>: The purpose of thyroid assessment is to determine the overall functionality of the pituitary-thyroid-metabolic axis, and therefore thyroid testing should be comprehensive and include TSH, free T4, free or total T3, and reverse T3, and the antibodies directed against thyroid peroxidase (anti-TPO) and thyroglobulin (anti-thyroglobulin). Overt or imminent hypothyroidism is suggested by TSH greater than 2 mU/L[96] or 3 mU/L[97], low T4 or T3, and/or the presence of anti-thyroid peroxidase antibodies.[98] Objective laboratory abnormality suggesting hypothyroidism in a patient with compatible clinical symptomatology or objective findings is sufficient justification to warrant a clinical trial of thyroid hormone supplementation provided that no contraindications are present and that the apparent hypothyroidism is not due to another cause such as hyperestrogenemia, which reduces thyroid hormone cellular bioavailability due to increased production of thyroxine binding globulin (TBG). Common clinical manifestations of hypothyroidism include fatigue, depression, cold hands and feet, dry skin, constipation, bradycardia, adult acne, hypertension, head hair loss, hypercholesterolemia, dysthymia/anhedonia, menstrual irregularities in women, and hypogonadism and subfertility in both men and women. Several approaches to the treatment of hypothyroidism are described in the section of *Therapeutic Considerations*.

---

[96] Weetman AP. Hypothyroidism: screening and subclinical disease. *BMJ*. 1997 Apr 19;314(7088):1175-8 http://bmj.bmjjournals.com/cgi/content/full/314/7088/1175

[97] "Now AACE encourages doctors to consider treatment for patients who test outside the boundaries of a narrower margin based on a target TSH level of 0.3 to 3.0. AACE believes the new range will result in proper diagnosis for millions of Americans who suffer from a mild thyroid disorder, but have gone untreated until now." American Association of Clinical Endocrinologists (AACE). 2003 Campaign Encourages Awareness of Mild Thyroid Failure, Importance of Routine Testing http://www.aace.com/pub/tam2003/press.php November 26, 2005

[98] Beers MH, Berkow R (eds). The Merck Manual. Seventeenth Edition. Whitehouse Station: Merck Research Laboratories; 1999. Page 96

- o <u>Other cardiovascular risk factors</u>: Lipids, homocysteine, high-sensitivity C-reactive protein (hsCRP) can also be assessed.
- o <u>Serum 25-hydroxy-vitamin D</u>: In 2004, Vasquez, Manso, and Cannell[99] proposed a "paradigm shift" for clinicians' appreciation of vitamin D that summarized new applications for the clinical use of this nutrient beyond its application in patients with osteoporosis or malabsorption. A novel concept at its time, our article admonished clinicians to use empiric supplementation and/or laboratory assessment of all patients seen in clinical practice. The goal with vitamin D supplementation is to get serum 25-hydroxy-vitamin D (25-OH-D) levels into the optimal range, as currently defined in the illustration. As the cardioprotective role of vitamin D becomes more clear, the peer-reviewed medical research increasingly advocates that **"vitamin D supplementation should be prescribed to patients with hypertension and 25-hydroxyvitamin D levels below target values."**[100]

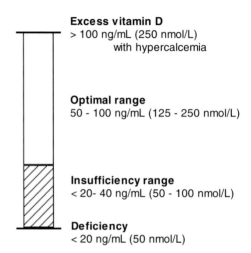

Excess vitamin D
> 100 ng/mL (250 nmol/L)
 with hypercalcemia

Optimal range
50 - 100 ng/mL (125 - 250 nmol/L)

Insufficiency range
< 20- 40 ng/mL (50 - 100 nmol/L)

Deficiency
< 20 ng/mL (50 nmol/L)

Interpretation of serum 25(OH) vitamin D levels. Modified from Vasquez et al, *Alternative Therapies in Health and Medicine* 2004 and Vasquez A. *Musculoskeletal Pain: Expanded Clinical Strategies* (Institute for Functional Medicine) 2008.

- o <u>Uric acid</u>: Many years ago uric acid was generally included in the standard chemistry/metabolic panel; these days it has to be ordered as a separate test. For at least a decade, "a strong, specific, stepwise, independent association of increasing serum uric acid and cardiac morbidity and mortality" has been noted[101], and recent research has shown that inhibition of uric acid production with allopurinol prevents fructose-induced urate-mediated metabolic disturbances that contribute to CVD, HTN, and the metabolic syndrome.[102] The roles of fructose and uric acid are discussed in greater detail in the following section on *Treatment Considerations*.
- o <u>Urine pH</u>: Urine pH can easily be monitored in-office or at home with the use of simple pH strips. Urine pH fluctuates throughout the day and therefore the most reliable evaluations are made with multiple daily assessments (easy and practical) and/or 24-h urine collections (cumbersome, inconvenient, and relatively impractical); an additional and important advantage to using multiple daily assessments of urine pH is that it allows the patient and doctor to observe how dietary and lifestyle fluctuations alter the whole-body biochemical-physiologic milieu. A urine pH of 7.0-8 is desirable as an indicator of dietary compliance and avoidance of the acidogenic Western diet, which is generally HTN-inducing due to its content of sodium, chloride, simple sugars and insufficiency of

[99] **Vasquez A**, Manso G, Cannell J. The clinical importance of vitamin D (cholecalciferol): a paradigm shift with implications for all healthcare providers. *Altern Ther Health Med*. 2004 Sep-Oct;10(5):28-36 http://optimalhealthresearch.com/cholecalciferol.html

[100] Pilz S, Tomaschitz A, Ritz E, Pieber TR; Medscape. Vitamin D status and arterial hypertension: a systematic review. *Nat Rev Cardiol*. 2009 Oct;6(10):621-30

[101] Alderman M. Uric acid in hypertension and cardiovascular disease. *Can J Cardiol* 1999 Nov;15 Suppl F:20F-2F

[102] News release from American Heart Association's 63rd High Blood Pressure Research Conference. High-sugar diet increases men's blood pressure; gout drug protective. Abstract P127. Sept. 23, 2009. http://americanheart.mediaroom.com/index.php?s=43&item=829 Accessed December 19, 2009

magnesium, potassium, calcium, and phytonutrients. Mild urinary alkalosis is the natural and optimal state of human physiology[103,104,105], and its induction is therefore simply a restoration of normalcy rather than an intervention or treatment per se. Caution might be employed when using this (or any other) treatment in patients with severe hepatorenal disease (who have lost the ability to buffer efficiently) and in patients with pre-existing electrolyte disturbances. Patients susceptible to urinary tract infections (UTIs) might experience an increased frequency of UTIs due to urinary alkalinization and may need to improve hygiene, supplement with additional ascorbic acid to prevent urine from becoming excessively alkaline, and/or correct gastrointestinal dysbiosis—this latter point is particularly important for women who experience recurrent UTIs, since urovaginal flora is strongly influenced by intestinal flora.[106]

o Urine sodium and potassium: Urine sodium (Na) and potassium (K) can be measured as markers for dietary intake and therefore as direct markers for compliance with dietary optimization. Urinary Na excretion ranges widely (thousand-fold) between human populations and individuals based mostly on dietary intake; among Yanomamo Indians in Brazil uNa is 0.2 mmol/24 h while among the northern Chinese the uNa is 242 mmol/24 h.[107] Very obviously, the general therapeutic goal in the treatment of HTN is to increase intake of potassium and reduce intake of sodium; the inverse ratio of these two cations positively correlates with blood pressure and other metabolic markers such as insulin sensitivity and endothelial function; thus measurement of urine sodium/potassium is more than a marker for nutritional compliance since is reflective and predictive of key aspects of cardiovascular health. Excepting sodium and potassium losses through perspiration, emesis, and diarrhea the urinary measurement of these minerals is clinically meaningful and correlates with dietary intake; the large Intersalt Study[108] involving 52 population samples in 32 countries for a total of 10,074 men and women aged 20-59 showed that higher urinary sodium excretion correlated positively and directly with systolic and diastolic blood pressures. While patient/physician-estimated potassium intake correlates with 24-h urinary K excretion, "patients tend to underestimate their sodium intake by 30% to 50%; therefore, urinary sodium excretion is more accurate to assess sodium intake."[109] Per the clinical trial by McCullough et al[110], patients on a low-Na diet (10 mEq/d) with excellent compliance have 24-hr Na excretion of approximately 4.6 - 13.4 mEq (outpatients and inpatients, respectively), compared with 24-hr Na excretion of 184.5 - 195.3 mEq for patients on a higher Na diet (200 - 250 mEq/d); the differences seen here in 24-hr Na excretion of approximately 9 mEq in low-Na groups

---

[103] Sebastian A, Frassetto LA, Sellmeyer DE, Merriam RL, Morris RC Jr. Estimation of the net acid load of the diet of ancestral preagricultural Homo sapiens and their hominid ancestors. *Am J Clin Nutr.* 2002 Dec;76(6):1308-16

[104] Maurer M, Riesen W, Muser J, Hulter HN, Krapf R. Neutralization of Western diet inhibits bone resorption independently of K intake and reduces cortisol secretion in humans. *Am J Physiol Renal Physiol.* 2003 Jan;284(1):F32-40

[105] Frassetto L, Morris RC Jr, Sellmeyer DE, Todd K, Sebastian A. Diet, evolution and aging--the pathophysiologic effects of the post-agricultural inversion of the potassium-to-sodium and base-to-chloride ratios in the human diet. *Eur J Nutr.* 2001 Oct;40(5):200-13

[106] Miles MR, Olsen L, Rogers A. Recurrent vaginal candidiasis. Importance of an intestinal reservoir. *JAMA.* 1977 Oct 24;238(17):1836-7

[107] Intersalt Cooperative Research Group. Intersalt: an international study of electrolyte excretion and blood pressure. Results for 24 hour urinary sodium and potassium excretion. Intersalt Cooperative Research Group. *BMJ.* 1988 Jul 30;297(6644):319-28

[108] Elliott P, Stamler J, Nichols R, Dyer AR, Stamler R, Kesteloot H, Marmot M. Intersalt revisited: further analyses of 24 hour sodium excretion and blood pressure within and across populations. Intersalt Cooperative Research Group. *BMJ.* 1996 May 18;312(7041):1249-53

[109] Leiba A, Vald A, Peleg E, Shamiss A, Grossman E. Does dietary recall adequately assess sodium, potassium, and calcium intake in hypertensive patients? *Nutrition.* 2005 Apr;21(4):462-6

[110] McCullough ML, Swain JF, Malarick C, Moore TJ. Feasibility of outpatient electrolyte balance studies. *J Am Coll Nutr.* 1991 Apr;10(2):140-8

compared to approximately 190 mEq in high-Na groups is plain to see, even for the mathematically impaired and those stalwart skeptics who continue to resist appreciating the ability of dietary modification to have measurable and meaningful effects. The urinary sodium:creatinine (uNa/uCr) ratio can be assessed; for example, in the study by Kwok et al[111] among 111 ambulatory vegetarians, hypertensives had uNa/uCr ratio of 32.6 compared with a ratio of 12.4 among normotensives. In this same study, the urinary sodium:potassium (uNa/uK) ratio was 4.7 for hypertensives and 3.4 for normotensives; blood pressure also correlated with calcium intake, and the review by Ruilope et al[112] showed that calcium increases renal excretion of sodium (in a prostaglandin-dependent mechanism). With this latter data in mind, a clinician might speculate that part of vitamin D3's HTN-ameliorating effect may be derived *in part* from its ability to increase intestinal absorption of calcium and thereby promote renal loss of sodium.

o   <u>Fasting serum insulin</u>: A direct relationship exists between elevated serum insulin, peripheral insulin resistance, and cardiovascular mortality.[113,114] Insulin promotes renal retention of sodium which leads to water retention and the subsequent volume overload and systemic hypertension. Clinicians can consider testing fasting serum insulin in patients likely to have hyperinsulinemia and insulin resistance; this can be used to tailor treatment, monitor benefit and compliance, and as a teaching aid for patients requiring or requesting additional details and insight. One of the largest medical laboratories in the US uses a reference range of "0.0-24.9 µIU/mL" (micro-IU [international units] per milliliter) for insulin.[115] Elevated fasting insulin concentration is generally defined as > 100 pmol/L (16.6 mU/L); however, leaning toward 60 pmol/L (10 mU/L)—or more conservatively 90 pmol/L (15 mU/L)—as the upper acceptable limits would provide for more sensitive detection of insulin resistance *as a marker for metabolic dysfunction* in appropriate clinical settings.[116] Per Vølund[117], the correct conversion factor for human insulin is 1 mU/L = 6 pmol/L.

o   <u>Hemoglobin A1c (Hgb-A1c)</u>: Hgb-A1c is also known as glycosylated hemoglobin, levels of which increase in direct proportion to average blood glucose levels. Thus, Hgb-A1c can be used on random blood samples to estimate blood glucose levels to establish or exclude a diagnosis of prediabetes or diabetes mellitus. Interpretation of Hgb-A1c levels is as follows: <u>Normal</u>: <5.7   <u>Prediabetic</u>: 5.7 - 6.4   <u>Diabetes mellitus</u>: >6.5 Treatment of diabetes mellitus and insulin resistance is reviewed in more detail in *Chiropractic and Naturopathic Mastery of Common Clinical Disorders*.[118]

---

[111] Kwok TC, Chan TY, Woo J. Relationship of urinary sodium/potassium excretion and calcium intake to blood pressure and prevalence of hypertension among older Chinese vegetarians. *Eur J Clin Nutr*. 2003 Feb;57(2):299-304

[112] "…calcium influences renal function and enhances renal sodium excretion. The intrarenal effects of low doses of calcium are dependent on the renal production of prostaglandins." Ruilope LM, Lahera V, AraqueA,SuarezC,RodicioJL,RomeroJC. Electrolyte excretion and sodium intake. *Am J Med Sci*. 1994;307 Suppl 1:S107-11

[113] "The magnitude and direction of the relationship between insulin concentration and incident CVD were similar. CONCLUSIONS: We found a significant association between HOMA-IR and risk of CVD after adjustment for multiple covariates." Hanley AJ, Williams K, Stern MP, Haffner SM. Homeostasis model assessment of insulin resistance in relation to the incidence of cardiovascular disease: the San Antonio Heart Study. *Diabetes Care*. 2002 Jul;25(7):1177-84

[114] "Hyperinsulinemia was associated with increased all-cause and cardiovascular mortality in Helsinki policemen independent of other risk factors,..." Pyörälä M, Miettinen H, Laakso M, Pyörälä K. Plasma insulin and all-cause, cardiovascular, and noncardiovascular mortality: the 22-year follow-up results of the Helsinki Policemen Study. *Diabetes Care*. 2000;23(8):1097-102

[115] Insulin. Test Number: 004333 CPT Code: 83525. https://www.labcorp.com Accessed November 24, 2010

[116] Personal communications, November 2010. I am grateful to Bill Beakey of Professional Laboratory Co-Op, James Bogash DC, Kara Fitzgerald ND, Dan Lukaczer, and Todd Lepine MD for their conversations with me about serum insulin.

[117] Vølund A. Conversion of insulin units to SI units. *Am J Clin Nutr*. 1993 Nov;58(5):714-5

[118] **Vasquez A**. <u>Chiropractic and Naturopathic Mastery of Common Clinical Disorders</u>. IBMRC 2009. http://optimalhealthresearch.com/clinical_mastery

o <u>Tests for lead accumulation</u>: In the United States, a consistent correlation has been found between body burden of lead and HTN, even when blood lead levels are well below the current US occupational exposure limit guidelines (40 microg/dl).[119] Harlan et al[120] analyzed data from the second National Health and Nutrition Examination Survey (1976-1980) and thereby found a direct relationship between blood lead levels and systolic and diastolic pressures for men and women and for white and black persons aged 12 to 74 years; they concluded, "Blood lead levels were significantly higher in younger men and women (aged 21 to 55 years) with high blood pressure, but not in older men or women (aged 56 to 74 years). In multiple regression analyses, the relationship of blood lead to blood pressure was independent of other variables for men, but not for women. Dietary calcium and serum zinc levels were inversely related to blood pressure." Schwartz and Stewart[121] contrasted blood lead, dimercaptosuccinic acid (DMSA)-chelatable lead, and tibial lead to find that blood lead was the assessment that most strongly correlated with HTN; they concluded, "**Systolic blood pressure was elevated by blood lead levels as low as 5 microg/dl**." Thus, clinicians might first measure blood lead levels, which do not measure total body burden but rather the lead that is mobile or *in transit* within the body and which appears to have the best correlation with HTN; the finding of normal blood lead results could then be followed with the more sensitive DMSA-provoked heavy metal testing before concluding that heavy metals are noncontributory to that particular patient's HTN. For heavy metal testing in various clinical scenarios, this author's preference is to use DMSA-provoked measurement of urine toxic metals. After a minimal test dose of DMSA (e.g., in the range of 50-100 mg) to screen for hypersensitivity, patients take oral DMSA 10 mg/kg as a single oral dose in the morning on an empty stomach after emptying the bladder and send a sample from the next urination for laboratory analysis; follow laboratory protocol if different from these instructions. Use of DMSA for lead and mercury chelation/detoxification and for diagnostic purposes is generally safe and effective[122,123,124,125,126]; detoxification procedures are reviewed in much greater detail in *Integrative Rheumatology*.[127]

o <u>Plasma aldosterone-to-renin ratio</u>: As the screening blood test for primary hyperaldosteronism, this test is indicated in any hypertensive patient with unexplained hypokalemia. When the plasma aldosterone measured in ng per dL is > 20 times the level of plasma renin activity in ng per mL per hour, hyperaldosteronism is suspected,

[119] Nash D, Magder L, Lustberg M, Sherwin RW, Rubin RJ, Kaufmann RB, Silbergeld EK. Blood lead, blood pressure, and hypertension in perimenopausal and postmenopausal women. *JAMA*. 2003 Mar 26;289(12):1523-32 http://jama.ama-assn.org/cgi/content/full/289/12/1523
[120] Harlan WR, Landis JR, Schmouder RL, Goldstein NG, Harlan LC. Blood lead and blood pressure. Relationship in the adolescent and adult US population. *JAMA*. 1985 Jan 25;253(4):530-4
[121] "Systolic blood pressure was elevated by blood lead levels as low as 5 microg/dl." Schwartz BS, Stewart WF. Different associations of blood lead, meso 2,3-dimercaptosuccinic acid (DMSA)-chelatable lead, and tibial lead levels with blood pressure in 543 former organolead manufacturing workers. *Arch Environ Health*. 2000 Mar-Apr;55(2):85-92
[122] Bradstreet J, Geier DA, Kartzinel JJ, Adams JB, Geier MR. A case-control study of mercury burden in children with autistic spectrum disorders. *Journal of American Physicians and Surgeons* 2003; 8: 76-79 http://www.jpands.org/vol8no3/geier.pdf
[123] Crinnion WJ. Environmental medicine, part three: long-term effects of chronic low-dose mercury exposure. *Altern Med Rev*. 2000 Jun;5(3):209-23 http://www.thorne.com/altmedrev/.fulltext/5/3/209.pdf
[124] Forman J, Moline J, Cernichiari E, Sayegh S, Torres JC, Landrigan MM, Hudson J, Adel HN, Landrigan PJ. A cluster of pediatric metallic mercury exposure cases treated with meso-2,3-dimercaptosuccinic acid (DMSA). *Environ Health Perspect*. 2000 Jun;108(6):575-7 http://ehp.niehs.nih.gov/docs/2000/108p575-577forman/abstract.html
[125] Miller AL. Dimercaptosuccinic acid (DMSA), a non-toxic, water-soluble treatment for heavy metal toxicity. *Altern Med Rev*. 1998 Jun;3(3):199-207 http://www.thorne.com/altmedrev/.fulltext/3/3/199.pdf
[126] DMSA. *Altern Med Rev*. 2000 Jun;5(3):264-7 http://thorne.com/altmedrev/.fulltext/5/3/264.pdf
[127] **Vasquez A**. Integrative Rheumatology. IBMRC 2006, 2007 and all future editions. http://optimalhealthresearch.com/rheumatology.html

confirmatory testing can be performed by an endocrinologist using an available salt-suppression test.[128]

o <u>Plasma and urine levels of epinephrine and norepinephrine</u>: Plasma and urine levels of epinephrine and norepinephrine can be measured while the patient is on a stable low-sodium diet. In a review and exemplary case report summarized in a following section, Morimoto *et al*[129] describe the use of plasma and urine epinephrine and norepinephrine as markers of sympathetic nervous system activity in a patient treated with neurovascular decompression (detailed later in this chapter); their strategy employed a sodium intake of 120 mmol/d with fasting blood samples taken via indwelling catheter at 7:30am after the patient had rested for 30 minutes in the supine position. Over the course of four months following surgical neurovascular decompression of the left ventrolateral medulla oblongata, Morimoto *et al* report the following:

> **Applied physiology**
>
> Epinephrine levels reflect activity of the adrenal medulla, while norepinephrine levels are a more general indicator of overall sympathetic nervous system activity. Post-intervention reductions in epinephrine and norepinephrine indicate reduced sympathetic activity, generally an important benefit in patients with hypertensive and cardiovascular diseases.

- <u>Plasma epinephrine</u>: Reduced from 0.22 to <0.05 (reference range <0.93 nmol/L).
- <u>Plasma norepinephrine</u>: Reduced from 0.95 to 0.30 (range 0.89 - 3.37 nmol/L).
- <u>Urine epinephrine</u>: Reduced from 83.5 to 26.2 (range 5.5 – 76.4 nmol/d).
- <u>Urine norepinephrine</u>: Reduced from 0.52 to 0.39 (range 0.06 – 0.024 mmol/d).

The importance of their case report is, among other considerations, that it shows that a post-intervention reduction in sympathetic nerve activity can be documented objectively, and that antihypertensive benefits can be significant and associated with *relative* reductions in catecholamine levels that may be *within* or *outside of* the normal reference range. With the awareness that reference ranges for plasma and urine levels of epinephrine and norepinephrine were established exclusively for the detection of *overt pathology* (i.e., autonomic failure at the bottom of the range and pheochromocytoma at the top of the range) rather than for *functional disorders* such as neurogenic hypertension, clinicians may judiciously utilize measurements of plasma and urine epinephrine and norepinephrine to assess for hypersympathotonia and to monitor patient's response to treatment by documenting reductions in catecholamine production after intervention.

- **Imaging**:
  o <u>Electrocardiography (ECG, EKG)</u>: To assess for injury or pathophysiologic adaptation, ECG is appropriate for patients with HTN[130] and those at high risk for or with evidence of CVD, MI, PVD, CHF, chest pain (CP, including angina), or shortness of breath (SOB).
  o <u>Upper cervical radiographs</u>: Clinicians highly skilled in manual manipulative therapeutics might choose to radiograph the upper cervical spine as a means to determine the appropriateness and application of spinal manipulative therapy to effect "marked and sustained reductions in BP similar to the use of two-drug combination

---

[128] Viera AJ, Neutze DM. Diagnosis of secondary hypertension: an age-based approach. *Am Fam Physician*. 2010 Dec 15;82(12):1471-8
[129] Morimoto S, Sasaki S, Takeda K, Furuya S, Naruse S, Matsumoto K, Higuchi T, Saito M, Nakagawa M. Decreases in blood pressure and sympathetic nerve activity by microvascular decompression of the rostral ventrolateral medulla in essential hypertension. *Stroke*. 1999 Aug;30(8):1707-10
[130] Bent S, Gensler LS, Frances C. Saint-Frances Guide: Clinical Clerkship in Outpatient Medicine. 2nd Edition. Philadelphia; Wolters Kluwer: 2008, 90

therapy."[131] Generally however, radiographs prior to spinal manipulative therapy are not advised unless indicated by specific clinical characteristics such as recent trauma, neurologic deficit, or increased possibility for congenital anomaly (e.g., Sprengel's deformity), atlantoaxial instability (e.g., Down syndrome, rheumatoid arthritis, ankylosing spondylitis), or underlying disease (e.g., suspicion of malignant disease).

o Other imaging: CT, US, and angiographic techniques are commonly used to assess for HTN-related tumors, vascular anomalies/occlusion, and renal abnormalities. More specifically, US or IV contrast CT assessment for abdominal aortic aneurysm is indicated for hypertensive patients with any history of smoking aged >65yo and patients with documented CAD/CVD.[132]

- **Biopsy/Procedure**: Tissue biopsy is generally not required except when investigating a specific pathoetiologic consideration. Angioplasty and stent placement for the treatment of renal artery stenosis, and aldosterone measurement in the adrenal vein to lateralize the side of an aldosterone-secreting tumor are examples of procedures used in some cases of HTN. Renal biopsy specifies type and severity of intrinsic renal disease when history, labs, and imaging are inconclusive.

- **Establishing the Diagnosis of Hypertension in Adults**: The diagnosis of adult hypertension is established after at least two measurements of blood pressure with either component greater than 140/90 mm Hg. Patients with systolic blood pressure 120-139 mm Hg or diastolic blood pressure 80-89 mm Hg are considered "prehypertensive"[133] and should be differentially diagnosed then treated with lifestyle and non-pharmacologic measures unless a *true primary cause* of the hypertension is discovered. Patients with diabetes mellitus, renal disease, or CVD should have their blood pressure controlled to ≤ 130/80 mm Hg. Patients with elevated systolic and normal diastolic pressures have **isolated systolic hypertension**, which in adults indicates an increased risk for stroke, heart failure, myocardial infarction, and overall mortality that can be ameliorated by effective intervention.[134] Given that mortality increases with chronic blood pressures greater than 115/75 mm Hg[135], progressive clinicians should appreciate 115/75 mm Hg as the upper end of the ideal range; from this perspective, the diagnostic threshold of 140/90 mm Hg for hypertension is appropriately seen as a great deviation from normal.

o Hypertension in infants, children, and adolescents: As previously mentioned, normal and abnormal values for blood pressure in infants and children are different from those of adults and are stratified based on age, gender, and height in a chart from the International Pediatric Hypertension Association. Please see their website at http://pediatrichypertension.org/ for downloadable charts and additional information helpful when dealing with childhood hypertension.

---

[131] Bakris G, Dickholtz M Sr, Meyer PM, Kravitz G, Avery E, Miller M, Brown J, Woodfield C, Bell B. Atlas vertebra realignment and achievement of arterial pressure goal in hypertensive patients: a pilot study. *J Hum Hypertens*. 2007 May;21(5):347-52

[132] "CONCLUSIONS: In-hospital screening of AAA is very efficient among patients with coronary artery disease. Therefore, patients with CAD may be considered for routine AAA screening." Monney P, Hayoz D, Tinguely F, Cornuz J, Haesler E, Mueller XM, von Segesser LK, Tevaearai HT. High prevalence of unsuspected abdominal aortic aneurysms in patients hospitalised for surgical coronary revascularisation. *Eur J Cardiothorac Surg*. 2004 Jan;25(1):65-8

[133] Bent S, Gensler LS, Frances C. Saint-Frances Guide: Clinical Clerkship in Outpatient Medicine. 2nd Edition. Philadelphia; Wolters Kluwer: 2008, 87

[134] Chobanian AV. Control of hypertension--an important national priority. *N Engl J Med*. 2001 Aug 16;345(7):534-5

[135] Benowitz NL. "Antihypertensive Agents." In Katzung BG (editor). Basic and Clinical Pharmacology. Tenth Edition. New York: McGraw Hill Medical; 2007, 159

Blood pressure description and clinical considerations

BP in mm Hg	Description and clinical considerations
<u>115/75</u> or slightly lower	<u>Optimal blood pressure</u>: "Starting at 115/75 mm Hg, cardiovascular risk doubles with each increment of 20/10 mm Hg throughout the blood pressure range."[136]
<u>120/80</u> to <u>139/89</u>	<u>Prehypertension</u>: Elevated risk for adverse cardiovascular outcomes; begin assessment and assertive lifestyle and nutritional interventions.
≤ <u>130/80</u>	<u>Blood pressure goal for patients with diabetes mellitus, renal disease, or CVD</u>: Patients with multiple risk factors for adverse cardiovascular outcomes must have each variable treated to more assertively than if only one risk factor was present.
<u>140/90</u> to <u>159/99</u>	<u>Stage 1 hypertension</u>: Implement effective treatment and management strategies and reviewed here and elsewhere. Drug-treated patients are generally started with **one** medication, most commonly hydrochlorothiazide. See the concise pharmacotherapy review at the end of this chapter for more information on drug therapy.
<u>160/100</u> or greater	<u>Stage 2 hypertension</u>: Implement effective treatment and management strategies and reviewed here and elsewhere. Drug-treated patients are generally started with **two** medications, most commonly hydrochlorothiazide plus another medication prescribed based on the patient's comorbidities and tolerance. See the concise pharmacotherapy review at the end of this chapter for more information on drug therapy. The *acute onset* of blood pressures greater than 160/100 – 160/110 must be treated as a potentially life-threatening emergency, because *acute onset* hypertension by definition of its acute onset poses a higher risk of complications because physiologic adaptations have not had time to accommodate the higher pressures. In inpatient hospital settings, sBP > 160 is commonly used as a threshold for use of hydralazine, generally administered as 10 mg IV PRN each 1-2 hours.
<u>200/120</u> or greater *without* complications	<u>Hypertensive urgency</u>: Severe HTN *without* symptoms or evidence of end-organ damage. These patients are appropriately treated in the emergency department with *orally administered* medications—see details that follow.
<u>200/120</u> or greater *with* complications	<u>Hypertensive emergency</u>: Severe HTN with symptoms or evidence of end-organ damage such as headache, blurred vision, chest pain, shortness of breath, or renal insufficiency. Must be treated in an intensive/critical care setting with *intravenous* antihypertensive medications—see details that follow.

---

[136] Benowitz NL. "Antihypertensive Agents." In Katzung BG (editor). <u>Basic and Clinical Pharmacology. Tenth Edition</u>. New York: McGraw Hill Medical; 2007, 159

Disease Complications:
- The increased morbidity and mortality of HTN can manifest as any of the following:
  - Congestive heart failure presenting with fatigue, lower extremity edema, rales, dyspnea or orthopnea
  - Retinopathy and visual impairment
  - Hypertensive nephropathy presenting as azotemia, edema, recalcitrant HTN
  - Stroke—hemorrhagic or ischemic
  - Atrial fibrillation due to atrial enlargement
  - Myocardial infarction or sudden death due to accelerated CVD complicated by cardiac hypertrophy (i.e., supply-demand mismatch)
  - Abdominal aortic aneurysm, especially with HTN plus tobacco smoking

Clinical Management: For routine outpatients, the obvious goal is to get the blood pressure down below 140/90 mm Hg as quickly, safely, and cost-effectively as possible while treating any primary underlying disorders; treatments that provide *collateral benefits* are preferred over those which cause *side effects*. Attention to naturopathic medicine's "hierarchy of therapeutics"[137] is important here in order to prioritize the implementation of therapeutic interventions. Correction of nutritional deficiencies (e.g., vitamin D, magnesium, potassium, calcium, phytonutrients), nutritional imbalances (e.g., insulin resistance and hyperglycemia, diet-induced metabolic acidosis), and hormonal imbalances (e.g., thyroid deficiency/excess, estrogen excess, aldosterone excess) should take precedence over the simple utilization of **antihypertensive drugs which suppress the manifestation of underlying dysfunction and thus allow it to perpetuate**; because of the latter, pharmacotherapy often abets rather than abates chronic disease. Following the exclusion of pathologic causes of HTN, the diagnosis of HTN should be explained to the patient as a sign of internal (e.g., nutritional, hormonal, metabolic, or structural) imbalance or otherwise as an opportunity to use this marker (blood pressure) as a barometer of overall health and compliance with a health-promoting lifestyle, including optimization of diet, exercise, relationships, and nutritional intake.

> **The physician's judgment remains paramount**
>
> "Positive experiences, trust in the clinician, and empathy improve patient motivation and satisfaction. This report serves as a guide, and the committee continues to recognize that the responsible physician's judgment remains paramount."
>
> The Seventh Report of the Joint National Committee on Prevention, Detection, Evaluation and Treatment of High Blood Pressure [JNC 7]

- Stratification of HTN management: Factors that direct the management of HTN include severity, manifestations of associated organ damage, and the patient's general condition and comorbidities.
  - Hypertensive emergency = >200/120 mm Hg *with evidence of end-organ damage* or *symptoms possibly attributable to the hypertension such as headache, blurred vision, chest pain, or shortness of breath*: Accompanying clinical manifestations may include renal failure, hematuria,

---

[137] The "hierarchy of therapeutics" is a guiding principle of naturopathic medicine that provides a conceptual framework for the prioritization and sequencing of therapeutic interventions. This is described in chapter 1 of *Integrative Orthopedics*, *Integrative Rheumatology*, and *Chiropractic and Naturopathic Mastery of Common Clinical Disorders* and is available on-line at http://OptimalHealthResearch.com/chapter1. Another resource available in January 2010 is Chapter 3 from *Textbook of Natural Medicine, 3rd Edition*: "A Hierarchy of Healing: The Therapeutic Order. The Unifying Theory of Naturopathic Medicine" available on-line: http://www.naturalmedtext.com/storedfiles/sample_Chapter%203%20-%20A%20Hierarchy%20of%20Healing%20-%20The%20Therapeutic%20Order.pdf?CFID=6826417&CFTOKEN=33445946

proteinuria, altered mental status, papilledema, retinal vascular changes, MI, angina, stroke, aortic dissection, and pulmonary edema. Treat in intensive/critical care setting with *intravenous* antihypertensive medications such as nitroprusside, nitroglycerine, esmolol, hydralazine, labetolol, nicardipine then transition to oral beta-blockers and ACEi (angiotensin converting enzyme inhibitor) drugs. Add diuretics such as furosemide/Lasix as needed to alleviate volume overload, pulmonary edema, HTN, and heart failure. The initial drop in blood pressure should not exceed 25% in order to prevent precipitation of organ ischemia due to reflexive arteriospasm.

o Hypertensive urgency = blood pressure >220/120 mm Hg[138] or >220/125 mm Hg[139] *without end-organ damage* and *without symptoms*: These patients are appropriately treated in the emergency department with *orally administered* medications such as nifedipine (oral, not sublingual), clonidine, and/or captopril. Patients can be discharged following normalization of blood pressure, but these patients require timely follow-up with a primary care provider. Complicating factors and concomitant disease may necessitate hospital admission.

o Acute-onset HTN: Acute HTN in a previously normotensive patient can lead to stroke and other complications at pressures of 160 mm Hg systolic or 110 mm Hg diastolic. Acute-onset HTN can cause stroke at pressures generally tolerated in chronic cases because in the latter vascular adaptations accommodate higher pressures. **Acute-onset HTN** *from any cause* **should be treated emergently/urgently when pressures approximate or exceed 160-180 mm Hg systolic or 110 mm Hg diastolic**, especially but not exclusively if accompanied by complications such as angina, shortness of breath, vision changes, papilledema, headache/confusion/seizures (which suggest cerebral edema or cerebral vasospasm), proteinuria, or edema of the face, peripheral extremities, or of the general body (anasarca, check for sacral edema and weight gain).

o Malignant HTN: Severe, intractable, and generally progressive HTN characterized by diastolic HTN > 130 mm Hg with clinical complications including renal failure, encephalopathy, or papilledema. Treat in hospital setting with intravenous antihypertensive medications (reviewed above for hypertensive emergency).

• Routine recommendations that should be communicated then documented in the patient's chart: These include ❶ encouragement of smoking cessation, ❷ a minimum of 30 minutes of exercise per day (for patients healthy enough to exercise), ❸ weight loss/optimization, ❹ limit alcohol intake to no more than 1-2 drinks per day, ❺ restrict sodium to ≤ 2,400 mg/d (i.e., ≤ 6 grams/d of sodium chloride), ❻ increase intake of fruits and vegetables, and ❼ reduce intake of total and saturated fat in order to promote weight loss and optimize serum lipids.[140] In the allopathic model, these lifestyle recommendations are used for three months before initiating drug treatment of HTN.

• Drug management and comanagement of HTN may be required. Drug management is appropriate in urgent situations, recalcitrant cases, patients with initial BP > 160/100 mm Hg, and for patients who are noncompliant with treatment. Patients and clinicians can facilitate progression through the "stages of change"[141] by appreciating the barriers and requirements

[138] Bent S, Gensler LS, Frances C. Saint-Frances Guide: Clinical Clerkship in Outpatient Medicine. 2nd Edition. Philadelphia; Wolters Kluwer: 2008, 89
[139] McPhee SJ, Papadakis MA (editors). Current Medical Diagnosis and Treatment. 2009. 48th Edition. New York; McGraw Hill Medical: 401
[140] Bent S, Gensler LS, Frances C. Saint-Frances Guide: Clinical Clerkship in Outpatient Medicine. 2nd Edition. Philadelphia; Wolters Kluwer: 2008, 90
[141] Prochaska, JO, Norcross, JC, and DiClemente, CC (1994). Changing for Good: A Revolutionary Six-Stage Program for Overcoming Bad Habits and Moving Your Life Positively Forward. NY, William Morrow and Company; 1994

that characterize the overcoming of each stage until the final stage of termination/integration is achieved. In common medical practice, lifestyle interventions, the processes of change, nutritional supplementation, and spinal manipulation are almost never given their full due consideration; thus, by default, drug treatment of hypertension is the allopathic standard of care because it is the only treatment given priority. Failure to discuss nondrug treatments with hypertensive patients is unethical because many nondrug treatments are superior in safety, affordability, and effectiveness when compared with drug treatments; failure to discuss nondrug treatments is also a violation of medical ethics' principles of beneficence, autonomy and informed consent.

> **Clinical insight**
> Patients with lifestyle-generated diseases should be coached in the reversal of the patterns that have caused their disease rather than being enabled to pursue their disease-promoting lifestyles while surrogate markers of metabolic-physiologic dysfunction (e.g., hypertension) are pharmacologically suppressed.

- Tailor treatment recommendations and goals to the patient's specific psychographics and BVG-LOC profile. More than 90-95% of HTN patients will be found to have no pathologic/medical cause of their HTN, thus implicating diet and lifestyle as the most responsible factors. In some situations, the resolution of the patient's HTN comes expeditiously through the simple and imperfect implementation of weight loss, diet modification, correction of nutritional deficiencies, and avoidance or reduced intake of infamous triggers such as tobacco, alcohol, and excess caffeine. **For many patients with HTN—especially when the HTN is part of a larger cluster of clinical findings such as type-2 diabetes mellitus or the metabolic syndrome (see chapter 13 of *Chiropractic and Naturopathic Mastery of Common Clinical Disorders*)—the successful management of their HTN will rely on the implementation of numerous changes in various aspects of "lifestyle" including diet, preparation/procurement of food, social interactions, core relationships, exercise involvement, time and money allocation, and— most importantly—changes in self image, and the establishment and "affirmation-through-action" of core values.** These issues can appear complex to the point of being "too complicated" for doctors and patients who are not personally accustomed to living consciously and for whom dispensing and consuming pills, respectively, are easier than the consciousness-raising and the self-disciplined and self-directed living required to advocate and manifest a health-centered life. Complexity and convenience should not be the determinants of care. Patients with lifestyle-generated diseases should be coached in the reversal of the patterns that have caused their disease rather than being enabled to pursue these disease-promoting lifestyles while surrogate markers of metabolic-physiologic dysfunction are pharmacologically suppressed. Therapeutic lifestyle changes must be merged with the patient's **beliefs** (important but changeable paradigms), **values** (subjective-objective rules), and **goals** (conscious and subconscious aspirations and trajectory). In order to facilitate this merger, the clinician must—first—understand the patient's position on these variables, then—second—deliver the treatment plan in such a way as to "speak to" the patient's beliefs, values, and goals. Most people do not have consciously-chosen and declarable beliefs, values, and goals for their lives; thus, this process of the physician's gaining an understanding of the patient's unconscious psychographic details is generally not completed on the first visit and may not be completed until the patient has done the requisite "homework" (perhaps facilitated by a professional therapist or lay counselor/coach) and has thereafter returned with a perceptible level of self-awareness. Clinicians who **seek first to understand, then to be understood**[142] will have advantages over clinicians who steamroll patients with lifestyle impositions and a "to do" list that is foreign to the patient's inner and previous experiences. With regard to psychographic information, clinicians are wise to remember the three tenets of evidence-based medicine, one of which rests upon this psychographic information: ❶ published research, ❷ the clinician's experience and expertise, and ❸ the patient's preferences and goals.

Psychographic profiling via "BVG-LOC"[143]

- <u>Beliefs</u>: What are the fundamental beliefs and expectations that the patient has for his/her future? Is life merely "suffering and toil" or is it meant to be "a well of delight"? Patients who expect misery are generally successful in its attainment unless they are guided and provoked toward a more positive life expectancy. The clinician can correct errors in thought and information.
- <u>Values</u>: What does the patient value? "*Autonomy and independence*"—will this manifest as resistance to the clinician's advice or as a willingness to comply with treatment so as to avoid future disability? "*Strength*"—will this be resistance to the plan or disciplined adherence to the plan? "*Love*"—is this self-sacrificing 'love' for other people or is it a wholesome and healthy love that includes the self? "*My family*"—does this include avoiding disability, being alive to support and encourage family members and upcoming generations? "*Nothing really*"—what are the mental barriers and painful experiences that have resulted in this emotional numbness; what would his/her life be like if he/she were to engage in life consciously and with purpose? The clinician assigns homework for the patient to clarify—and later commit to in action—a list of personal values.
- <u>Goals</u>: What are the patient's social, physical, professional, personal, and spiritual goals? Is the current lifestyle and health/disease trajectory consistent with the attainment and extended enjoyment of these goals? Are the goals too limited, and has the patient accommodated small goals with small effort and the resulting lackluster results that reinforce self-depreciation and low self-esteem, thus perpetuating a vicious cycle? Goals are a reflection of core values and one's intimate belief about what is possible and what levels of success, love, and happiness are appropriate for one's life.
- <u>Locus of Control</u>: Does the patient view the world as chaotic and menacing (external locus of control), or as understandable and thus worthy of meaningful engagement (internal locus of control)? If the patient views him/herself as a victim, then compliance will be low because every and any excuse will serve as a rationalization for why he/she "couldn't" exercise, eat right, and take medications or nutrients as prescribed. Patients who experience their health problems as incomprehensible and "idiopathic" are less likely to engage in purposeful health activities and are more likely to be noncompliant with treatment(s) and more passive in their willingness to rely on "doctor's orders" and drug treatments. Physicians should encourage the best self-image in and self-efficacy from patients by reminding them by either Socratic-dialectic education or direct verbalization that the patient has the power and thus the "response-ability" to strongly influence his/her health outcomes via positive health expectations and behaviors.

- <u>Patients must receive instruction on at-home blood pressure monitoring and/or follow-up in-office assessments</u>: At the time of diagnosis, patients are instructed of the importance of proper treatment and follow-up visits (ranging from weekly to biweekly to monthly) to

---

[142] Covey SR. <u>The Seven Habits of Highly Effective People</u> (1989); see also <u>The 8th Habit: From Effectiveness to Greatness</u> (2004).
[143] The "BVG-LOC" acronym was created by Dr Alex Vasquez and originally published in: **Vasquez A**. <u>Chiropractic Management of Chronic Hypertension</u> in 2010; that text is the foundation for this current work.

facilitate compliance and monitor treatment effectiveness. HTN must never be taken lightly by the clinician or the patient as it represents and indicates a significant departure from optimal health and the failure of internal homeostatic mechanisms; more concretely, HTN is generally a silent and progressive disorder which prematurely undercuts health and vitality and which tends to culminate in unnecessary morbidity (e.g.., pain, suffering, loss of function, renal dialysis, and stroke) and early death. Patients can use office-calibrated home blood pressure monitoring equipment to self-monitor compliance, lifestyle effects, and effectiveness of treatment; patients are advised that at-home monitoring does not substitute for in-office visits and that in-office blood pressure measurements are the standard by which treatment decisions are made. "White coat hypertension" (WCH) is explained as an exaggerated stress response to innocuous stimuli that has parallels in other areas of the patient's life and is therefore not an excuse for normal at-home readings; accordingly, studies have shown that patients with WCH show increased risk for cardiovascular complications.[144,145] Depending on HTN severity and the protocol being followed, patients might be seen in the office for a quick follow-up assessment once every 2-7 days, or less frequently if BP checks are occurring reliably at home. Patients with metabolic syndrome, obesity, or who are likely to be noncompliant are followed-up more frequently than medically indicated in order to promote compliance and patient-physician alliance. Generally, after the normalization of blood pressure with treatment, patients are reevaluated every 3-6 months in the office. Laboratory tests are performed at least annually and can be performed on an as needed basis with any evidence or suspicion of problems such as nephropathy, dyslipidemia, DM, or drug side effects.

- <u>Patients already taking antihypertensive medications are likely to require a dosage adjustment or medication discontinuation after using diet, lifestyle, and nutritional interventions</u>. Clinicians should anticipate this benefit and inform the patient and prescribing doctor appropriately. Failure to anticipate the normalization of blood pressure and to adjust medications appropriately may result in hypotension, most commonly manifested by fatigue and/or (pre)syncope.

- <u>Document everything</u>: Document all relevant clinical findings, laboratory/imaging results, treatments with rationale, patient education, plan of scheduled follow-up, and referal/comanagment. Ensure that chart notes document education, consent to treatment, and that "patient verbalizes understanding; all questions are answered and concerns addressed."

Clinical management of HTN
1. **Assessment** for urgency and end-organ damage
2. **Differential diagnosis** and comprehensive assessment
3. **Effective treatment** or appropriate referral
4. **Patient education**
5. **Scheduled follow-up**
6. **Monitor** for compliance, treatment effectiveness, adverse effects, and new complications
7. **Document all of the above in the patient chart**

---

[144] "CONCLUSIONS: Coronary disease may be more severe among patients with WCH than among those without." Kostandonis D, Papadopoulos V, Toumanidis S, Papamichael C, Kanakakis I, Zakopoulos N. Topography and severity of coronary artery disease in white-coat hypertension. *Eur J Intern Med*. 2008 Jun;19(4):280-4

[145] "Our findings also further stress the interest, for clinicians, of assessing the presence of a white-coat effect as a means to further identify patients at increased cardiovascular risk and guide treatment accordingly." Bochud M, Bovet P, Vollenweider P, Maillard M, Paccaud F, Wandeler G, Gabriel A, Burnier M. Association Between White-Coat Effect and Blunted Dipping of Nocturnal Blood Pressure. *Am J Hypertens*. 2009 Oct;22(10):1054-61

Treatment Considerations for "Primary" Hypertension—An Evidence-based Article-by-Article Review with Commentary: Reviewed here are the most successful and/or most common treatments for HTN; these treatments can generally be categorized as **dietary** (i.e., foods consumed), **nutritional** (i.e., foods consumed plus the use of nutritional supplements), **hormonal** (e.g., correction of hypothyroidism, hyperaldosteronism, hyperparathyroidism), **surgical** (reviewed here: microvascular decompression of the left ventrolateral medulla oblongata), **manipulative** (reviewed here: spinal and paraspinal soft tissue manipulation), and **lifestyle intervention**, with the latter being a large general category that includes but is not limited to exercise, weight optimization (generally weight *loss* for the treatment of HTN), Qigong, controlled breathing, meditation, and acupuncture. Readers will be better able to appreciate the clinical significance of the blood pressure reductions achieved if they are aware that ❶ most blood-pressure-lowering drugs used chronically on an outpatient basis achieve reductions in the magnitude of approximately 12/6 mm Hg while reductions of 20/10 mm Hg generally require combination (i.e., at least two drugs) therapy[146], ❷ the vast majority (more than 70%) of medically-treated HTN patients take at least two blood-pressure-lowering drugs to achieve or approach their BP goal, and ❸ the criteria to establish efficacy of an antihypertensive effect as defined by the US Food and Drug Administration for approval of a new antihypertensive drug requires proof of both efficacy and safety in a blinded-design study; proof of efficacy is defined as a placebo-subtracted reduction in diastolic BP of 4-5 mm Hg or more, and "…most single agent antihypertensive [drugs] yield an 8 mm Hg drop in pressure in people with Stage 1 hypertension…"[147] Upon close reading of the following sections, readers will note that most of the nonpharmacologic therapeutics reviewed can achieve reductions greater than 5 mm Hg in BP.

- **The supplemented Paleo-Mediterranean Diet**: The health-promoting diet of choice for the majority of people is a diet based on abundant consumption of fruits, vegetables, seeds, nuts, omega-3 and monounsaturated fatty acids, and lean sources of protein such as lean meats, fatty cold-water fish, soy and whey proteins. This diet prohibits and obviates overconsumption of chemical preservatives, artificial sweeteners, and carbohydrate-dominant foods such as candies, pastries, breads, potatoes, grains, and other foods with a high glycemic load and high glycemic index. This "Paleo-Mediterranean Diet"—first detailed by Vasquez[148,149] in 2005—is a combination of the "Paleolithic" or "Paleo diet" and the well-known "Mediterranean diet", both of which are well described in peer-reviewed journals and the lay press. The Paleo-Mediterranean Diet is wholly consistent with the "polymeal"—a multicomponent cardioprotective diet plan characterized by emphasis on phytonutrient-rich foods including fish, red wine, garlic, almonds, dark chocolate, and most (low-carbohydrate) fruits and vegetables—which is estimated to have the potential to lower the incidence of CVD by 76%.[150]

---

[146] Magill MK, Gunning K, Saffel-Shrier S, Gay C. New developments in the management of hypertension. *Am Fam Physician*. 2003 Sep 1;68(5):853-8 http://www.aafp.org/afp/20030901/853.html

[147] "The criteria used in this study to establish efficacy of an antihypertensive effect are those defined by the Food and Drug Administration for approval of a new antihypertensive drug. Specifically, it would require a blinded design with a placebo-subtracted reduction in diastolic BP of 5 mm Hg or more and be free of serious side effects to be approvable." Bakris G, Dickholtz M Sr, Meyer PM, et al. Atlas vertebra realignment and achievement of arterial pressure goal in hypertensive patients: a pilot study. *J Hum Hypertens*. 2007 May;21(5):347-52. See also information from the US FDA website (http://fda.gov/RegulatoryInformation/Guidances/ucm129461.htm, accessed June 12, 2010) which states, "…because the effect of active drugs is often small (diastolic blood pressure change of 4-5 mm Hg more than placebo), studies conducted in a blinded fashion and with placebo controls are essential."

[148] **Vasquez A**. The Importance of Integrative Chiropractic Health Care in Treating Musculoskeletal Pain and Reducing the Nationwide Burden of Medical Expenses and Iatrogenic Injury and Death. *Original Internist* 2005; 12(4): 159-182

[149] **Vasquez A**. A Five-Part Nutritional Protocol that Produces Consistently Positive Results. *Nutritional Wellness* 2005 Sept

[150] Franco OH, Bonneux L, de Laet C, Peeters A, Steyerberg EW, Mackenbach JP. The Polymeal: a more natural, safer, and probably tastier (than the Polypill) strategy to reduce cardiovascular disease by more than 75%. *BMJ*. 2004 Dec 18;329(7480):1447-50

In the subsections that follow, various studies related to dietary intervention for hypertension will be summarized; these dietary patterns can be viewed in a continuum ranging from the ❶ SAD diet to ❷ the DASH diet to ❸ the Paleo-Mediterranean diet. Also included is the fourth most common dietary pattern, that of ❹ the vegetarian diet and its related variants of veganism, pescovegetarianism, and lacto-ovo-vegetarianism. Combining the Paleo-Mediterranean diet with multivitamin/multimineral supplementation (including physiologic doses of vitamin D3 to optimize serum levels), with balanced combination fatty acid (ALA, GLA, EPA, DHA) supplementation and probiotics forms the "supplemented Paleo-Mediterranean diet" (sPMD)[151], the five basic components of which are outlined below:

1. Paleo-Mediterranean Diet: The most nutrient-dense diet available; more amenable to social integration and greater nutrient content compared to vegetarianism; provides sufficient protein to promote satiety and therefore reduced caloric intake.

2. Multivitamin and multimineral supplementation: Routine vitamin and mineral supplementation is warranted because dietary intake (based on SAD) is generally insufficient to provide sufficient vitamins and minerals[152]; supranutritional doses of vitamins and minerals stimulates variant/defective enzymes with decreased coenzyme binding affinity (increased K[m]).[153]

3. Vitamin D3 in physiologic doses to optimize serum 25-OH-D levels: Vitamin D3 deficiency and insufficiency are common in the general population and are causatively and/or epidemiologically associated with HTN, CVD, CHF, type-1 and type-2 diabetes mellitus, mental depression and schizophrenia, systemic inflammation, and various cancers and autoimmune disorders. The physiologic requirement for vitamin D3 is approximately 4,000 IU per day for adult men. Dosages should be sufficient to effect serum 25-OH-D levels within the optimal range of 50-100 ng/ml.

4. Balanced combination fatty acid supplementation with ALA, GLA, EPA, DHA, with dietary oleic acid: Patients consuming the SAD may be presumed to have numerous fatty acid imbalances (e.g., excess arachidonate and *trans* fatty acids) along with insufficiencies of ALA, GLA, EPA, DHA, and oleic acid. Hunter-gather intake of omega-3 fatty acids is approximately 7 grams per day contrasted to 1 gram per day provided by Westernized/industrialized diets. Fatty acid imbalances/deficiencies commonly seen in patients consuming Westernized/industrialized/SAD diets—similar to and probably additive to if not synergistic with vitamin D deficiency/insufficiency—contributes to HTN, CVD, CHF, type-1 and type-2 diabetes mellitus, mental depression and schizophrenia, systemic inflammation, and various cancers and autoimmune disorders.

5. Probiotics: Probiotics are safe and effective anti-inflammatory, immunoenhancing, and immunomodulating agents[154,155] and are—based on published research and clinical experience—suitable for routine use, ideally as a rotating combination of yogurts, kefir, other fermented foods, and—particularly for dairy-intolerant patients—supplements.

---

[151] **Vasquez A**. The Importance of Integrative Chiropractic Health Care in Treating Musculoskeletal Pain and Reducing the Nationwide Burden of Medical Expenses and Iatrogenic Injury and Death. *Original Internist* 2005; 12(4): 159-182

[152] Fletcher RH, Fairfield KM.Vitamins for chronic disease prevention in adults: clinical applications. *JAMA*. 2002 Jun 19;287(23):3127-9

[153] Ames BN, Elson-Schwab I, Silver EA. High-dose vitamin therapy stimulates variant enzymes with decreased coenzyme binding affinity (increased K(m)): relevance to genetic disease and polymorphisms. *Am J Clin Nutr*. 2002 Apr;75(4):616-58

[154] Neish AS. Microbes in gastrointestinal health and disease. Gastroenterology. 2009 Jan;136(1):65-80

[155] Galdeano CM, de Moreno de LeBlanc A, Vinderola G, Bonet ME, Perdigón G. Proposed model: mechanisms of immunomodulation induced by probiotic bacteria. *Clin Vaccine Immunol*. 2007 May;14(5):485-92

The Four Main Food-Consumption Patterns

Diet pattern	Characteristics
❶ SAD: Standard American Diet	▪ Food choices in this diet are based on convenience, recent advertisements, coupons and cost, popular trends, social pressure, and instant gratification at the expense of the feeling of health or its authentic attainment. ▪ This diet tends to be high in sucrose, fructose, sodium, chloride, and chemical colorants, preservatives, and artificial flavors. It is generally low in essential fatty acids, minerals, vitamins in their natural form, fiber and phytonutrients. ▪ This diet is largely responsible for the modern epidemics of *overconsumption malnutrition* which causes obesity, hypertension, cardiovascular disease, and increased risk for various cancers and other chronic diseases. ▪ Because the foods tend to be mass-produced, of low quality, and of durable shelf life due to lack of nutritional value, chemical preservatives, and packaging, the economics of these products is that of low cost for consumers and high profit for producers and sellers. Tertiary profitability is enjoyed by drug companies, so-called "health insurance" corporations, and hospital and clinic systems that have to implement the damage control and rescue remedies necessary to sustain life following long-term consumption of this diet. ▪ If not for the SAD dietary pattern and the physical inactivity that generally accompanies it, hypertension would not exist as the epidemic that it currently is, and antihypertensive medications would be *orphan drugs*. ▪ Because of the characteristic incorporation of "flavor enhancers" such as monosodium glutamate and carrageenan, and because of the high content of sodium and sugars, the *supranormal* stimulation provided to taste receptors downregulates the subtle perception of taste so that consumers become accustomed to (i.e., *addicted to*) the supranormal stimulation and are thereby disinclined to consume a normal natural diet due to its comparatively "bland" taste. ***Clinical pearl***: Generally, 1-2 weeks are required following discontinuation of the SAD diet before gustatory sensitivity is restored so that foods in their natural state can be appreciated. Patients need to lean toward going "cold turkey" (pun intended) and thereby avoiding excess sugar, sodium, flavor-enhancers and other supranormal stimulation for 1-2 weeks so that they can thereafter consume and enjoy a *natural* whole foods diet.
❷ DASH: Dietary Approaches to Stop Hypertension	▪ *Better* food choices than the SAD diet, with emphasis placed on: ▪ *Reduced* consumption of saturated fat, cholesterol, and total fat, red meat, sweets, added sugars, and sugar-containing beverages compared to the SAD. ▪ *Increased* consumption of fruits, vegetables, and fat-free or low-fat milk and milk products, whole grain products, fish, poultry, and nuts. ▪ Compared to the SAD, DASH provides more potassium, magnesium, calcium, protein, and fiber and less sodium and sugars such as sucrose and fructose. ▪ In sum, the DASH diet a *better* diet pattern compared to the random and nonlogical convenience- and pleasure-based eating habits followed by most Americans and others seduced by the convenience, low cost, and supranormal stimulation of the SAD or "Westernized" diet. However, the inclusion of grains and excess carbohydrates makes it suboptimal, particularly when compared to diets based on vegetables, nuts, berries, seeds.

The Four Main Food-Consumption Patterns — *continued*

Diet pattern	Characteristics
❸ **Paleo-Mediterranean Diet**	▪ The Paleo-Mediterranean diet consists almost exclusively of unprocessed and as-fresh-as-possible and as-raw-as-possible fruits, vegetables, nuts, seeds, berries and lean sources of protein, especially fish, poultry, and lean grass-fed meats and game meats. A modern modification allows the inclusion of whey and soy protein isolates for their functional benefits beyond the mere provision of protein to include functionally active proteins, peptides, amino acid profiles, whey immunoglobulins and lactoferrin, and the soy phytonutrients genistein, daidzeinm, and beta-sitosterol. Dark chocolate, olive oil, and red wine are also accepted staples of this dietary pattern. ▪ The Mediterranean diet as commonly described also includes "whole grains" such as wheat and starchy vegetables such as potatoes; these are best avoided. Knowledgeable clinicians will appreciate that the modern notion of "whole grains" is a farce because of mechanical processing which pulverizes the husk and bran of the grain into oblivion, rendering its natural-state physiochemical properties powerless. ▪ In its highest form (i.e., excluding grains and other mechanically processed and overcooked food items), the Paleo-Mediterranean diet is the most nutrient-dense and physiologically appropriate diet for human beings with the greatest promise of health optimization and disease prevention.[156]
❹ **Vegetarian diet, and related variants**	▪ Plant-based diets *should* consist of fruits, vegetables, nuts, seeds, berries consumed as raw and as fresh as possible; this might seem obvious except that many (pseudo)vegetarians rely on grains and processed foods and are thus only vegetarians to the extent that they avoid meat (perhaps "acarneists") and not to the extent that they rely on vegetables, as the term *vegeta*rianism implies. Consumption of legumes for their relatively higher protein content is common. Avoidance of grains due to their allergenicity and low phytonutrient and micronutrient content is advised. ▪ The lack of sufficient vitamin B-12 along with the relatively higher content of anti-nutrients such as phytic acid makes a purely vegetarian diet of tenuous durability for the unskilled, unknowledgeable, and undisciplined consumer. Many people adopt a so-called vegetarian diet for sociopolitical reasons without becoming aware of its proper implementation; such persons can consume a protein-deficient diet consistent with "breaditarianism"[157]—which is basically equal to or worse than the SAD diet due to its lack of adequate protein and overreliance on simple carbohydrates ▪ <u>Vegan</u> = exclusive consumption of plant foods only. ▪ <u>Vegetarian</u> = reliance upon plant foods, with the occasional inclusion of diary, eggs, and fish. ▪ <u>Pescovegetarian</u> = consumption of plants and fish. ▪ <u>Lacto-ovo-vegetarian</u> = consumption of plants, milk, eggs (i.e., animal protein without the killing of animals).

---

[156] Cordain L, Eaton SB, Sebastian A, Mann N, Lindeberg S, Watkins BA, O'Keefe JH, Brand-Miller J. Origins and evolution of the Western diet: health implications for the 21st century. *Am J Clin Nutr*. 2005 Feb;81(2):341-5 http://www.ajcn.org/cgi/content/full/81/2/341
[157] O'Keefe JH Jr,Cordain L.Cardiovascular disease resulting from a diet and lifestyle at odds with our Paleolithic genome.*Mayo Clin Proc* 2004;79:101-8

Most of the studies reviewed in the following section pertain to the Paleo-Mediterranean diet (PMD) and its optimized expression in the supplemented Paleo-Mediterranean diet (sPMD). Studies on the DASH diet generally showed benefit when contrasted to the SAD eating pattern which is the norm for most Americans and increasingly among other nationalities. In this text, the DASH diet is advocated only insofar as it is an improvement over the SAD eating pattern; it is secondary to the PMD and tertiary to the sPMD in its effectiveness for disease treatment and prevention.

o Small clinical trial: Metabolic and physiologic improvements from consuming a Paleolithic, hunter-gatherer type diet (*European Journal of Clinical Nutrition*, Feb 2009): Despite the small subject size (n = 9), this study demonstrates safety and beneficial effectiveness of the Paleolithic diet in addressing several of the perturbations that characterize the metabolic syndrome and lifestyle-induced predisposition to CVD. "Results: Compared with the baseline (usual) diet, we observed (a) **significant reductions in BP** associated with improved arterial distensibility; (b) **significant reduction in plasma insulin** vs time AUC [area under the curve], during the OGTT [oral glucose tolerance testing]; and (c) large significant reductions in total cholesterol, low-density lipoproteins (LDL) and triglycerides (-0.8, -0.7 and -0.3 mmol/l respectively). In all these measured variables, either **eight or all nine participants had identical directional responses when switched to Paleolithic type diet, that is, near consistently improved status of circulatory, carbohydrate and lipid metabolism/physiology."**[158]

o Randomized 3-month cross-over pilot study: Beneficial effects of a Paleolithic diet on cardiovascular risk factors in type 2 diabetes (*Cardiovascular Diabetology*, Jul 2009): Although small (n=13), this study is impressive because it shows not only the benefits of the Paleolithic diet but also its superiority over the commonly recommended "diabetic diet" which is advocated by conventional-standard-mainstream-government and medical groups that claim to advocate health and victory in the so-called war against obesity and diabetes mellitus. "Compared to the diabetes diet, the Paleolithic diet resulted in lower mean values of HbA1c (-0.4% units), triacylglycerol (-0.4 mmol/L), **diastolic blood pressure (-4 mmHg),** weight (-3 kg), BMI (-1 kg/m2) and waist circumference (-4 cm), and higher mean values of high density lipoprotein cholesterol (+0.08 mmol/L)."[159]

Clinical benefits from a Paleolithic hunter-gatherer diet
☑ **Significant reductions in blood pressure**,
☑ Improved arterial distensibility,
☑ **Significant reduction in plasma insulin**,
☑ Large significant reductions in total cholesterol, low-density lipoproteins (LDL) and triglycerides,
☑ Consistently improved status of circulatory, carbohydrate and lipid metabolism/physiology.

"Conclusions: Even **short-term consumption of a paleolithic type diet improves BP and glucose tolerance, decreases insulin secretion, increases insulin sensitivity and improves lipid profiles without weight loss in healthy sedentary humans.**"

Frassetto LA, Schloetter M, Mietus-Synder M, Morris RC Jr, Sebastian A. Metabolic and physiologic improvements from consuming a paleolithic, hunter-gatherer type diet. *Eur J Clin Nutr.* 2009 Feb 11

---

[158] Frassetto LA, Schloetter M, Mietus-Synder M, Morris RC Jr, Sebastian A. Metabolic and physiologic improvements from consuming a paleolithic, hunter-gatherer type diet. *Eur J Clin Nutr.* 2009 Feb 11.
[159] Jonsson T, Granfeldt Y, Ahren B, Branell UC, Palsson G, Hansson A, Soderstrom M, Lindeberg S. Beneficial effects of a Paleolithic diet on cardiovascular risk factors in type 2 diabetes: a randomized cross-over pilot study. *Cardiovasc Diabetol.* 2009;8:35. http://cardiab.com/content/8/1/35

o Randomized controlled trial with n=144: Effects of the Dietary Approaches to Stop Hypertension (DASH) diet alone and in combination with exercise and caloric restriction on insulin sensitivity and lipids (*Hypertension*, May 2010): In this study lead by Blumenthal[160] published in 2010, the authors examined the effects of the DASH diet on insulin sensitivity and lipids in a randomized controlled trial with 144 overweight (BMI: 25 to 40) men (n=47) and women (n=97) with BP up to 159/99 mm Hg. Study subjects were randomly assigned for 4 months to one of three groups with the following results (table below), respectively. Of important note is the worsening of glucose control and insulin sensitivity on the DASH diet; this suggests that the DASH diet may ultimately promote development of metabolic syndrome despite appearing to be cardioprotective based on short-term reductions in blood pressure. Note that the weight loss induced by *caloric restriction + exercise* of 19 lbs over 4 months equates to 4.75 lbs per month; this is consistent with what clinicians should expect in clinical practice, namely patients' weight loss of 4-8 lbs per month with dietary optimization plus increased physical activity.

Intervention	*Results*
DASH diet alone	☺ Weight loss: Imperceptible, only -0.3 kg ☺ Exercise capacity: No improvement ☹ Glucose control: Slight worsening of glucose levels after the oral glucose load; fasting serum insulin actually increased from 16.6 to 17.6 mcu/ml ☹ Lipids: No change; slight worsening of triglycerides ☺ Blood pressure: Clinically significant reductions in blood pressure
DASH diet *with* aerobic exercise *and* caloric restriction *Per this study, this is the closest of the 3 options to the foundational diet (sPMD is more strict) and lifestyle protocol advocated in this textbook.*	☺ Weight loss: Clinically and statistically significant at -8.7 kg (-19.2 lbs) ☺ Exercise capacity: Significant increase in aerobic capacity ☺ Glucose control: Lower fasting glucose; lower glucose levels after the oral glucose load; improved insulin sensitivity; fasting serum insulin reduced from 18.1 to 12.5 mcu/ml ☺ Lipids: Meaningful reductions in total cholesterol, triglycerides, and low-density lipoprotein cholesterol (LDL) ☺ Blood pressure: Clinically significant reductions in blood pressure
Usual control (UC) diet	☹ Weight *gain*: +0.9 kg ☺ Exercise capacity: no improvement ☺ Glucose control: no improvement ☺ Lipids: no improvement ☺ Blood pressure: no improvement

---

[160] Blumenthal JA, Babyak MA, Sherwood A, Craighead L, Lin PH, Johnson J, Watkins LL, Wang JT, Kuhn C, Feinglos M, Hinderliter A. Effects of the dietary approaches to stop hypertension diet alone and in combination with exercise and caloric restriction on insulin sensitivity and lipids. *Hypertension*. 2010 May;55(5):1199-205

o   <u>Randomized clinical trial: Effects of the dietary approaches to stop hypertension diet, exercise, and caloric restriction on neurocognition in overweight adults with high blood pressure</u> (*Hypertension*, Jun 2010): In this clinical trial, 124 subjects with either prehypertension or stage 1 hypertension (sBP 130 to 159 mm Hg or dBP 85 to 99 mm Hg) who were sedentary and overweight or obese (BMI: 25 to 40) were randomized to the DASH diet alone, DASH with exercise and caloric restriction, or a usual control (UC) diet group. Subjects completed tests of executive function, memory, and learning and psychomotor speed at baseline and at the end of the 4-month trial. Results showed the following: "Participants on the DASH diet combined with a behavioral weight management program exhibited greater improvements in executive function-memory-learning and psychomotor speed, and DASH diet alone participants exhibited better psychomotor speed compared with the usual diet control. Neurocognitive improvements appeared to be mediated by increased aerobic fitness and weight loss. ... In conclusion, combining aerobic exercise with the DASH diet and caloric restriction improves neurocognitive function among sedentary and overweight/obese individuals with prehypertension and hypertension."[161] Specific to changes in blood pressure, the following results were noted (per Table 2 of the original article):

Intervention & BP changes in mm HG	*Initial BP*	*Final BP*	*BP change*
DASH diet alone	137.5/87.2	127.8/79.5	-9.7/-7.7
DASH diet *with* aerobic exercise *and* caloric restriction	138.6/85.4	125.1/77.2	**-13.5/-8.2**
Usual control (UC) diet	138.6/85.7	136.2/82.7	-2.2/-3

Thus, as we should expect, dietary improvement plus caloric restriction and exercise resulted in greater reductions in BP than diet improvement alone, which was better than no change at all. The neurocognitive improvements associated with improved diet and increased exercise are consistent with the previously documented neurogenic/neuroprotective/synaptogenic effects of exercise[162], as well as improved neuronal function seen with increased phytonutrient intake.[163] *Consider the implications.*

What might be the cumulative additive/synergistic neuro-intellectual results—on a personal, interpersonal, social, and national level—of dietary optimization, frequent exercise, decided application of one's efforts and abilities, and habitual exposure to complex neurointellectual phenomena—for example, highly structured music[164,165]? Synergism of these events would likely elevate humanity toward its positive potential.

---

[161] Smith PJ, Blumenthal JA, Babyak MA, Craighead L, Welsh-Bohmer KA, Browndyke JN, Strauman TA, Sherwood A. Effects of the dietary approaches to stop hypertension diet, exercise, and caloric restriction on neurocognition in overweight adults with high blood pressure. *Hypertension*. 2010 Jun;55(6):1331-8
[162] Cotman CW, Berchtold NC, Christie LA. Exercise builds brain health: key roles of growth factor cascades and inflammation. *Trends Neurosci*. 2007 Sep;30(9):464-72
[163] Spencer JP. The impact of fruit flavonoids on memory and cognition. *Br J Nutr*. 2010 Oct;104 Suppl 3:S40-7 and Spencer JP. Flavonoids and brain health: multiple effects underpinned by common mechanisms. *Genes Nutr*. 2009 Dec;4(4):243-50
[164] Suda M, Morimoto K, Obata A,Koizumi H, Maki A.Cortical responses to Mozart's sonata enhance spatial-reasoning ability.*Neurol Res* 2008;30:885-8
[165] Jausovec N, Jausovec K, Gerlic I. The influence of Mozart's music on brain activity in the process of learning. *Clin Neurophysiol*. 2006;117:2703-14

o Randomized controlled trial: Effects of the DASH diet alone and in combination with exercise and weight loss on blood pressure and cardiovascular biomarkers in men and women with high blood pressure (*Archives of Internal Medicine*, Jan 2010): This publication reports results of a randomized controlled clinical trial among 144 overweight/obese hypertensive patients for 4 months; intervention was either DASH diet alone, DASH diet with a weight management program, or usual control diet.

Intervention	Results
DASH diet alone	☺ BP was reduced by -11.2/-7.5 mm Hg
DASH diet *with* aerobic exercise *and* caloric restriction	☺ BP was reduced by **-16.1/-9.9** mm Hg ☺ Greater improvement was noted in this group than with DASH alone for pulse wave velocity, baroreflex sensitivity, and left ventricular mass
Usual control (UC) diet	☺ Nonsignificant BP reduction of -3.4/-3.8 mm Hg

The authors reported the results and conclusion as follows: "Clinic-measured BP was reduced by 16.1/9.9 mm Hg (DASH plus weight management); 11.2/7.5 mm (DASH alone); and 3.4/3.8 mm (usual diet controls). ... Greater improvement was noted for DASH plus weight management compared with DASH alone for pulse wave velocity, baroreflex sensitivity, and left ventricular mass. CONCLUSION: For overweight or obese persons with above-normal BP, the addition of exercise and weight loss to the DASH diet resulted in even larger BP reductions, greater improvements in vascular and autonomic function, and reduced left ventricular mass."[166]

o Review: Effects of exercise, diet and weight loss on high blood pressure (*Sports Medicine*, 2004): The authors of this review note that HTN "is a major health problem in the US, affecting more than 50 million people" and that "anti-hypertensive medications are not effective for everyone, and may be costly and result in adverse effects that impair quality of life and reduce adherence. Moreover, abnormalities associated with high BP, such as insulin resistance and hyperlipidaemia, may persist or may even be exacerbated by some anti-hypertensive medications." Thereafter, their expert review of the literature may be summarized as follows:

Intervention	Blood pressure reduction
Exercise alone: without intentional weight loss or diet intervention	-3.5/-2.0 mm Hg
DASH diet	-5.5/-3.0 mm Hg
Weight loss of 17.6 lbs (8 kg)	-8.5/-6.5 mm Hg
Combined exercise and weight loss	**-12.5/-7.9 mm Hg**

[166] Blumenthal JA, Babyak MA, Hinderliter A, et al. Effects of the DASH diet alone and in combination with exercise and weight loss on blood pressure and cardiovascular biomarkers in men and women with high blood pressure: the ENCORE study. *Arch Intern Med.* 2010 Jan 25;170(2):126-35

The benefits of exercise and weight loss extend beyond BP reduction to include reductions in left ventricular mass and wall thickness (i.e., reductions in left ventricular hypertrophy), reduced arterial stiffness and improved endothelial function.[167]

o The 2009 Canadian Hypertension Education Program recommendations for the management of hypertension: Part 2—therapy (*Canadian Journal of Cardiology*, May 2009): These are very conventional and standard recommendations from the medical community which are included here for the sake of completeness so that doctors have a recent reference guideline from which they can move beyond in the delivery of superior clinical care. "RECOMMENDATIONS: For lifestyle modifications to prevent and treat hypertension, restrict dietary sodium to less than 2300 mg (100 mmol)/day (and 1500 mg to 2300 mg [65 mmol to 100 mmol]/day in hypertensive patients); perform 30 min to 60 min of aerobic exercise four to seven days per week; maintain a healthy body weight (body mass index 18.5 kg/m(2) to 24.9 kg/m(2)) and waist circumference (smaller than 102 cm for men and smaller than 88 cm for women); limit alcohol consumption to no more than 14 units [drinks] per week in men or nine units per week in women; follow a diet that is reduced in saturated fat and cholesterol, and that emphasizes fruits, vegetables and low-fat dairy products, dietary and soluble fiber, whole grains and protein from plant sources; and consider stress management in selected individuals with hypertension."[168] These guidelines would have been better if they had advised complete avoidance of grains (sources of generally acidogenic phytonutrient-poor carbohydrates) and other sources of simple carbohydrate including candies and soft drinks in general and those pseudofoods laden with high-fructose corn syrup in particular.

> **Lifestyle recommendations from the Canadian Hypertension Education Program**
> - Restrict dietary sodium to less than 2300 mg (100 mmol)/day (and 1500 mg to 2300 mg [65 mmol to 100 mmol]/day in hypertensive patients).
> - Perform 30 min to 60 min of aerobic exercise four to seven days per week.
> - Maintain a healthy body weight (body mass index 18.5 kg/m(2) to 24.9 kg/m(2)) and waist circumference (< 102 cm for men and < 88 cm for women).
> - Limit alcohol consumption to no more than 14 units per week in men or nine units per week in women.
> - Follow a diet that is reduced in saturated fat and cholesterol.
> - Follow a diet that emphasizes fruits, vegetables and low-fat dairy products, dietary and soluble fiber, whole grains and protein from plant sources.
> - Consider stress management in selected individuals with hypertension.
>
> Khan NA, Hemmelgarn B, Herman RJ, et al. The 2009 Canadian Hypertension Education Program recommendations for the management of hypertension: Part 2—therapy. *Can J Cardiol*. 2009 May;25(5):287-98

o Meta-analysis: Adherence to Mediterranean diet and health status (*British Medical Journal*, Sep 2008): "Greater adherence to a Mediterranean diet is associated with a significant

---

[167] Bacon SL, Sherwood A, Hinderliter A, Blumenthal JA. Effects of exercise, diet and weight loss on high blood pressure. *Sports Med*. 2004;34:307-16

[168] Khan NA, Hemmelgarn B, Herman RJ, Bell CM, Mahon JL, Leiter LA, Rabkin SW, Hill MD, Padwal R, Touyz RM, Larochelle P, Feldman RD, Schiffrin EL, Campbell NR, Moe G, Prasad R, Arnold MO, Campbell TS, Milot A, Stone JA, Jones C, Ogilvie RI, Hamet P, Fodor G, Carruthers G, Burns KD, Ruzicka M, DeChamplain J, Pylypchuk G, Petrella R, Boulanger JM, Trudeau L, Hegele RA, Woo V, McFarlane P, Vallée M, Howlett J, Bacon SL, Lindsay P, Gilbert RE, Lewanczuk RZ, Tobe S; Canadian Hypertension Education Program. The 2009 Canadian Hypertension Education Program recommendations for the management of hypertension: Part 2—therapy. *Can J Cardiol*. 2009 May;25(5):287-98

improvement in health status, as seen by a **significant reduction in overall mortality** (-9%), mortality from **cardiovascular diseases** (-9%), incidence of or mortality from **cancer** (-6%), and incidence of **Parkinson's disease and Alzheimer's disease** (-13%). These results seem to be clinically relevant for public health, in particular for **encouraging a Mediterranean-like dietary pattern for primary prevention of major chronic diseases.**"[169] The results of this meta-analysis have major implications for clinical practice and public health policy.

> **Clinical Pearl: lowering plasma glucose → lower insulin levels → less sodium-water retention → alleviation of hypertension**
>
> Treatments that lower plasma glucose levels, either via reduced intake of carbohydrates or by increasing glucose disposal (i.e., increasing insulin sensitivity) have an anti-hypertensive effect via lowering insulin levels. **Because insulin promotes sodium-water retention, any treatment that lowers glucose-insulin levels will help correct the contribution of hyperinsulinemia to hypertension.** Likewise, avoidance of dietary fructose is now known to avoid the fructose-induced elevations in serum uric acid which contribute to endothelial dysfunction, hypertension, and the metabolic syndrome.

- **Short-term water-only fasting**: The anti-hypertensive and anti-diabetic benefits of low-carbohydrate diets and short-term fasting have been substantiated in the research literature for several decades. However, the chiropractic physician Alan Goldhamer deserves credit for the most recent revival of short-term fasting as a therapeutic tool for chronic hypertension and diabetes mellitus.

  o Open clinical trial: Chiropractic-supervised water-only fasting in the treatment of hypertension (*Journal of Manipulative Physiological Therapeutics*, Jun 2001): In this open trial, 174 consecutive hypertensive patients were treated in an inpatient setting under clinician supervision. The treatment program began with a short prefasting period (approximately 2 to 3 days on average) during which food consumption was limited to fruits and vegetables, followed by supervised water-only fasting (approximately 10 to 11 days on average) and a refeeding period (approximately 6 to 7 days on average) introducing a low-fat, low-sodium, vegan diet. "RESULTS: Almost 90% of the subjects achieved blood pressure less than 140/90 mm Hg by the end of the treatment program. **The average reduction in blood pressure was 37/13 mm Hg**, with the greatest decrease being observed for subjects with the most severe hypertension. **Patients with stage 3 hypertension (those with systolic blood pressure greater than 180 mg Hg, diastolic blood pressure greater than 110 mg Hg, or both) had an average reduction of 60/17 mm Hg at the conclusion of treatment**. All of the subjects who were taking antihypertensive medication at entry (6.3% of the total sample) successfully discontinued the use of medication. CONCLUSION: Medically supervised water-only fasting appears to be a safe and effective means of normalizing blood pressure and may assist in motivating health-promoting diet and lifestyle changes."[170]

---

[169] Sofi F, Cesari F, Abbate R, Gensini GF, Casini A. Adherence to Mediterranean diet and health status: meta-analysis. *BMJ*. 2008 Sep 11;337:a1344
[170] Goldhamer A, Lisle D, Parpia B, Anderson SV, Campbell TC. Medically supervised water-only fasting in the treatment of hypertension. *J Manipulative Physiol Ther* 2001 Jun;24(5):335-9 http://www.healthpromoting.com/Articles/335-339Goldhamer115263.QXD.pdf

o Open clinical trial: Chiropractic-supervised water-only fasting in the treatment of borderline hypertension (*Journal of Alternative and Complementary Medicine*, Oct 2002): 68 consecutive patients with borderline hypertension were treated in an inpatient setting under professional supervision. The treatment program consisted of a short prefasting period (approximately 1-2 days on average) during which food consumption was limited to fruits and vegetables followed by supervised water-only fasting (approximately 13.6 days on average). Fasting was followed by a refeeding period (approximately 6.0 days on average). The refeeding program consisted of a low-fat, low-sodium, plant-based, vegan diet. "RESULTS: Approximately 82% of the subjects achieved BP at or below 120/80 mm Hg by the end of the treatment program. **The mean BP reduction was 20/7 mm Hg,** with the greatest decrease being observed for subjects with the highest baseline BP. A linear regression of BP decrease against baseline BP showed that the estimated BP below which no further decrease would be expected was 96.0/67.0 mm Hg at the end of the fast and 99.2/67.3 mm Hg at the end of refeeding. These levels are in agreement with other estimates of the BP below which stroke events are eliminated, thus suggesting that these levels could be regarded as the "ideal" BP values. CONCLUSION: Medically supervised water-only fasting appears to be a safe and effective means of normalizing BP and may assist in motivating health-promoting diet and lifestyle changes."[171]

o Retrospective cost-effectiveness and clinical effectiveness analysis for short-term fasting in the treatment of hypertension and diabetes mellitus: Initial cost of care results in medically supervised water-only fasting for treating high blood pressure and diabetes (*Journal of Alternative and Complementary Medicine*, Dec 2002): In this brief report, Dr Goldhamer again reports success with the short-term fasting program in hypertensive patients as well as diabetic patients. Here, Goldhamer reports that the **average reduction in systolic blood pressure was 30/11 mm Hg at the completion of the program and 28/11 mm Hg on follow-up.** "Weight loss averaged 26 pounds after the program and was 28 pounds below baseline on follow-up. The average cost of medical care and drugs was $5,784.00 per year in the year(s) prior to participation and $3,000.00 in the year after participation for an average reduction of $2,784.00 per subject in the first year alone. This exceeded the cost of the entire program and compound savings are expected in the years to follow."[172]

- **Specific food items to be avoided or reasonably minimized**: Clinicians and patients should be aware that dietary intake of food allergens, fructose, sodium chloride, and arachidonic acid can contribute to the development, perpetuation, and therapeutic recalcitrance of chronic HTN.

  o **Food allergen avoidance, customized per patient (*The Lancet*, May 1979)**: According to a clinical study of migraineurs (n = 60) published in *The Lancet*, identification and avoidance of food allergens can generally normalize blood pressure in migraine patients who have concomitant hypertension[173]; findings of this study included, "The commonest foods causing reactions were wheat (78%), orange (65%), eggs (45%), tea and coffee (40% each), chocolate and milk (37%) each), beef (35%), and corn, cane sugar, and yeast (33%

---

[171] Goldhamer AC, Lisle DJ, Sultana P, Anderson SV, Parpia B, Hughes B, Campbell TC. Medically supervised water-only fasting in the treatment of borderline hypertension. *J Altern Complement Med*. 2002 Oct;8(5):643-50 http://www.healthpromoting.com/Articles/articles/study%202/acmpaper5.pdf
[172] Goldhamer AC. Initial cost of care results in medically supervised water-only fasting for treating high blood pressure and diabetes. *J Altern Complement Med*. 2002 Dec;8(6):696-7 http://www.healthpromoting.com/Articles/pdf/Study%2032.pdf
[173] Grant EC. Food allergies and migraine. *Lancet*. 1979 May 5;1(8123):966-9

each). When an average of **ten common foods** was avoided there was a dramatic fall in the number of headaches per month, 85% of patients becoming headache-free. The 25% of patients with hypertension became normotensive."

o **Minimization of dietary sodium chloride**: Excess sodium (Na) promotes water retention and subsequent volume expansion, while also contributing to vasoconstriction and arterial stiffness via enhanced adrenergic reactivity and via promotion of "**intracellular hypercalcinosis**" (per Vasquez[174]) possibly due to enhanced sodium-calcium exchange.[175] When consumed in common table salt, the chloride (Cl) anion promotes acidosis which results in the progression of CAD/CVD morbidity and mortality and the exacerbation of HTN with increased renal losses of magnesium, potassium, and calcium. These effects justify the advice for HTN patients to avoid dietary NaCl and also justify the use of drug diuretics that enhance Na excretion by the kidney. Clinical responsiveness to low-sodium diets ranges from clinically insignificant to a maximum reduction in the range of -22/-14 to -16/-9.[176] Contraindications to low-sodium diet are uncommon (e.g., hyponatremia); **low-sodium/NaCl diets should generally be a component of all anti-hypertensive treatment plans.** Approximately 20% of patients will show antihypertensive benefit from sodium restriction.[177] As previously noted, Canadian guidelines published in 2009 support the restriction of dietary sodium to less than 2300 mg (100 mmol)/day and to less than 1500-2300 mg [65 mmol to 100 mmol]/day in hypertensive patients.[178] One might hope that readers would appreciate that human physiology developed over millennia wherein the addition of manufactured table salt was a logistical impossibility; in an excellent paradigm-shifting compilation and integration of research, Cordain and his pioneering expert co-authors[179] noted, "the addition of manufactured salt to the food supply and the displacement of traditional potassium-rich foods by foods introduced during the Neolithic and Industrial periods caused a 400% decline in the potassium intake while simultaneously initiating a 400% increase in sodium ingestion. The inversion of potassium and sodium concentrations [dietary sodium-potassium ratio] in hominin diets had no evolutionary precedent and now plays an integral role in eliciting and contributing to numerous diseases of civilization." Adverse effects of NaCl can be at least partly offset by administration of calcium, vitamin D, magnesium, potassium, bicarbonate and citrate.

[174] **Vasquez A**. Intracellular Hypercalcinosis: A Functional Nutritional Disorder with Implications Ranging from Myofascial Trigger Points to Affective Disorders, Hypertension, and Cancer. *Naturopathy Digest* 2006 Previously published in-print and on-line at http://www.naturopathydigest.com/archives/2006/sep/vasquez.php and included at the end of this chapter.
[175] Benowitz NL. "Antihypertensive Agents." In Katzung BG (editor). Basic and Clinical Pharmacology. Tenth Edition. New York: McGraw Hill Medical; 2007, 163
[176] "The average fall in blood pressure from the highest to the lowest sodium intake was 16/9 mm Hg." MacGregor GA, Markandu ND, Sagnella GA, Singer DR, Cappuccio FP. Double-blind study of three sodium intakes and long-term effects of sodium restriction in essential hypertension. *Lancet.* 1989 Nov 25;2(8674):1244-7
[177] Domino FJ (editor in chief). The 5-Minute Clinical Consult. 2010. 18th Edition. Philadelphia; Wolters Kluwer: 2009, 656-7
[178] Khan NA, Hemmelgarn B, Herman RJ, Bell CM, Mahon JL, Leiter LA, Rabkin SW, Hill MD, Padwal R, Touyz RM, Larochelle P, Feldman RD, Schiffrin EL, Campbell NR, Moe G, Prasad R, Arnold MO, Campbell TS, Milot A, Stone JA, Jones C, Ogilvie RI, Hamet P, Fodor G, Carruthers G, Burns KD, Ruzicka M, DeChamplain J, Pylypchuk G, Petrella R, Boulanger JM, Trudeau L, Hegele RA, Woo V, McFarlane P, Vallée M, Howlett J, Bacon SL, Lindsay P, Gilbert RE, Lewanczuk RZ, Tobe S; Canadian Hypertension Education Program. The 2009 Canadian Hypertension Education Program recommendations for the management of hypertension: Part 2—therapy. *Can J Cardiol.* 2009 May;25(5):287-98
[179] Cordain L, Eaton SB, Sebastian A, Mann N, Lindeberg S, Watkins BA, O'Keefe JH, Brand-Miller J. Origins and evolution of the Western diet: health implications for the 21st century. *Am J Clin Nutr.* 2005 Feb;81(2):341-5 http://www.ajcn.org/cgi/content/full/81/2/341

o **Fructose avoidance for caloric moderation and uric acid reduction (American Heart Association, news release Sep 2009)**: Production of uric acid is stimulated by ingestion of fructose (most notoriously in the form of high-fructose corn syrup, common in many processed foods and cola drinks), and uric acid directly contributes to the development of insulin resistance and HTN and other classic features of the metabolic syndrome. **In a clinical trial published in September 2009, 74 adult men added fructose 200 g/d to their regular diet (typical American diet averages 50-70 g/d of fructose) for 2 weeks and experienced a 6/3 elevation in BP, elevations in serum triglycerides and LDL cholesterol, and a more than doubling of the incidence of metabolic syndrome from approximately 20% to 50% as determined by two sets of international criteria.** The authors logically concluded, **"These results suggest that fructose may be a cause of metabolic syndrome. They also suggest that excessive fructose intake may have a role in the worldwide epidemic of obesity and diabetes."**[180] Men in this trial who were randomized to receive the xanthine oxidase inhibitor allopurinol (dose not reported; common adult amount is 200-600 mg/d in divided doses, preferably with food) did not develop adverse effects from the increased fructose ingestion, thus clearly implicating fructose-induced hyperuricemia as the biochemical pathway involved. Clinicians should appreciate that the rapid (within 2 weeks) development of HTN and a doubling of the incidence of metabolic syndrome by the addition of fructose to the diet is of undeniably major importance as it clearly implicates high-fructose corn syrup as a major culprit in the burgeoning epidemics of HTN, type-2 diabetes mellitus, and the metabolic syndrome. In a study[181] involving adolescents with elevated uric acid levels (serum uric acid levels > or = 6 mg/dL), allopurinol 200 mg twice daily resulted in a reduction in blood pressure of approximately -7/-5 mm Hg (compared to approximately -2/-2 for placebo); this was a proof-of-concept study (i.e., that uric acid contributes to HTN) and not necessarily an endorsement to use allopurinol for the treatment of HTN. Adverse effects due to allopurinol can include skin rash that may be followed by more severe hypersensitivity reactions such as "exfoliative, urticarial and purpuric lesions as well as Stevens-Johnson syndrome (erythema multiforme exudativum) and/or generalized vasculitis, irreversible hepatotoxicity and on rare occasions, death."[182] **Adherence to the Paleo-Mediterranean Diet in general and a low-fructose diet in particular can help reduce elevated serum uric acid levels without the use of drugs because this dietary profile is low in fructose and promotes urinary alkalinization**; alkalinizing the urine via avoidance of acidogenic foodstuffs such as dairy and sodium chloride and by increased intake of fruits and vegetables (or supplemental forms of citrate and bicarbonate[183]) promotes renal excretion of uric acid, thus lessening the adverse metabolic effects of uric acid on insulin resistance and endothelial dysfunction. Clinicians should note that, as a

---

[180] News release from American Heart Association's 63rd High Blood Pressure Research Conference. High-sugar diet increases men's blood pressure; gout drug protective. Abstract P127. Sept. 23, 2009. http://americanheart.mediaroom.com/index.php?s=43&item=829 Accessed December 19, 2009
[181] "Allopurinol, 200 mg twice daily for 4 weeks,... For casual BP, the mean change in systolic BP for allopurinol was -6.9 mm Hg vs -2.0 mm Hg for placebo, and the mean change in diastolic BP for allopurinol was -5.1 mm Hg vs -2.4 for placebo. CONCLUSIONS: In this short-term, crossover study of adolescents with newly diagnosed hypertension, treatment with allopurinol resulted in reduction of BP." Feig DI, Soletsky B, Johnson RJ. Effect of allopurinol on blood pressure of adolescents with newly diagnosed essential hypertension: a randomized trial. *JAMA*. 2008 Aug 27;300(8):924-32
[182] Brinker AD. Allopurinol and the role of uric acid in hypertension. [letter] *JAMA*. 2009 Jan 21;301(3):270
[183] "The treatment of uric acid stones should focus on alkalinization of the urine with citrate or bicarbonate salts." Liebman SE, Taylor JG, Bushinsky DA. Uric acid nephrolithiasis. *Curr Rheumatol Rep*. 2007 Jun;9(3):251-7

result of the manufacturing process, high-fructose corn syrup contains mercury[184], a toxic metal for which no known "safe" and free-from-harm dose exists; adverse effects of mercury exposure include renal damage and clinical hypertension, the latter is promoted by the former while also being generated independently by increased catecholamine release (according to case reports[185]). Per the 2009 review by Houston[186], **"The clinical consequences of mercury toxicity include hypertension**, CHD, MI, increased carotid IMT [intima media thickness] and obstruction, CVA, generalized atherosclerosis, and renal dysfunction with proteinuria." Mercury contamination of corn syrup ranks among the better examples of how industrialization of the food supply causes untoward [i.e., unexpected and negative] effects; it also exemplifies how one problem (overconsumption of processed "junk" food which contains pro-hypertensive fructose in nonphysiologic/unnatural concentrations) can lead/contribute to other types of problems (adverse effects of mercury, neurotoxicity, nephrotoxicity, and chronic overstimulation of the sympathetic nervous system). Rapid induction of hypertension and the metabolic syndrome in humans by fructose consumption is almost certainly *not* mediated by the mercury content; the extent to which mercury from corn syrup contributes to hypertension is not known, but facts that are already established include the following: ❶ mercury is a known immunotoxin, nephrotoxin, and neurotoxin, ❷ mercury can cause hypertension in humans, ❸ mercury causes hypertension in humans via at least two mechanisms—inhibition of catecholamine breakdown, and induction of renal damage, ❹ corn syrup contains two agents known to cause hypertension in humans: mercury and fructose.

- o **Arachidonate avoidance**: Arachidonate promotes intracellular calcium accumulation which promotes the development of HTN. Avoidance of arachidonic acid helps restore intracellular ion homeostasis and results in reduction of elevated BP. Restoration of fatty acid balance via simultaneous reduced intake of arachidonate and increased intake of oleic acid (found in olive oil), gamma-linolenic acid (found in borage seed oil, hemp seed oil, black currant seed oil, and evening primrose oil), and eicosapentaenoic acid (EPA) and docosahexaenoic acid (DHA) (both from cold-water fish oil) helps reduce intracellular hypercalcinosis that promotes chronic HTN in addition to effecting beneficial changes in inflammatory, hemorrheologic, and coagulation indices.

- **Fish oil or combination fatty acid supplementation**: The cardioprotective benefits of fish oil are insufficiently represented by the minimal numerical reduction in blood pressure that is achieved with this intervention. Despite only lowering blood pressure by a few points (if at all), n-3 fatty acids are safer, less expensive, and more effective than statin and fibrate

---

[184] "Average daily consumption of high fructose corn syrup is about 50 grams per person in the United States. With respect to total mercury exposure, it may be necessary to account for this source of mercury in the diet of children and sensitive populations." Dufault R, LeBlanc B, Schnoll R, Cornett C, Schweitzer L, Wallinga D, Hightower J, Patrick L, Lukiw WJ. Mercury from chlor-alkali plants: measured concentrations in food product sugar. *Environ Health*. 2009 Jan 26;8:2. See also: "High fructose corn syrup has been shown to contain trace amounts of mercury as a result of some manufacturing processes, and its consumption can also lead to zinc loss." Dufault R, Schnoll R, Lukiw WJ, Leblanc B, Cornett C, Patrick L, Wallinga D, Gilbert SG, Crider R. Mercury exposure, nutritional deficiencies and metabolic disruptions may affect learning in children. *Behav Brain Funct*. 2009 Oct 27;5:44.

[185] "Because of the clinical presentation [severe hypertension in children] and the finding of elevated catecholamines, most of the patients were first studied for possible pheochromocytoma. Subsequently, elevated levels of mercury were found." Torres AD, Rai AN, Hardiek ML. Mercury intoxication and arterial hypertension: report of two patients and review of the literature. *Pediatrics*. 2000 Mar;105(3):E34

[186] Houston MC. The role of mercury and cadmium heavy metals in vascular disease, hypertension, coronary heart disease, and myocardial infarction. *Altern Ther Health Med*. 2007 Mar-Apr;13(2):S128-33

antihypercholesterolemic drug treatment for reducing total and cardiovascular mortality.[187] Thus, **combination fatty acid supplementation should be used for its pronounced cardioprotective benefits regardless of its modest ability to reduce elevated blood pressure.** The combination of EPA+DHA from fish oil and GLA from borage oil (or other source) in a ratio of approximately 2:1 (e.g., daily intake of 4 grams EPA+DHA along with 2 grams GLA) appears to provide the best cardioprotective benefit based on favorable changes in serum lipids, according to a speculative prospective clinical trial by Laidlaw and Holub.[188]

- **Correction of vitamin D deficiency**: Vitamin D3 (cholecalciferol)—with or without calcium supplementation—can reduce blood pressure in cholecalciferol-deficient hypertensive patients as effectively as the use of antihypertensive medication. As I have discussed in extensive detail elsewhere, a reasonable dose of vitamin D3 for adults is in the range of 4,000-10,000 IU per day, and doctors new to vitamin D therapy should read our clinical monograph published in 2004 and available on-line.[189] The most important drug interaction with vitamin D3 is seen with hydrochlorothiazide (HCTZ), a commonly-used antihypertensive diuretic that promotes hypercalcemia. Vitamin D supplementation in patients taking HCTZ must be implemented slowly, with professional supervision, and with laboratory monitoring of serum calcium at days 10, 30, and 60 following the use of combined cholecalciferol-HCTZ treatment. The goal of vitamin D3 supplementation is for serum 25-OH-vitamin D3 levels to reach the optimal range of 50-100 ng/ml, as shown in the diagram.

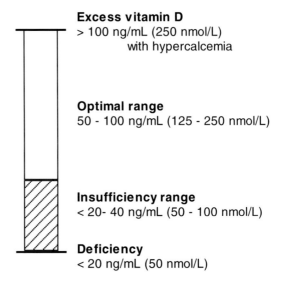

Excess vitamin D
> 100 ng/mL (250 nmol/L)
  with hypercalcemia

Optimal range
50 - 100 ng/mL (125 - 250 nmol/L)

Insufficiency range
< 20- 40 ng/mL (50 - 100 nmol/L)

Deficiency
< 20 ng/mL (50 nmol/L)

Interpretation of serum 25(OH) vitamin D levels. Modified from Vasquez et al, *Alternative Therapies in Health and Medicine* 2004 and Vasquez A. *Musculoskeletal Pain: Expanded Clinical Strategies* (Institute for Functional Medicine) 2008.

  - Controlled clinical trial: Effects of short-term calcium supplementation with or without vitamin D3 supplementation on blood pressure and parathyroid hormone levels in elderly women. (*Journal of Clinical Endocrinology and Metabolism*, Apr 2001): In an 8-week study of 148 elderly women (average age 74 years) with a 25-hydroxycholecalciferol (25OHD(3)) level <20 ng/ml (<50 nmol/l), **daily administration of 1200 mg calcium plus**

[187] "Compared with control groups, risk ratios for overall mortality were 0.87 for statins, 1.00 for fibrates, 0.84 for resins, 0.96 for niacin, 0.77 for n-3 fatty acids, and 0.97 for diet. Compared with control groups, risk ratios for cardiac mortality indicated benefit from statins (0.78), resins (0.70) and n-3 fatty acids (0.68)." Studer M, Briel M, Leimenstoll B, Glass TR, Bucher HC. Effect of different antilipidemic agents and diets on mortality: a systematic review. *Arch Intern Med.* 2005 Apr 11;165(7):725-30

[188] "A mixture of 4 g EPA+DHA and 2 g GLA favorably altered blood lipid and fatty acid profiles in healthy women. On the basis of calculated PROCAM values, the 4:2 group was estimated to have a 43% reduction in the 10-y risk of myocardial infarction." Laidlaw M, Holub BJ. Effects of supplementation with fish oil-derived n-3 fatty acids and gamma-linolenic acid on circulating plasma lipids and fatty acid profiles in women. *Am J Clin Nutr.* 2003 Jan;77(1):37-42

[189] **Vasquez A**, Manso G, Cannell J. The clinical importance of vitamin D (cholecalciferol): a paradigm shift with implications for all healthcare providers. *Altern Ther Health Med.* 2004 Sep-Oct;10(5):28-36 http://optimalhealthresearch.com/cholecalciferol.html

800 IU vitamin D3 (note: very low dose of vitamin D) was superior to 1200 mg calcium without vitamin D. Vitamin D plus calcium resulted in an increase in serum 25OHD(3) of 72%, a decrease in serum PTH of 17%, a decrease in heart rate of 5.4%, and a **decrease in blood pressure of approximately -13/-7 mm Hg**.[190] These results are clinically important because of the significant alleviation of hypertension that is noted, even despite the low dose of vitamin D3 that was used. Collateral benefits in muscle strength, mood, cognition, balance (and reduced falling), and enhanced resistance to infection are commonly noted with vitamin D3 supplementation; such benefits are not seen with antihypertensive drug use.

o Placebo-controlled clinical trial: Vitamin D improves endothelial function and reduces blood pressure in patients with Type 2 diabetes mellitus and low vitamin D levels (*Diabetic Medicine*, Mar 2008): In a double-blind, parallel group, placebo-controlled randomized trial, **a single dose of 100,000 IU vitamin D2 (note the use of ergocalciferol, the less effective form of vitamin D compared with cholecalciferol, vitamin D3)** or placebo was administered to patients with Type-2 diabetes mellitus (DM-2) who were vitamin D deficient with an average baseline 25-hydroxyvitamin D level <20 ng/ml (<50 nmol/l). Benefits of vitamin D supplementation included significantly improved flow mediated vasodilatation (FMD) of the brachial artery by 2.3% and **significantly decreased systolic blood pressure by -14 mmHg** compared with placebo.[191] Total reduction in blood pressure for vitamin D compared to placebo (per Table 2 of the original article) was -13.9/-4.5 mm Hg.

- **Exercise**: Current guidelines indicate that everyone should obtain 30-60 minutes of exercise 4-7 times per week unless specific contraindications exist. Patients with or at risk for CAD should receive baseline and stress/exercise ECG before commencing vigorous exercise; if ECG abnormalities are detected or if angina is reported, then stress echocardiography and/or perfusion scan should be considered.

- **Weight optimization**: All patients *and doctors* should maintain a healthy body weight. Canadian guidelines published in 2009 specify a body mass index 18.5-24.9 and waist circumference (<102 cm [40.2 inches] for men and <88 cm [34.6 inches] for women).[192] In most

> **Weight loss provides numerous psychosocial and physical benefits**
>
> "With a substantial weight loss of 35 kg and 42% loss of excessive weight, and correction of disturbed metabolic parameters, they significantly improved in general well-being, health distress, and perceived attractiveness, approaching halfway the values of a normal-weight reference group. ... In physical activity, they bypassed the reference group. Days of sick leave decreased to the level of the reference group. **Improvements in HRQL [health-related quality-of-life] paralleled the rate of weight loss.**"
>
> Mathus-Vliegen EM, de Weerd S, de Wit LT. Health-related quality-of-life in patients with morbid obesity after gastric banding for surgically induced weight loss. *Surgery*. 2004 May;135(5):489-97

---

[190] "A short-term supplementation with vitamin D(3) and calcium is more effective in reducing SBP than calcium alone. Inadequate vitamin D(3) and calcium intake could play a contributory role in the pathogenesis and progression of hypertension and cardiovascular disease in elderly women." Pfeifer M, Begerow B, Minne HW, Nachtigall D, Hansen C. Effects of a short-term vitamin D(3) and calcium supplementation on blood pressure and parathyroid hormone levels in elderly women. *J Clin Endocrinol Metab*. 2001 Apr;86(4):1633-7

[191] Sugden JA, Davies JI, Witham MD, Morris AD, Struthers AD. Vitamin D improves endothelial function in patients with Type 2 diabetes mellitus and low vitamin D levels. *Diabet Med*. 2008 Mar;25(3):320-5

[192] Khan NA, Hemmelgarn B, Herman RJ, Bell CM, Mahon JL, Leiter LA, Rabkin SW, Hill MD, Padwal R, Touyz RM, Larochelle P, Feldman RD, Schiffrin EL, Campbell NR, Moe G, Prasad R, Arnold MO, Campbell TS, Milot A, Stone JA, Jones C, Ogilvie RI, Hamet P, Fodor G, Carruthers G, Burns KD, Ruzicka M, DeChamplain J, Pylypchuk G, Petrella R, Boulanger JM, Trudeau L, Hegele RA, Woo V, McFarlane P, Vallée M, Howlett J,

patients and clinical situations, body weight and body mass can be used as an indicator of compliance with a health-promoting diet and plan of regular *sufficiently intense* exercise. Exercise sufficiency can be assessed by the ability of the activity to produce mild breathlessness, diaphoresis, and changes in or favorable maintenance of body composition and optimal weight.

- **Coenzyme Q-10 (CoQ-10 or CoQ10) with doses ranging from 100-300 mg per day**: Average dietary intake of CoQ-10 is 2-5 mg/d. CoQ-10 is made endogenously; however, some patients—particularly those with migraines, asthma, hypertension, allergies, heart failure and idiopathic dilated cardiomyopathy—may have an inborn or acquired error of metabolism that prevents them from making sufficient amounts of this vitally important substance. Hypertensive patients generally have lower serum CoQ-10 levels than normotensive persons. **Typical blood levels of CoQ-10 range from 0.7-1 mcg/ml; however clinical benefit in CVD may require serum levels of 2-3 and up to 4 mcg/ml to attain maximal clinical benefit.**[193] Testing of serum CoQ-10 levels is not necessary before starting treatment; however, patients who do not benefit as expected should have their CoQ-10 levels measured and supplementation increased to attain optimal serum levels before deciding that treatment is inefficacious. While clinical benefit may occur within the first week of supplementation, maximal improvement generally takes 4-8 weeks in order to obtain tissue saturation and beneficial changes in cell physiology. CoQ-10 is clearly one of the most powerful and broadly-beneficial nutritional supplements on the nutrition-healthcare market; research literature shows clinically meaningful benefit of CoQ-10 supplementation in patients with myocardial infarction, HTN, heart failure, renal failure, allergies, asthma, migraine, Parkinson's disease, and chronic viral infections such as HIV. CoQ-10 has generally been produced and studied in its oxidized form as "ubiquinone" however more current research and clinical trends suggest that the reduced form "ubiquinol" is better absorbed (perhaps 3x); a small clinical trial (n=7) showed impressive improvements in serum CoQ10 and clinical status followed by ubiquinol treatment compared to ubiquinone treatment in CHF patients with malabsorption-inducing bowel wall edema.[194] Whether ubiquinol has clinical advantage over ubiquinone to such an extent that the higher cost is justified in other clinical scenarios—especially those which are not associated with malabsorption and/or the bowel wall edema seen in severe heart failure—remains to be determined. **In hypertensive patients, CoQ-10 doses of 60-120 mg/d can typically lower BP by about -15/-9 mm Hg.** CoQ-10 can be safely used with antihypertensive medications and is generally safer than all antihypertensive medications. CoQ-10 may rarely interfere with coumadin/warfarin action in some patients; a cross-over study of 24 patients on chronic warfarin showed that neither CoQ-10 nor *Ginkgo biloba* affected coagulation indices nor warfarin dosage.[195] More frequent monitoring of INR is

Bacon SL, Lindsay P, Gilbert RE, Lewanczuk RZ, Tobe S; Canadian Hypertension Education Program. The 2009 Canadian Hypertension Education Program recommendations for the management of hypertension: Part 2—therapy. *Can J Cardiol.* 2009 May;25(5):287-98

[193] Kumar A, Kaur H, Devi P, Mohan V. Role of coenzyme Q10 (CoQ10) in cardiac disease, hypertension and Meniere-like syndrome. *Pharmacol Ther.* 2009 Dec;124(3):259-68

[194] "Patients with CHF, NYHA class IV, often fail to achieve adequate plasma CoQ10 levels on supplemental ubiquinone at dosages up to 900 mg/day. These patients often have plasma total CoQ10 levels of less than 2.5 microg/ml and have limited clinical improvement. It is postulated that the intestinal edema in these critically ill patients may impair CoQ10 absorption. ... Ubiquinol has dramatically improved absorption in patients with severe heart failure and the improvement in plasma CoQ10 levels is correlated with both clinical improvement and improvement in measurement of left ventricular function." Langsjoen PH, Langsjoen AM. Supplemental ubiquinol in patients with advanced congestive heart failure. *Biofactors.* 2008;32(1-4):119-28

[195] "The study indicated that Coenzyme Q10 and Ginkgo biloba do not influence the clinical effect of warfarin." Engelsen J, Nielsen JD, Hansen KF. [Effect of Coenzyme Q10 and Ginkgo biloba on warfarin dosage in patients on long-term warfarin treatment. A randomized, double-blind, placebo-controlled cross-over trial]. [Article in Danish] *Ugeskr Laeger.* 2003 Apr 28;165(18):1868-71. See also Engelsen J, Dalsgaard NJ, Winther K. The healthcare products coenzyme Q10 and ginko biloba do not interact with warfarin. Abstracdt P796. *Thrombosis and Haemostasis.* 2001: July Presented at Eighteenth Congress of the International Society on Thrombosis and Haemostasis, July 6-12, 2001 in Paris, France.

routinely advised following any change in diet or medication. CoQ-10 supplementation provides numerous collateral benefits; research literature shows clinically meaningful benefit of CoQ-10 supplementation in patients with myocardial infarction, HTN, heart failure, renal failure, allergies, asthma, migraine, gingivitis, male infertility/subfertility, Parkinson's disease, and chronic viral infections.

In a personal communication by email in which the current author corresponded with world-renowned CoQ-10 researcher Peter Langsjoen MD FACC (citations[196,197]) about CoQ-10's mechanism of action in the treatment of hypertension, the following reply was received, quoted here with permission:

Personal communication from Peter H. Langsjoen, MD, FACC
January 25, 2011
Dear Alex, In regards to the antihypertensive effect of coenzyme Q10, I do have a couple of thoughts. The first theory is that coenzyme Q10 (CoQ10) has some influence on endothelial function, which may thereby have some benefit in hypertension. There is one thing that is quite clear, and that is that CoQ10 cannot have any direct vasodilator function because we never see a decrease in blood pressure in patients who already have low-normal blood pressures. My own theory on this subject is that the decrease in blood pressure from CoQ10 supplementation is a secondary phenomenon. We have observed that patients with established hypertension quite frequently have underlying diastolic dysfunction and it is clear that CoQ10 supplementation improves diastolic function because this is in large part an active process requiring a large amount of ATP to re-establish calcium gradients such that the actin and myosin fibrils can uncouple. When diastolic function improves, there is a secondary gradual decrease in hypertension. The theory is that the diastolic dysfunction actually occurs first as a result of CoQ10 decrease, which occurs beginning in early-middle age and can certainly be aggravated by a variety of factors including stress and poor diet. One of the first adaptive responses that we have from impairment in the filling phase, or diastole phase, of the cardiac cycle is an increase in catecholamines, and these patients almost always have a tendency for an increase in both blood pressure and heart rate. It is my theory that when we improve the diastolic dysfunction, the adaptive high catecholamine state gradually subsides, and with this, there is frequently a decrease in blood pressure and a decreased need for antihypertensive medication. … Additional correspondence February 17, 2011: "QH (ubiquinol) is 2-3x better absorbed than QX (ubiquinone). Some promotional materials have exaggerated this. Also, since QX is promptly reduced to QH after absorption, there is no difference in antioxidant effect of supplemental QH vs QX. The only difference is the improved absorption." … My very best regards, Peter Peter H. Langsjoen, MD, FACC

---

[196] Langsjoen PH, Langsjoen AM. Supplemental ubiquinol in patients with advanced congestive heart failure. *Biofactors*. 2008;32(1-4):119-28

[197] Langsjoen P, Langsjoen P, Willis R, Folkers K. Treatment of essential hypertension with coenzyme Q10. *Mol Aspects Med*. 1994;15 Suppl:S265-72

CoQ-10's safety and efficacy in the treatment of hypertension are very well established, and the mechanism(s) of action are manifold rather than singular. CoQ-10 has been shown to improve glycemic control, reduce serum insulin levels, promote beneficial redistribution of adipose, provide anti-inflammatory and anti-allergy benefits, and to improve mitochondrial bioenergetics. Peer-reviewed articles on the use of CoQ-10 for cardiovascular health are reviewed and summarized in the sections that follow.

o Correlational study: CoQ-10 is an independent predictor of mortality in chronic heart failure (*Journal of the American College of Cardiology*, Oct 2008): Plasma samples from 236 patients admitted to the hospital with heart failure were assayed for LDL and total cholesterol, and total CoQ-10. "CONCLUSIONS: Plasma CoQ-10 concentration was an independent predictor of mortality in this cohort. The **CoQ-10 deficiency might be detrimental to the long-term prognosis of CHF [chronic heart failure],** and there is a rationale for controlled intervention studies with CoQ-10."[198]

o Review: Role of coenzyme Q10 (CoQ10) in cardiac disease, hypertension and Meniere-like syndrome (*Pharmacology and Therapeutics*, Dec 2009): In this excellent review that covers the role of CoQ-10 in the treatment of cardiovascular diseases—heart failure, HTN, myocardial infarction, arrhythmia—and Meniere syndrome and hearing loss, Kumar et al[199] review the literature to conclude that CoQ-10 provides major clinical benefit in all of these conditions and without adverse effects. Cardioprotective properties of CoQ-10 include its role as an antioxidant, vasodilator, and membrane stabilizer in addition to its ability to decrease blood viscosity, proinflammatory cytokines, endothelial dysfunction, insulin resistance, and to promote proper diastolic and systolic function of the myocardium. Additional functions of CoQ-10 specific to its benefit in HTN appear related to the ability of CoQ-10 to antagonize aldosterone and/or angiotensin; if confirmed, these functions would support the concept that CoQ10 functions in part like an aldosterone antagonist (such as spironolactone) and/or an angiotensin 2 receptor blocker (such as losartan). **Typical blood pressure reduction with use of CoQ10 can be as high as -18/-11 mm Hg,** depending on dose, attained serum levels; other common nutritional deficiencies such as magnesium, potassium, and vitamin D can also be addressed to improve efficacy. Maximal improvement might take 4-8 weeks; however, some patients will respond more quickly—within the first week—and this observation underscores the importance of frequent BP monitoring and the need to adjust doses of antihypertensive drugs as needed to avoid hypotension and its complications such as syncope.

o Randomized, double-blind, placebo-controlled trial of coenzyme Q10 in isolated systolic hypertension (*Southern Medical Journal*, Nov 2001): Twice daily administration of 60 mg of oral CoQ-10 was given to 46 men and 37 women with isolated systolic hypertension in a 12-week randomized, double-blind, placebo-controlled trial. "**RESULTS: The mean reduction in systolic blood pressure of the CoQ-treated group was 17.8 mm Hg.** None of the patients exhibited orthostatic blood pressure changes. CONCLUSIONS: Our

---

[198] Molyneux SL, Florkowski CM, George PM, Pilbrow AP, Frampton CM, Lever M, Richards AM. Coenzyme Q10: an independent predictor of mortality in chronic heart failure. *J Am Coll Cardiol*. 2008 Oct 28;52(18):1435-41

[199] Kumar A, Kaur H, Devi P, Mohan V. Role of coenzyme Q10 (CoQ10) in cardiac disease, hypertension and Meniere -like syndrome. *Pharmacol Ther*. 2009 Dec;124(3):259-68

results suggest CoQ may be safely offered to hypertensive patients as an alternative treatment option."[200]

o Open clinical trial: Coenzyme Q-10 in essential hypertension (*Molecular Aspects of Medicine*, 1994): In this open trial with no comparative placebo group, 26 patients with essential hypertension received oral CoQ10 50 mg twice daily for 10 weeks.[201] Results of this study showed the following:
  - Systolic BP decreased from 164.5 to 146.7 mmHg (reduction of -17.8 mmHg).
  - Diastolic BP decreased from 98.1 to 86.1 mmHg (reduction of -12 mmHg).
  - Plasma CoQ-10 values increased from 0.64 mcg/ml to 1.61 mcg/ml. Of particular note is that eight of 26 patients (30%) had baseline values of plasma CoQ-10 that were subnormal before treatment and which normalized with supplementation.
  - Serum total cholesterol decreased from 222.9 mg/dl to 213.3 mg/dl.
  - Serum HDL cholesterol increased slightly from 41.1 mg/dl to 43.1 mg/dl.
  - Plasma renin activity, urinary aldosterone, serum and urinary sodium and potassium, plasma endothelin, electrocardiographic and echocardiographic findings and did not change.
  - In a subgroup of 5 patients tested, peripheral vascular resistances were 2,283 dyne·s·cm−5 before treatment and 1,627 dyne·s·cm−5 after treatment, thus indicating a clear reduction in peripheral resistance by CoQ-10. The authors concluded that the antihypertensive effect of CoQ-10 is probably mediated by reduction in peripheral resistance.

These anti-hypertensive results, the collateral benefits, and the absence of adverse effects make CoQ-10 appear superior to drug treatment for the treatment of chronic HTN.

o Clinical trial with water-soluble CoQ-10: Effect of hydrosoluble coenzyme Q10 on blood pressures and insulin resistance in hypertensive patients with coronary artery disease (*Journal of Human Hypertension*, Mar 1999): In this randomized double-blind placebo-controlled trial among patients receiving antihypertensive medication and with coronary artery disease (n=59: 30 in treatment group, 29 in placebo group), patients received oral coenzyme Q10 (60 mg twice daily) for 8 weeks. **In the coenzyme Q10 group, beneficial reductions were noted in systolic and diastolic blood pressures (average 168/106 reduced to 152/97 [-16/-9] mm Hg),** heart rate, **waist–hip ratio**, fasting and 2-h plasma insulin and glucose levels, triglyceride levels and angina; CoQ-10 supplementation raised HDL-cholesterol. The authors concluded, "These findings indicate that treatment with coenzyme Q10 decreases blood pressure possibly by decreasing oxidative stress and insulin response in patients with known hypertension receiving conventional antihypertensive drugs."[202]

o Open trial using average dose of CoQ-10 225 mg/d for the treatment of essential hypertension (*Molecular Aspects of Medicine*, 1994): This study was one of the first to use dosage adjustments to **attain serum CoQ10 levels of at least 2 mcg/ml**. "A total of 109

[200] Burke BE, Neuenschwander R, Olson RD. Randomized, double-blind, placebo-controlled trial of coenzyme Q10 in isolated systolic hypertension. *South Med J*. 2001 Nov;94(11):1112-7

[201] Digiesi V, Cantini F, Oradei A, Bisi G, Guarino GC, Brocchi A, Bellandi F, Mancini M, Littarru GP. Coenzyme Q10 in essential hypertension. *Mol Aspects Med*. 1994;15 Suppl:s257-63

[202] Singh RB, Niaz MA, Rastogi SS, Shukla PK, Thakur AS. Effect of hydrosoluble coenzyme Q10 on blood pressures and insulin resistance in hypertensive patients with coronary artery disease. *J Hum Hypertens*. 1999 Mar;13(3):203-8

patients with symptomatic essential hypertension presenting to a private cardiology practice were observed after the addition of CoQ10 (average dose, 225 mg/day by mouth) to their existing antihypertensive drug regimen. … A definite and gradual improvement in functional status was observed with the **concomitant need to gradually decrease antihypertensive drug therapy within the first one to six months**. Thereafter, clinical status and cardiovascular drug requirements stabilized with a **significantly improved systolic and diastolic blood pressure**. Overall New York Heart Association (NYHA) functional class improved from a mean of 2.40 to 1.36

NYHA Stages of Heart Failure
1. <u>Class 1</u>: Comfortable at all times. No limitation of physical activity. Ordinary activity does not cause undue fatigue, palpitation, dyspnea or anginal pain.
2. <u>Class 2</u>: Comfortable at rest. Slight limitation of physical activity. Ordinary activity causes fatigue, palpitation, dyspnea, or anginal pain.
3. <u>Class 3</u>: Comfortable at rest. Marked limitation of physical activity. Less than ordinary activity causes fatigue, palpitation, dyspnea or anginal pain.
4. <u>Class 4</u>: Symptomatic at rest. Cannot perform any physical activity without progressive discomfort.
American Heart Association. 1994 Revisions to Classification of Functional Capacity and Objective Assessment of Patients With Diseases of the Heart. http://www.americanheart.org Accessed Nov 2010.

(P < 0.001) and 51% of patients came completely off of between one and three antihypertensive drugs at an average of 4.4 months after starting CoQ10. … In the 9.4% of patients with echocardiograms both before and during treatment, we observed a highly significant improvement in left ventricular wall thickness and diastolic function."[203]

- **<u>Potassium supplementation, preferably via fruits, vegetables, and their juices</u>**: Antihypertensive mechanisms of potassium include vasodilator activity, diuretic and naturietic effects, and suppression of renin, angiotensin, and adrenergic tone.[204] In February 2004, the Institute of Medicine (IOM) set the Adequate Intake of potassium for adults at 4.7 grams a day—more than double previous recommendations; more than 90% of American adults do not meet these recommendations. If 90% of the population is not meeting recommended intakes of potassium, and these recommendations from the IOM come after an extensive review of the scientific literature, then potassium assessment and supplementation should be routine components of patient care; furthermore, this shows to the inadequacy of current laboratory assessments for evaluating potassium status and potassium balance.

An irony exists in the observations that 1) metabolic syndrome is a very common lethal condition with a hypertensive component, and 2) thiazide diuretics are first-line treatment for most cases of hypertension, and 3) thiazide diuretics exacerbate many CVD-inducing aspects of the metabolic syndrome, such as insulin resistance and dyslipidemia. A 2007 experimental study published in Journal of the American Society of Nephrology showed that potassium supplementation—alone or in combination with treatment to reduce fructose-induced hyperuricemia—can ameliorate exacerbation of metabolic syndrome caused by thiazide diuretics.[205] This is yet another example of nutritional intervention being used to

[203] Langsjoen P, Langsjoen P, Willis R, Folkers K. Treatment of essential hypertension with coenzyme Q10. *Mol Aspects Med.* 1994;15 Suppl:S265-72
[204] Patki PS, Singh J, Gokhale SV, Bulakh PM, Shrotri DS, Patwardhan B. Efficacy of potassium and magnesium in essential hypertension: a double-blind, placebo controlled, crossover study. *BMJ.* 1990 Sep 15;301(6751):521-3
[205] Reungjui S, Roncal CA, Mu W, Srinivas TR, Sirivongs D, Johnson RJ, Nakagawa T. Thiazide diuretics exacerbate fructose-induced metabolic syndrome. *J Am Soc Nephrol.* 2007 Oct;18(10):2724-31 http://jasn.asnjournals.org/content/18/10/2724.full.pdf

treat the primary disease as well as alleviate the secondary metabolic disturbances caused by the current drug-of-choice.

True to what is to be expected from studies conducted by researchers with little or no previous training in clinical nutrition, most studies of potassium supplementation for the treatment of HTN have been methodologically flawed due to ❶ utilization of potassium in the form of potassium chloride (KCl), ❷ failure to simultaneously reduce intake of dietary NaCl so as to normalize the K:Na ratio and ❸ also reduce total Cl intake; furthermore, ❹ the notion that "potassium intake from foods is associated with reduced blood pressure and that potassium supplementation (e.g., KCl) could be equivalent to potassium intake from food" is a *colossal failure* to appreciate the manifold cardioprotective benefits of the phytonutrients *consumed along with potassium* when obtained from its richest natural food sources—fruits, vegetables, nuts, seeds, berries. Furthermore, reverence for KCl reveals ignorance of the cardiovasculotoxic and acidogenic effects of chloride.

Respective amounts of potassium per serving of food or juice (1 cup = 8 fluid ounces =240 milliliters) are provided in the table below.

> ## The importance of potassium
> "Adults should consume at least 4.7 grams of potassium per day to lower blood pressure, blunt the effects of salt, and reduce the risk of kidney stones and bone loss. However, most American women 31 to 50 years old consume no more than half of the recommended amount of potassium, and men's intake is only moderately higher. There was no evidence of chronic excess intakes of potassium in apparently health individuals and thus no UL [upper limit of intake] was established."
>
> Food and Nutrition Board of the Institute of Medicine of the National Academies. "Dietary Reference Intakes: Water, Potassium, Sodium, Chloride, and Sulfate." Released: February 11, 2004
> http://www.iom.edu/Reports/2004/Dietary-Reference-Intakes-Water-Potassium-Sodium-Chloride-and-Sulfate.aspx

Potassium content of common foods

Food serving	*Potassium in mg (sodium as available)*
One papaya	780
One cup of mixed vegetable juice	740 (35 mg sodium, up to 630 mg sodium)
One cup of prune juice	700
One cup of carrot juice	520 (160 mg sodium)
One cup plain low-fat yogurt	510 (150 mg sodium)
One cup of cantaloupe	490
One cup of orange juice	470
One small banana	465
One cup of honeydew melon	460
One-third cup of raisins	365
One cup of carrot-orange juice	360 (35 mg sodium)
One medium mango	320
One medium kiwi	250
One small orange	240
One medium pear	210

Note again that the physiologic effect of potassium is influenced by the potassium:sodium ratio (sodium reduces effectiveness and retention of potassium), potassium:chloride ratio (chloride reduces effectiveness and retention of potassium), and the overall pH acid-base balance of the human host (i.e., metabolic acidosis reduces effectiveness and retention of potassium, while an alkaline state improves retention and effectiveness of potassium). Importantly, magnesium status is an important positive-direct determinant of potassium status, particularly in patients with recalcitrant hypokalemia and/or hyperaldosteronism.[206]

o   Double-blind, placebo controlled, crossover study: Efficacy of potassium and magnesium in essential hypertension (*British Medical Journal*, Sep 1990): The authors conducted a double-blind randomized placebo-controlled crossover trial of 32 weeks' duration among 37 adults with mild hypertension (diastolic blood pressure less than 110 mm Hg); patients received either placebo or potassium 60 mmol/day (approximately 2,250 mg/d) alone or in combination with magnesium 20 mmol/day (approximately 480 mg/d) in a crossover design without other intervention. More specifically, patients were treated with either placebo, K alone, or K+Mg for 8 weeks each with a 2-week washout period between treatments. While blood pressure in the placebo group did not change after 8 weeks of treatment, BP in the K group dropped from 157/101 to 143/85 (drop of **-14/-16 mm Hg**) and from 154/99 to 146/88 (drop of -8/-11) in the K+Mg group. The reduction in serum cholesterol was from the initial value of 7.5 mmol/l (290 mg/dL) to 6.0 mmol/l (232 mg/dL) and 6.1 mmol/l (235 mg/dL) in the K and K+Mg groups, respectively. The authors wrote, "RESULTS: **Potassium alone or in combination with magnesium produced a significant reduction in systolic and diastolic blood pressures** (p less than 0.001) and a **significant reduction in serum cholesterol concentration** (p less than 0.05); other biochemical variables did not change. Magnesium did not have an additional effect. ... The drug was well tolerated and compliance was satisfactory. CONCLUSION-- Potassium 60 mmol/day lowers arterial blood pressure in patients with mild hypertension. Giving magnesium as well has no added advantage."[207] While the reduction in blood pressure by potassium is to be expected, two surprising findings in this study are 1) the reduction in serum cholesterol and 2) the lack of additive benefit by the magnesium supplementation, particularly when other studies have shown antihypertensive benefit of magnesium when used alone. In this study, both the potassium and the magnesium were provided in a liquid form as KCl and MgCl, respectively; better sources would have been the citrate or malate chelates for alkalinization and enhanced bioavailability. Attentive readers might have also noted one additional curious finding from this study: none of the 37 patients were reported to have developed diarrhea or loose stools from the magnesium 480 mg/d; this may or may not be significant to the credibility of the study; in clinical practice, some patients will report loose stools with magnesium doses as low as 200 mg per day.

o   Meta-analysis: Potassium supplementation for the management of primary hypertension in adults (*Cochrane Database of Systematic Reviews*, Jul 2006): Using reasonable inclusion/exclusion criteria, the authors of this meta-analysis found that "Six RCT's

---

[206] "Magnesium deficiency is frequently associated with hypokalemia. Concomitant magnesium deficiency aggravates hypokalemia and renders it refractory to treatment by potassium. Herein is reviewed literature suggesting that magnesium deficiency exacerbates potassium wasting by increasing distal potassium secretion. A decrease in intracellular magnesium, caused by magnesium deficiency, releases the magnesium-mediated inhibition of ROMK channels and increases potassium secretion. Magnesium deficiency alone, however, does not necessarily cause hypokalemia. An increase in distal sodium delivery or elevated aldosterone levels may be required for exacerbating potassium wasting in magnesium deficiency." Huang CL, Kuo E. Mechanism of hypokalemia in magnesium deficiency. *J Am Soc Nephrol*. 2007 Oct;18(10):2649-52

[207] Patki PS, Singh J, Gokhale SV, Bulakh PM, Shrotri DS, Patwardhan B. Efficacy of potassium and magnesium in essential hypertension: a double-blind, placebo controlled, crossover study. *BMJ*. 1990 Sep 15;301(6751):521-3

(n=483), with eight to 16 weeks follow-up, met our inclusion criteria. Meta-analysis of five trials (n=425) with adequate data indicated that potassium supplementation compared to control resulted in a large but statistically non-significant reductions in **SBP** (mean difference: **-11.2**, 95% CI: -25.2 to 2.7) and **DBP** (mean difference: **-5.0**, 95% CI: -12.5 to 2.4)."[208] The conclusion that potassium supplementation resulted in "large but statistically non-significant reductions" would appear to be an example of *statistical methodology* trumping *clinical practicality* insofar as a reduction of -11/-5 mm Hg is indeed clinically significant and also meets criteria for drug efficacy/approval per the US FDA (assuming that the difference is placebo subtracted). The authors reviewed "two high quality trials (n=138)" showing blood pressure reductions of **-7.1/-5.5** mm Hg but again concluded that these findings represented "non-significant reductions in blood pressure." Given the safety and *essentiality* of potassium, its inadequate consumption from Westernized diets, its facilitated urinary excretion due to consumption of salt/sugar/caffeine/alcohol and many diuretic drugs, and its demonstrated efficacy, clinicians are justified in utilizing potassium in the treatment of HTN especially when sourced from *natural whole foods* and fruit/vegetable juices; indeed, a recent clinical trial[209] utilizing the DASH diet (described previously) in all subjects showed that blood pressure reductions were enhanced among the subset of subjects consuming 8-16 ounces of vegetable juice daily, even when the sodium:potassium ratio was nonphysiologic at >1 since 8 ounces of the juice contained 480 mg of sodium and 470 mg of potassium.

o Randomized trial with 1-year follow-up and a title that says it all: Increasing the dietary potassium intake reduces the need for antihypertensive medication (*Annals of Internal Medicine*, Nov 1991): The stated purpose of this study[210] was "To determine whether an increase in dietary potassium intake from natural foods reduces the need for antihypertensive medication in patients with essential hypertension." Forty-seven patients with medication-controlled hypertension completed one year of dietary treatment (or control nonintervention) and follow-up; the dietary intervention focused on increasing intake of potassium-rich foods, with compliance monitored by 3-day food records and by measuring 24-hour urinary potassium excretion. Results showed the following: "After 1 year, the average drug consumption (number of pills per day) relative to that at baseline was 24% in group 1 (potassium-rich diet) and 60% in group 2 (control diet) (P less than 0.001). By the end of the study, blood pressure could be controlled using less than 50% of the initial therapy in 81% of the patients in group 1 compared with 29% of the patients in group 2 (P = 0.001). Patients in group 1 ended the study with a lower number of reported symptoms compared with patients in the control group (P less than 0.001). CONCLUSION: Increasing the dietary potassium intake from natural foods is a feasible and effective measure to reduce antihypertensive drug treatment." With powerful results such as these, world-wise clinicians will not be surprised that US National Heart, Lung, and Blood Institute (NHLBI)'s endorsed dietary program "Stay

---

[208] Dickinson HO, Nicolson DJ, Campbell F, Beyer FR, Mason J. Potassium supplementation for the management of primary hypertension in adults. *Cochrane Database Syst Rev*. 2006 Jul 19;3:CD004641

[209] Shenoy SF, Kazaks AG, Holt RR, Chen HJ, Winters BL, Khoo CS, Poston WS, Haddock CK, Reeves RS, Foreyt JP, Gershwin ME, Keen CL. The use of a commercial vegetable juice as a practical means to increase vegetable intake: a randomized controlled trial. *Nutr J*. 2010 Sep 17;9:38

[210] Siani A, Strazzullo P, Giacco A, Pacioni D, Celentano E, Mancini M. Increasing the dietary potassium intake reduces the need for antihypertensive medication. *Ann Intern Med*. 1991 Nov 15;115(10):753-9

Young at Heart: Cooking the Heart-Healthy Way"[211] is notably low in potassium; this will be reviewed in a section toward the end of this chapter.

- **Magnesium (Mg) dosed at 600 mg per day or to bowel tolerance**: Given the safety and low cost of magnesium, along with the high prevalence of magnesium deficiency in the general population, routine oral magnesium supplementation is warranted. The standard replacement dose for oral magnesium supplementation is 600 mg per day; some patients may tolerate less or need more, with a typical range of 200-1,800 mg/d being used in clinical practice. Insufficient doses are inefficacious, while excess doses are generally benign (causing only transient loose stools). Renal insufficiency and/or treatment with the magnesium-retaining diuretic spironolactone indicate the need for cautious dosing and more frequent clinical and laboratory monitoring. Measurement of *intracellular* Mg levels in erythrocytes or leukocytes is more accurate than is measurement of *serum* Mg levels.

  o Clinical trial: Oral magnesium supplementation reduces ambulatory blood pressure in patients with mild hypertension (*American Journal of Hypertension*, Oct 2009): For a 12-week period, 48 patients with mild uncomplicated hypertension were assigned either to treatment with 600 mg (25 mmol) of magnesium pidolate orally twice a day for 12 weeks + lifestyle recommendations (n=24) or to treatment with lifestyle recommendations only. "RESULTS: In the Mg(2+) supplementation group, **small but significant reductions in mean 24-h systolic and diastolic BP levels were observed**, in contrast to control group (-**5.6** vs. -1.3 mm Hg, and **-2.8** vs. -1 mm Hg, respectively). These effects of Mg(2+) supplementation were consistent in both daytime and night-time periods. Serum Mg(2+) levels and urinary Mg(2+) excretion were significantly increased in the intervention group. Intracellular Mg(2+) and K(+) levels were also increased, while intracellular Ca(2+) and Na(+) levels were decreased in the intervention group. None of the intracellular ions were significantly changed in the control group. CONCLUSION: This study suggests that oral Mg(2+) supplementation is associated with small but consistent ambulatory BP reduction in patients with mild hypertension."[212] Readers should note that magnesium supplementation in this study was shown to reduce intracellular calcium and to increase intracellular potassium simultaneously with the reduction in BP. These findings are consistent with my proposal for treatment of intracellular hypercalcinosis[213] published in 2006 and with the fact that magnesium sufficiency is mandatory for the intracellular uptake of potassium; **any patient with chronic hypokalemia**

> **Key concept: Subphysiologic doses of nutrients are generally subtherapeutic**
>
> In order to obtain a physiologic effect and an optimal clinical benefit from nutritional supplementation, the supplementation must be of adequate *duration*, *dose*, and *bioavailability* to optimally supply cellular processes. *Cofactors*, *co-nutrients*, and the *proper biochemical milieu* (pH in particular) are also required for optimal effectiveness of the nutritional intervention.
>
> Vasquez A. **Subphysiologic doses of vitamin D are subtherapeutic**: comment on the study by The Record Trial Group. *The Lancet*. Published online May 6, 2005 http://optimalhealthresearch.com/lancet

[211] US National Heart, Lung, and Blood Institute (NHLBI). Stay Young at Heart: Cooking the Heart-Healthy Way. http://www.nhlbi.nih.gov/health/public/heart/other/syah/index.htm Accessed December 2009 and re-reviewed in November 2010.
[212] Hatzistavri LS, Sarafidis PA, Georgianos PI, Tziolas IM, Aroditis CP, Zebekakis PE, Pikilidou MI, Lasaridis AN. Oral magnesium supplementation reduces ambulatory blood pressure in patients with mild hypertension. *Am J Hypertens*. 2009 Oct;22(10):1070-5
[213] **Vasquez A**. Intracellular Hypercalcinosis: A Functional Nutritional Disorder with Implications Ranging from Myofascial Trigger Points to Affective Disorders, Hypertension, and Cancer. *Naturopathy Digest* 2006 Previously published in-print and on-line at http://www.naturopathydigest.com/archives/2006/sep/vasquez.php and included at the end of this chapter.

should be tested and/or treated for magnesium insufficiency. *How do we translate "600 mg (25 mmol) of magnesium pidolate orally twice a day" into an understanding of the clinical dosage which is generally expressed in milligrams of elemental Mg?* The physiologic action of magnesium supplements depends upon their content of magnesium ion. Magnesium pidolate is the magnesium salt of pidolic acid (pyroglutamic acid), which is only 8.7% Mg by weight. Thus, "600 mg (25 mmol) of magnesium pidolate orally twice a day" provides 1,200 mg of magnesium pidolate which provides 8.7% of 600 mg of elemental magnesium, which is only 104 mg of elemental Mg per day. Given that the standard replacement dose for Mg is 600 mg per day of elemental Mg, we see that the dose used in this study was suboptimally therapeutic (only 17% of the standard dose of Mg) and that therefore the clinical results are less impressive than those which would have been obtained if the study subjects had used a more substantial amount of Mg.

- **Acetyl-L-carnitine and L-carnitine**: Acetyl-L-carnitine (ALC) first made its impression on clinicians when it was found to be effective treatment for Alzheimer's disease; later research found application for this nutrient in the treatment of hepatic coma, Peyronie's disease, male sexual dysfunction, various types of peripheral neuropathy, dysthymia, fibromyalgia, and various types of physical and mental fatigue. Common therapeutic doses are 1,500-3,000 mg per day of either or both of ALC and/or L-carnitine, taken orally, between meals; clinicians should appreciate that amino acid therapy is generally administered between meals to avoid problems arising from competitive blockade among amino acids as they are absorbed/utilized. L-carnitine and ALC can be administered together; use of one does not necessarily preclude use of the other. For example in the study by Cavallini et al[214] among aging men, L-carnitine 2 g/day plus acetyl-L-carnitine 2 g/day proved significantly more effective than testosterone in improving nocturnal penile tumescence and International Index of Erectile Function score.

  o <u>Review: Carnitine insufficiency caused by aging and overnutrition compromises mitochondrial performance and metabolic control</u> (*Journal of Biological Chemistry*, Jun 2009): The authors wrote, "...we hypothesized that **carnitine insufficiency might contribute to mitochondrial dysfunction and obesity-related impairments in glucose tolerance**. Consistent with this prediction, whole body carnitine diminution was identified as a common feature of insulin resistant states such as advanced age, genetic diabetes and diet-induced obesity."[215] This impressive study documented that carnitine deficiency is noted in patients with obesity and insulin resistance; thus, carnitine supplementation—either as L-carnitine or acetyl-L-carnitine, or a combination of the two—appears warranted in such groups simply from the standpoint of correcting this nutrient deficiency/insufficiency.

  o <u>Clinical trial: Ameliorating hypertension and insulin resistance in subjects at increased cardiovascular risk. Effects of acetyl-L-carnitine therapy</u> (*Hypertension*, Sep 2009): In a previous trial, acetyl-L-carnitine infusion acutely ameliorated insulin resistance in type-2 diabetics. In this sequential off-on-off pilot study, the authors prospectively evaluated the

---

[214] Cavallini G, Caracciolo S, Vitali G, Modenini F, Biagiotti G. Carnitine versus androgen administration in the treatment of sexual dysfunction, depressed mood, and fatigue associated with male aging. *Urology*. 2004 Apr;63(4):641-6

[215] Noland RC, Koves TR, Seiler SE, Lum H, Lust RM, Ilkayeva O, Stevens R, Hegardt FG, Muoio DM. Carnitine Insufficiency Caused by Aging and Overnutrition Compromises Mitochondrial Performance and Metabolic Control. *J Biol Chem*. 2009 Jun 24. [Epub ahead of print]

effects of 24-week oral acetyl-L-carnitine (1 g twice daily) therapy on the glucose disposal rate (GDR), assessed by hyperinsulinemic euglycemic clamps, and components of the metabolic syndrome in nondiabetic subjects at increased cardiovascular risk. "Acetyl-L-carnitine increased GDR from 4.89+/-1.47 to 6.72+/-3.12 mg/kg per minute (P=0.003, Bonferroni-adjusted) and improved glucose tolerance in patients with GDR </=7.9 mg/kg per minute, whereas it had no effects in those with higher GDRs. ... **Systolic blood pressure decreased from 144.0 to 135.1 mm Hg and from 130.8 to 123.8 mm Hg in the lower and higher GDR groups, respectively... Acetyl-L-carnitine safely ameliorated arterial hypertension**, insulin resistance, impaired glucose tolerance, and **hypoadiponectinemia** in subjects at increased cardiovascular risk. Whether these effects may translate into long-term cardioprotection is worth investigating."[216] Total adiponectin increased from 4.7 to 6.0 meq/L, while HMW adiponectin increased from 2.2 to 3.0 meq/L (p<0.05 for both changes). The finding of relative carnitine deficiency in patients with

> ### Acetyl-L-carnitine increases adiponectin: clinical significance and mechanism of action against hypertension
>
> Discovered in 1996, adiponectin is a beneficial protein hormone secreted from adipose tissue, and as such it is an adipokine (adipocyte-derived hormone). Adiponectin is secreted in two forms: a low molecular weight form and a more metabolically active high molecular weight (HMW) multimer. Adiponectin is unique among adipokines in that its effects are largely beneficial; it has anti-diabetic, anti-atherogenic, and anti-inflammatory properties. Another unique feature of adiponectin is that—even though it is made in adipose tissue—its production is inversely proportional to the total load of visceral fat. Per Matsuzawa: "Hypoadiponectinemia induced by visceral fat accumulation is closely associated with type 2 diabetes, lipid disorders, **hypertension** and also certain inflammatory diseases."
>
> Metabolic effects of adiponectin include:
> - decreases gluconeogenesis and reduces serum glucose,
> - increases peripheral glucose uptake, indicating improved insulin sensitivity,
> - enhances β-oxidation of fatty acids, promotes triglyceride clearance,
> - protects from endothelial dysfunction and atherosclerosis,
> - promotes weight loss.
>
> Matsuzawa Y. Adiponectin: a key player in obesity related disorders. *Curr Pharm Des.* 2010 Jun;16(17):1896-901

HTN and DM along with the finding that acetyl-L-carnitine supplementation raises adiponectin in these patient groups suggests that the hypoadiponectinemia in HTN and DM may be a direct result from hypocarnitinemia.

o Randomized placebo-controlled double-blind crossover study: Effect of combined treatment with alpha-lipoic acid (400 mg/d) and acetyl-L-carnitine (1,000 mg/d) on vascular function and blood pressure in patients with documented coronary artery disease (*Journal of Clinical Hypertension*, Apr 2007): The authors note that mitochondria produce reactive oxygen species that may contribute to vascular dysfunction, and that both oxidative stress and mitochondrial dysfunction can be ameliorated by alpha-lipoic acid and acetyl-L-carnitine. Among 36 subjects with coronary artery disease, active

---

[216] Ruggenenti P, Cattaneo D, Loriga G, Ledda F, Motterlini N, Gherardi G, Orisio S, Remuzzi G. Ameliorating Hypertension and Insulin Resistance in Subjects at Increased Cardiovascular Risk. Effects of Acetyl-L-Carnitine Therapy. *Hypertension*. 2009 Sep;54(3):567-74

treatment for 8 weeks increased brachial artery diameter by 2.3%, consistent with reduced arterial tone. "Active treatment **decreased systolic blood pressure** for the whole group and had a significant effect in the subgroup with blood pressure above the median (151 to 142 mm Hg) and in the subgroup with the metabolic syndrome (139 to 130 mm Hg)."[217] Although this study used low-modest doses of acetyl-carnitine and lipoic acid, it showed that antihypertensive benefits were greatest in patients with systolic blood pressure >135 mm Hg—blood pressure was reduced by approximately -9/-5 mm Hg—and in patients with metabolic syndrome—blood pressure was reduced by approximately -7/-3 mm Hg. More significant results probably would have been obtained with higher doses, but these results are still statistically and clinically significant.

- **L-Arginine**: L-arginine (Arg) is the amino acid precursor for the formation of vasodilating nitric oxide (NO) produced via the action of endothelial nitric oxide synthase. A significant number of hypertensive patients have impaired conversion of Arg into NO, and a subset of these patients benefit from oral Arg supplementation. As usual, amino acid supplementation is delivered between meals (empty stomach) to facilitate absorption, and coadministration of simple carbohydrate can facilitate insulin-mediated cellular amino acid uptake. Recently, asymmetric dimethylarginine (ADMA) has been identified as an independent cardiovascular risk factor; per the excellent review by Böger[218], clinicians should appreciate that ADMA—formed from degradation of methylated proteins and an endogenous competitive inhibitor of NO synthase (NOS)—is a vasoconstrictor found in elevated levels among patients with hypercholesterolemia, atherosclerosis, hypertension, chronic renal failure, chronic heart failure, hyperthyroidism, hyperhomocysteinemia and folate deficiency. As expected, administration of Arg has demonstrated antihypertensive benefit, particularly among patients with high ADMA levels; indeed, elevated ADMA may identify which patients are likely to respond to Arg supplementation via a more favorable Arg:ADMA ratio. Laboratory testing for ADMA is available now from some research centers (such as Baylor[219]) and will surely become more widely available in the future. The predictable clinical take-home messages are that ❶ intravenous Arg administration generally produces a greater response than does oral administration, ❷ the hypotensive benefits of Arg supplementation are short-lived, ❸ the hypotensive benefits of Arg are more consistently seen in the groups expected to have high ADMA levels as previous listed, and ❹ younger patients (with less atherosclerosis and arterial calcification) are more likely to respond. **Clinicians should appreciate that the cardioprotective benefits of Arg extend beyond and are not entirely dependent upon its antihypertensive benefit; other benefits include decreased platelet aggregation and adhesion, decreased monocyte adhesion, antiproliferative effects on vascular smooth muscle, and improved endothelium-dependent vasodilation which can occur locally and systemically without an accompanying hypotensive effect.** Very importantly, concomitant administration of the amino acid N-acetyl-cysteine (NAC) appears to enhance the

[217] McMackin CJ, Widlansky ME, Hamburg NM, Huang AL, Weller S, Holbrook M, Gokce N, Hagen TM, Keaney JF Jr, Vita JA. Effect of combined treatment with alpha-Lipoic acid and acetyl-L-carnitine on vascular function and blood pressure in patients with coronary artery disease. *J Clin Hypertens* (Greenwich). 2007 Apr;9(4):249-55

[218] Böger RH. Asymmetric dimethylarginine, an endogenous inhibitor of nitric oxide synthase, explains the "L-arginine paradox" and acts as a novel cardiovascular risk factor. *J Nutr.* 2004 Oct;134(10 Suppl):2842S-2847S http://jn.nutrition.org/cgi/content/full/134/10/2842S

[219] Institute of Metabolic Disease at Baylor Research Institute. Asymmetric dimethylarginine (ADMA). http://www.baylorhealth.edu/imd/researchtests/asymmetric.htm Accessed December 2009

cardioprotective efficacy of Arg according to recent research.[220] Aside from the possibility of promoting reactivation of herpes simplex outbreaks, Arg is remarkably safe and is commonly used in immunonutrition formulas as a life-saving treatment in critically ill patients; Zhou and Martindale[221] recently noted, "The numerous potential beneficial effects of arginine in the critically ill patient include: 1) stimulation of immune function via its influence on lymphocyte, macrophage, and dendritic cells; 2) improved wound healing; 3) increased net nitrogen balance; 4) **increased blood flow to key vascular beds**; and 5) decreased clinical infections and length of hospital stay." The doses employed have ranged widely from 1,200 mg/d to 30,000 mg/d, (i.e., 1.2-30 g/d) and have included both oral and intravenous administration. Of course, Arg can be used with other dietary and nutritional interventions and with drug treatments with the caveat that common sense is employed to minimize the risk of hypotension by not initiating too many new treatments simultaneously in a given patient. While oral administration of L-arginine is generally considered beneficial at best and benign at worst, a report published in 2009 by Jahangir et al[222] showed that L-arginine supplementation at 9 grams per day for 4 days did not alter vascular reactivity but did increase methylation demand (shown by increased homocysteine to methionine ratio); this study and its implications (namely that methylation factors such as folate, betaine, pyridoxine, and cobalamin might be coadministered with L-arginine to optimize vascular health and endothelial function) are reviewed at the end of this section on L-arginine.

- o Open clinical trial: The effects of sustained-release L-arginine on blood pressure and vascular compliance in 29 healthy individuals (normotensives and hypertensives) treated for one week (*Alternative Medicine Review*, Mar 2006): Miller[223] used 2.1 g/d Arg administered in two divided doses in a sustained release preparation to find that approximately 65% of hypertensive patients responded favorably with an average reduction of -4/-3.7 mm Hg for the group as a whole that included normotensives and hypertensives. **Among patients who were "borderline or hypertensive" the average BP reduction was -11/-4.9 mm Hg.** Vascular elasticity assessed by digital pulse wave analysis showed a significant increase in large artery compliance (mean 23% improvement). Given the low dose, the short duration, and the low cost and absence of adverse effects, these results are worthy of clinical consideration and additional study. Consistent with many studies in clinical nutrition, the intervention provided an alterative, homeostatic effect in that—in contrast to the effects of pharmaceutical drugs—the effects are benign and rather minimal in healthy-normotensive persons and are clinically significant and therapeutic in patients with the index disease.

- o Randomized placebo-controlled trial with 123 patients: Effect of L-arginine on blood pressure in pregnancy-induced hypertension (*Journal of Maternal-Fetal and Neonatal Medicine*, May 2006): Inclusion criteria for this trial included maternal age range 16-45 years, diagnosis of gestational hypertension without proteinuria (patients normotensive

[220] Martina V, Masha A, Gigliardi VR, et al. Long-term N-acetylcysteine and L-arginine administration reduces endothelial activation and systolic blood pressure in hypertensive patients with type 2 diabetes. *Diabetes Care*. 2008 May;31(5):940-4 http://care.diabetesjournals.org/content/31/5/940.long

[221] "The numerous potential beneficial effects of arginine in the critically ill patient include: 1) stimulation of immune function via its influence on lymphocyte, macrophage, and dendritic cells; 2) improved wound healing; 3) increased net nitrogen balance; 4) increased blood flow to key vascular beds; and 5) decreased clinical infections and length of hospital stay." Zhou M, Martindale RG. Arginine in the critical care setting. *J Nutr*. 2007 Jun;137(6 Suppl 2):1687S-1692S http://jn.nutrition.org/cgi/content/full/137/6/1687S

[222] Jahangir E, Vita JA, Handy D, Holbrook M, Palmisano J, Beal R, Loscalzo J, Eberhardt RT. The effect of L-arginine and creatine on vascular function and homocysteine metabolism. *Vasc Med*. 2009 Aug;14(3):239-48

[223] Miller AL. The effects of sustained-release-L-arginine formulation on blood pressure and vascular compliance in 29 healthy individuals. *Altern Med Rev*. 2006 Mar;11(1):23-9 http://www.thorne.com/altmedrev/.fulltext/11/1/23.pdf

until the 20th week), and gestational age ranging between 24 and 36 weeks. Subjects were allocated to receive either Arg 20 g/500 mL intravenously or placebo treatment through an i.v. line. Treatment or placebo was administered in the morning from 8-10 a.m. and was repeated for four consecutive days. The final analysis was performed on 62 women in the Arg group and 61 in the placebo group. "RESULTS: Maternal clinical features such as age, height, weight, and gestational age at inclusion were similar between groups. Both systolic and diastolic blood pressures were reduced by treatment, the effect of L-arginine being significantly higher than that of the placebo (systolic values F = 8.59, p < 0.005; diastolic values F = 3.36; p < 0.001). … CONCLUSIONS: In conclusion, these data support the use of L-Arg as an antihypertensive agent for gestational hypertension especially in view of the other beneficial effects nitric oxide donors display in pregnancy. Further, L-Arg seems well tolerated since in this sample none of the patients reported adverse effects requiring study interruption."[224] According to Figure 4 of the article, **BP reductions due to arginine supplementation were approximately -5/-8 mm Hg**.

o Double-blind placebo-controlled clinical trial: Long-term N-acetylcysteine and L-arginine administration reduces endothelial activation and systolic blood pressure in hypertensive patients with type 2 diabetes (*Diabetes Care*, May 2008): This double-blind trial included 24 male patients with type-2 DM and HTN divided into two groups of 12 patients that randomly received either placebo or NAC 1,200 mg/d and ARG 1,200 mg/d orally for 6 months. "RESULTS—The NAC + ARG treatment caused a reduction of both systolic and diastolic mean arterial blood pressure, total cholesterol, LDL cholesterol, oxidized LDL, high-sensitive C-reactive protein, intracellular adhesion molecule, vascular cell adhesion molecule, nitrotyrosine, fibrinogen, and plasminogen activator inhibitor-1, and an improvement of the intima-media thickness during endothelial postischemic vasodilation. HDL cholesterol increased. No changes in other parameters studied were observed. CONCLUSIONS—NAC + ARG administration seems to be a potential well-tolerated antiatherogenic therapy because it improves endothelial function in hypertensive patients with type 2 diabetes by improving NO bioavailability via reduction of oxidative stress and increase of NO production. Our study's results give prominence to its potential use in primary and secondary cardiovascular prevention in these patients."[225] The **BP change in the treatment group was -5/-5 mm Hg**; the results of this study are remarkable considering the low dose of Arg employed and the manifold biochemical benefits attained.

o Review: L-arginine and cardiovascular system (*Pharmacological Reports*, Jan-Feb 2005): "The majority of experimental and clinical studies clearly show a beneficial effect of L-arginine on endothelium in conditions associated with its hypofunction and thus with reduced NO synthesis. Some clinical studies involving healthy volunteers or patients suffering from hypertension and diabetes indicate that it may also regulate vascular hemostasis."[226] The full text of this article goes on to itemize several clinical trials (at

---

[224] Neri I, Jasonni VM, Gori GF, Blasi I, Facchinetti F. Effect of L-arginine on blood pressure in pregnancy-induced hypertension: a randomized placebo-controlled trial. *J Matern Fetal Neonatal Med*. 2006 May;19(5):277-81

[225] Martina V, Masha A, Gigliardi VR, et al. Long-term N-acetylcysteine and L-arginine administration reduces endothelial activation and systolic blood pressure in hypertensive patients with type 2 diabetes. *Diabetes Care*. 2008 May;31(5):940-4 http://care.diabetesjournals.org/content/31/5/940.long

[226] Cylwik D, Mogielnicki A, Buczko W. L-arginine and cardiovascular system. *Pharmacol Rep*. 2005 Jan-Feb;57(1):14-22 http://www.if-pan.krakow.pl/pjp/pdf/2005/1_14.pdf

variable level of detail), the majority of these synopses related to HTN are summarized here:

- Placebo controlled trial of 30 g (thirty grams) Arg infused intravenously over 30 minutes to healthy volunteers: Diastolic BP was "markedly reduced" more than was systolic BP; another study conducted in women found similar results.
- Consumption of an Arg-enriched diet by healthy volunteers: BP reduction.
- Oral administration of 21g daily to healthy young men for 3 days: No correlation of Arg with blood pressure.
- Oral administration of 20g daily to healthy men for 28 days: No reduction in BP.
- Oral administration of 9g daily to healthy subjects for 6 months: No reduction in BP; however, "long-term administration of this amino acid had a favorable effect on endothelium, improving its function and reducing concentration of endothelin." (Endothelins are peptides that constrict blood vessels and contribute to HTN.)
- Intravenous Arg given at a dose of 500 mg/kg in patients with primary and secondary hypertension: "Considerable reduction both in systolic and diastolic pressure in all the cases."
- Intravenous Arg given at a dose of 30g over 60 minutes in patients with treated/untreated HTN: Previously untreated HTN patients had the best clinical response, followed by ACEi-treated patients, and a slight BP reduction in normal volunteers.
- Oral Arg 5.6 or 12.6 g/day for 6 weeks in patients with heart failure: Reduction in arterial blood pressure.
- Oral Arg 21 g for 3 days to young men with coronary artery disease: No changes in blood pressure despite improvement in brachial artery dilation.
- Intravenous bolus of 3g Arg to healthy subjects and patients with insulin-independent diabetes, hypercholesterolemia and primary hypertension: Best response was seen in young healthy patients (response inverse to age), then hypertensives, and lastly in patients with hypercholesterolemia and DM.
- Oral Arg 21 g/d for 4 weeks in young patients with hypercholesterolemia: Improved endothelium-dependent dilatation.
- Intravenous infusion of Arg 30 g for 60 minutes in patients with limb ischemia: "Marked reduction in diastolic and systolic pressure and an increased blood flow in the femoral artery."

o Randomized placebo-controlled clinical trial: The effect of L-arginine and creatine on vascular function and homocysteine metabolism (*Vascular Medicine*, Aug 2009): The authors[227] introduce their study by noting that studies with L-arginine supplementation have shown inconsistent effects on endothelial function (readers will have noted this from the studies reviewed above). The authors point out that, while L-arginine is a nitric oxide precursor, it is also the precursor to guanidinoacetate (GAA), which leads to the formation of creatine and the consumption of methionine to produce homocysteine, thereby utilizing methyl groups and increasing methylation demand. The purpose of this study was to investigate the effect of supplementation with L-arginine and creatine (alone or in combination) on vascular function and methylation/homocysteine

---

[227] Jahangir E, Vita JA, Handy D, Holbrook M, Palmisano J, Beal R, Loscalzo J, Eberhardt RT. The effect of L-arginine and creatine on vascular function and homocysteine metabolism. *Vasc Med*. 2009 Aug;14(3):239-48

metabolism. Patients with documented CAD (n=109) were randomized to receive L-arginine (9gm/d), creatine (21gm/day), L-arginine plus creatine, or placebo for 4 days (n=26–29 per group); brachial artery flow-mediated dilation and plasma levels of L-arginine, creatine, homocysteine, methionine, and GAA were measured at baseline and follow up. Results of this study showed that L-arginine and creatine supplementation had no effects on vascular function; we could argue that 4 days is insufficient duration to produce changes in physiologic function. L-arginine increased GAA (P<0.01) and the ratio of homocysteine to methionine (from 0.7 to 0.9; P<0.01) suggesting increased methylation demand. Supplementation with L-arginine increased plasma homocysteine from 11.1 micromol/L to 11.2 micromol/L (P=0.006); one could easily argue that such a minute change is clinically insignificant, while one could also argue that a negative change within the span of 4 days of supplementation portends a potentially hazardous trend if carried out for months and years. More important than the change in homocysteine levels is the more sensitive increase in the ratio of homocysteine to methionine, indicating increased methylation demand which is likely to have adverse effects in various metabolic pathways; the authors note, "Thus, it remains possible that L-arginine metabolism imposes a methylation demand that counterbalances the effects of NO generated despite the absence of a change in measured plasma homocysteine." The average GFR of patients in this study was 68 ml/min by the Cockcroft–Gault formula (consistent with stage 2—almost stage 3—kidney disease), and previous studies have shown that patients with kidney disease are less likely to respond to treatments that improve endovascular health, including L-arginine, due in part to higher levels of circulating ADMA and homocysteine. The combination of creatinine and L-arginine did not suppress GAA production or prevent the increase in homocysteine-to-methionine ratio. Unexpectedly, the authors found that creatine supplementation (alone or in combination with L-arginine) was associated with an 11 to 20% increase in plasma homocysteine; other studies *of longer duration* using *lower doses of creatine* (<5.5 gm/d for 4 weeks) have shown the opposite effect—namely that creatine supplementation lowers plasma homocysteine.

L-arginine conversion to nitric oxide and effect on methionine-homocysteine metabolism

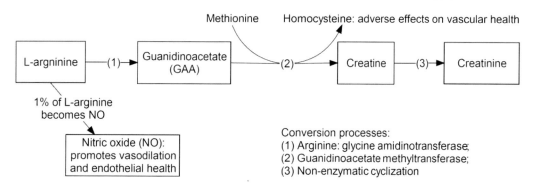

Altogether, these findings raise the possibility that L-arginine's effects on vascular function may be dependent on the patient's methylation ability; patients with poor methylation ability may experience exacerbation of endothelial dysfunction via L-arginine's conversion to GAA and the increased production of homocysteine. When L-arginine is used, supplementation with methyl donors and homocysteine-lowering nutrients such as folic acid, pyridoxine, cobalamin, betaine, and N-acetyl-cysteine may improve the efficacy of L-arginine supplementation while additively or

Adverse effects of elevated homocysteine
1. Activation of coagulation,
2. Stimulation of monocyte adhesion,
3. Enhanced oxidation of low density lipoprotein (LDL),
4. Impairment of NO-mediated vascular responses (vasodilation),
5. Adverse effects on bone health and increased risk for osteoporosis.

synergistically improving vascular reactivity and endothelial health; this underscores the importance of dietary optimization and foundational multivitamin/multimineral supplementation (as a component of the "5-part nutritional protocol" described previously in this text) and the general need to avoid single-intervention treatment approaches.

- **Vitamin C (ascorbic acid) 3 g/d or bowel tolerance**: Since ascorbic acid is biochemically synthesized from glucose, these molecules remain structurally similar; not surprisingly therefore, an excess of glucose (i.e., as in hyperglycemia) reduces cellular uptake of ascorbic acid, leading to a relative "cellular scurvy" even in the absence of the classic presentation of scurvy. "In neutrophils from different volunteers, glucose inhibited uptake and accumulation of ascorbic acid by both transport activities 3-9-fold. ... Glucose-induced inhibition of both ascorbic acid transport activities occurred in neutrophils of all donors tested and was fully reversible."[228]

  o Clinical trial: Vitamin C for refractory hypertension in elderly patients (*Arzneimittelforschung*, 2006): Treatment with ascorbic acid 600 mg/d for 6 months was evaluated for effects on blood pressure and levels of C-reactive protein, 8-isoprostane, and malondialdehyde-modified low-density lipoproteins among 12 elderly patients (average age 78.3y) and 12 adult patients (average age 54.6y) with refractory hypertension. **Treatment with ascorbic acid markedly reduced systolic blood pressure in the elderly group from 154.9 to 134.8 mmHg (p < 0.001); pulse pressure reduced from 79.1 to 63.4. These benefits of vitamin C supplementation were accompanied by an increase in the serum levels of ascorbic acid and decreases in the levels of C-reactive protein, 8-isoprostane, and malondialdehyde-modified low-density lipoproteins**. In contrast, ascorbic acid did not affect blood pressure in the adult nonelderly group. These results suggest that ascorbic acid is useful for controlling blood pressure in elderly patients with refractory hypertension."[229] Clinicians should appreciate that elevated systolic blood pressure is an important predictor of cardiovascular mortality in elderly patients, and that its ascorbate-induced reduction by -20 mmHg is highly clinically significant.

---

[228] Washko P, Levine M. Inhibition of ascorbic acid transport in human neutrophils by glucose. *J Biol Chem*. 1992 Nov 25;267(33):23568-74
[229] Sato K, Dohi Y, Kojima M, Miyagawa K, Takase H, Katada E, Suzuki S. Effects of ascorbic acid on ambulatory blood pressure in elderly patients with refractory hypertension. *Arzneimittelforschung*. 2006;56(7):535-40

- **Urinary alkalinization**: In non-pathologic states, the pattern of dietary intake is the single most important determinant of systemic/urine acid-base balance.[230] The two main classes of acids of physiologic importance are 1) carbonic acid—formed when carbon dioxide (CO_2) from metabolism of carbohydrates and fatty acids combines with water (H_2O) to form carbonic acid (H_2CO_3), and 2) noncarbonic acids—these are primarily generated from the oxidation of sulfur-containing amino acids which results in the formation of sulfuric acid (H_2SO_4); avoidance of the former is mostly achieved via respiration (i.e., removal of CO_2) while elimination of the latter requires bicarbonate and renal excretion.[231] Average urine pH among societies consuming a Paleo-Mediterranean diet and obtaining daily physical exercise is 7.5-9; clearly this very alkaline state reflects a diet high in fruits and vegetables, and provides physiologic benefits including increased excretion of xenobiotics[232] and renal retention of potassium, magnesium, and calcium. For example, among New Guinean hunter-gatherer tribal groups living in the *primitive feral condition*, "urine pH of adults was usually between 7.5 and 9.0 because of potassium bicarbonate and carbonate excretion."[233] Excess urine alkalinity can predispose to urinary tract infections; thus some clinicians may be more comfortable with a urine pH goal of approximately 7.5-8.0.

  o Clinical trial: Neutralization of Western diet inhibits bone resorption independently of K intake and reduces cortisol secretion in humans (*American Journal of Physiology - Renal Physiology*, Jan 2003): Acid-base neutralization by substituting equimolar amounts of sodium bicarbonate and potassium bicarbonate for NaCl and KCl "induced a significant cumulative calcium retention (10.7 +/- 0.4 mmol) and significantly reduced the urinary excretion of deoxypyridinoline, pyridinoline, and n-telopeptide. Mean daily plasma cortisol decreased from 264 +/- 45 to 232 +/- 43 nmol/l (P = 0.032), … An acidogenic Western diet results in mild metabolic acidosis in association with a state of cortisol excess, altered divalent ion metabolism, and increased bone resorptive indices. Acidosis-induced increases in cortisol secretion and plasma concentration may play a role in mild acidosis-induced alterations in bone metabolism and possibly in osteoporosis associated with an acidogenic Western diet."[234] Clinicians should appreciate that long-term reductions in cortisol along with renal retention of calcium would be expected to have a favorable effect on blood pressure.

  o Review: Diet, evolution and aging—the pathophysiologic effects of the post-agricultural inversion of the potassium-to-sodium and base-to-chloride ratios in the human diet (*European Journal of Nutrition*, Oct 2001): This excellent review article discusses the changes in mineral intake (i.e., less potassium complicated by more sodium) and the shift from a plant-based alkalinizing diet to a pseudo-food acidifying diet and the physiological ramifications of these dietary changes. Note their conclusion in the following quote which states that any level of acidosis may be unacceptable and that

---

[230] "Nutrition has long been known to strongly influence acid-base balance. Recently, we have shown that it is possible to appropriately estimate the renal net acid excretion (NAE) of healthy subjects from the composition of their diets." Remer T. Influence of nutrition on acid-base balance--metabolic aspects. *Eur J Nutr*. 2001 Oct;40(5):214-20

[231] Rennke HG, Denker BM. Renal Physiology: The Essentials. Second Edition. Philadelphia: Lippincott Williams and Wilkins; 2007, 129

[232] "Urine alkalinization is a treatment regimen that increases poison elimination by the administration of intravenous sodium bicarbonate to produce urine with a pH > or = 7.5." Proudfoot AT, Krenzelok EP, Vale JA. Position Paper on urine alkalinization. *J Toxicol Clin Toxicol*. 2004;42(1):1-26

[233] Sebastian A, Frassetto LA, Sellmeyer DE, Merriam RL, Morris RC Jr. Estimation of the net acid load of the diet of ancestral preagricultural Homo sapiens and their hominid ancestors. *Am J Clin Nutr*. 2002 Dec;76(6):1308-16

[234] Maurer M, Riesen W, Muser J, Hulter HN, Krapf R. Neutralization of Western diet inhibits bone resorption independently of K intake and reduces cortisol secretion in humans. *Am J Physiol Renal Physiol*. 2003 Jan;284(1):F32-40

(conversely) a state of alkalinization is the normal and ideal human condition: "We argue that any level of acidosis may be unacceptable from an evolutionarily perspective, and indeed, that **a low-grade metabolic alkalosis may be the optimal acid-base state for humans.**"[235]

o   Clinical trial: Urine alkalization facilitates uric acid excretion (*Nutrition Journal*, Oct 2010): Highly consistent with and positively affirming of the protocol and paradigm advocated in this text, this clinical trial published in *Nutrition Journal* in October 2010, authors of this study note that "Increase in the incidence of hyperuricemia associated with gout as well as hypertension, renal diseases and cardiovascular diseases has been a public health concern." Their clinical trial therefore sought to increase renal excretion of uric acid by altering urine pH via dietary improvement, moving in the direction of a more plant-based and more Paleo-Mediterranean diet. The authors made recipes consisting of "protein-rich and less vegetable-fruit food materials" (acid diet) and of "less protein but vegetable-fruit rich food materials" (alkali diet). Urine pH reached a steady state 3 days after switching from ordinary daily diets to specified regimens. Results showed that H+ (acidity) in urine is directly affected by the metabolic degradation of food materials, and that uric acid and excreted urine pH retained a linear relationship; the higher the pH (more alkaline), the greater the uric acid excretion. The authors concluded, "We conclude that alkalization of urine by eating nutritionally well-designed food is effective for removing uric acid from the body."[236] Given the increasing evidence that intracellular urate directly contributes to microvascular disease and the anticipated pathological complications in the brain, kidneys, and cardiovascular system[237], reducing the total body load of uric acid (i.e., the composite load in intracellular and extracellular/plasma compartments) is justified and warranted.

> **Diet optimization is the "safest and most economical" intervention to lower the total body load of uric acid**
>
> "This study has clarified that alkalization of urine by the manipulation of food materials promotes the removal of uric acid. When one pays enough attention to the construction of a nutritionally balanced menu, dietary intervention becomes the safest and the most economical way for the prevention of hyperuricemia."
>
> Kanbara A, Hakoda M, Seyama I. Urine alkalization facilitates uric acid excretion. *Nutrition Journal* 2010, 9:45 http://www.nutritionj.com/content/9/1/45

*   **Mind-Body Approaches including Qigong, controlled breathing, transcendental meditation, and acupuncture**: Traditional therapeutics and lifestyle activities such as Qigong, controlled breathing, meditation, and acupuncture can effect statistically and clinically significant reductions in BP among hypertensive patients. Mechanisms of action include induction of beneficial neurohormonal responses (e.g., increased dehydroepiandrosterone and melatonin levels following meditation) as well as induction of a relaxed state. Avoidance of physiological stressors can play a role in blood pressure control and should be implemented on an as-appropriate basis. Sympathetic neural activity via beta-

---

[235] Frassetto L, Morris RC Jr, Sellmeyer DE, Todd K, Sebastian A. Diet, evolution and aging—the pathophysiologic effects of the post-agricultural inversion of the potassium-to-sodium and base-to-chloride ratios in the human diet. *Eur J Nutr*. 2001 Oct;40(5):200-13
[236] "We conclude that alkalization of urine by eating nutritionally well-designed food is effective for removing uric acid from the body." Kanbara A, Hakoda M, Seyama I. Urine alkalization facilitates uric acid excretion. *Nutrition Journal* 2010, 9:45 http://www.nutritionj.com/content/9/1/45
[237] "...dietary intake of sugars rich in fructose may be driving the development of microvascular disease as a consequence of raising intracellular uric acid." Kanbay M, Sánchez-Lozada LG, Franco M, Madero M, Solak Y, Rodriguez-Iturbe B, Covic A, Johnson RJ. Microvascular disease and its role in the brain and cardiovascular system: a potential role for uric acid as a cardiorenal toxin. *Nephrol Dial Transplant*. 2010 Oct 8. [Epub ahead of print]

adrenergic receptors in the kidney stimulates release of renin, which is a peptidase enzyme that converts angiotensinogen to angiotensin-1 and thereby expedites the formation of angiotensin-2 in the lungs; angiotensin-2 is a vasoconstrictor and stimulates aldosterone production which increases sodium resorption and thus water retention.[238]; Thus, the net effect of sympathetic nervous activation is increased volume within a constricted vasculature, thus causing HTN. Data on therapeutic interventions in the following four subsections are derived from the review by Nahas[239] (*Canadian Family Physician*, Nov 2008) unless otherwise noted.

- Qigong: A Chinese medicine form of movement, breathing, and meditation: As a part of traditional Chinese medicine (TCM), Qigong incorporates movement, breathing, and meditation. Two systematic reviews involving hundreds of patients (n = > 900 to > 1,200 subjects) have examined the role of Qigong in the treatment of hypertension. Despite some methodological shortcomings, evidence shows that Qigong can reduce BP among hypertensives by -12 to -17 mm Hg systolic and -8.5 to -10 mm Hg diastolic. Thus, the BP-lowering results obtained by Qigong are comparable to drug treatment of HTN.
- Controlled breathing: Most studies (4 of 5) using slow controlled breathing have shown an antihypertensive benefit presumably mediated through increased parasympathetic and reduced sympathetic activity; as expected, diabetics with autonomic dysfunction tend to receive less benefit.
- Transcendental meditation: Twice-daily sessions of sitting quietly while repeating a specific mantra can effect a BP-lowering effect of approximately -4.7/-3.2 mm Hg.
- Acupuncture: Acupuncture is difficult to study in a placebo-controlled manner due to the physical, individualized, and experiential nature of the treatment. Antihypertensive benefits of acupuncture have ranged from no different from the so-called placebo to reductions of -6 to -14 mm Hg for systolic BP and -3 to -7 mm Hg for diastolic BP.

- **Whey peptides, casokinins, and lactokinins**: Yet another benefit of whey protein consumption is the salutary effect on blood pressure, probably mediated by whey protein's anti-stress, anti-oxidant/pro-glutathione, and ACE-inhibiting properties. Very interestingly, the anti-hypertensive effects of milk peptides may depend on their specific hydrolysation by lactic acid producing bacteria in the intestines; thus, clinical anti-hypertensive benefit of milk/whey peptides may require establishment of eubiosis, eradication of intestinal dysbiosis, and/or co-supplementation with probiotics. (For extensive reviews on the clinical consequences of dysbiosis and the [re]establishment of eubiosis, see monographs[240] and book chapters[241] by Vasquez). Whey protein is commonly consumed in doses that provide 20-80 grams of protein per day; individual antihypertensive responses will, of course, vary.
  - Clinical trial: The long-term effects of whey protein isolate on blood pressure, vascular function, and inflammatory markers in overweight individuals. (*Obesity*, Jul 2010): This study evaluated the effects of whey protein isolate (27 grams twice daily) on blood

[238] Benowitz NL. "Antihypertensive Agents." In Katzung BG (editor). Basic and Clinical Pharmacology. Tenth Edition. New York: McGraw Hill Medical; 2007, 161
[239] Nahas R. Complementary and alternative medicine approaches to blood pressure reduction: An evidence-based review. *Can Fam Physician*. 2008 Nov;54(11):1529-33 http://www.cfp.ca/cgi/content/full/54/11/1529
[240] **Vasquez A**. Reducing Pain and Inflammation Naturally - Part 6: Nutritional and Botanical Treatments Against "Silent Infections" and Gastrointestinal Dysbiosis, Commonly Overlooked Causes of Neuromusculoskeletal Inflammation and Chronic Health Problems. *Nutritional Perspectives* 2006; 29 (January): 5-21
[241] Chapter Four in: **Vasquez A**. Integrative Rheumatology. IBMRC 2006, 2007. http://optimalhealthresearch.com/rheumatology.html

pressure, vascular function and inflammatory markers compared to the effects of casein and glucose (control) supplementation in overweight/obese individuals. Seventy men and women with average BMI of 31.3 completed this 12-week study. Blood pressure reductions due to whey protein isolate were noted at 6 weeks and were significant for systolic and diastolic pressures at 12 weeks of supplementation. No significant changes in inflammatory markers were noted. This study demonstrated that supplementation with whey protein improves blood pressure and vascular function (assessed by the augmentation index) in overweight and obese individuals. Systolic blood pressure (SBP) decreased significantly by 3% at week 6 (115.5 mm Hg) and by 4% at week 12 (114.5 mm Hg) compared to baseline (119.3 mm Hg) in the whey protein group. A significant decrease of 3.3% in diastolic blood pressure (DBP) at week 12 (62.0 mm Hg) compared with baseline (64.1 mm Hg) in the whey protein group was noted. Thus, the total BP reduction by whey protein isolate in this study is approximately -4.8/-2.1 mm Hg.[242]

o Clinical trial: Effects of whey protein isolate on body composition, lipids, insulin and glucose in overweight and obese individuals. (*British Journal of Nutrition*, Sep 2010): Whey protein isolate supplementation in 70 men and women with a mean age of 48.4 years and a mean BMI of 31.3 for 12 weeks in a parallel study design resulted in no significant change in body composition or serum glucose at 12 weeks compared with the control (glucose) or casein group. A significant decrease in total cholesterol and LDL cholesterol at week 12 in the whey protein isolate group compared with the casein and control groups was noted. Fasting insulin levels and homeostasis model assessment of insulin resistance scores were also significantly decreased in the whey protein isolate group compared with the control group. The present study demonstrated that supplementation with whey protein isolate improves fasting lipids and insulin levels in overweight and obese individuals.[243]

o Randomized cross-over clinical trial: The acute effects of four protein meals on insulin, glucose, appetite, and energy intake in lean men. (*British Journal of Nutrition*, Oct 2010: The authors note that different dietary proteins vary in their ability to influence satiety and reduce food intake. The present study compared the effects of four protein meals—whey, tuna, turkey, and egg albumin—on postprandial glucose and insulin concentrations as well as on appetite measures and energy intake in 22 lean healthy men. Results showed that blood glucose response after the consumption of the test meal measured as area under the curve (AUC) was significantly lower with the whey meal and tuna meal than with the turkey and egg meals. The AUC blood insulin was significantly higher with the whey meal than with the tuna, turkey and egg meals; however, the AUC rating of hunger was significantly lower with the whey meal than with the tuna, turkey, and egg meals. Mean energy intake at the ad libitum meal following the protein meal was significantly lower with the whey meal than with the tuna, egg, and turkey meals. Results showed that whey protein meal produced a greater acute insulin response, reduced appetite and decreased ad libitum energy intake at a subsequent meal compared with the other protein meals, indicating a potential for

---

[242] Pal S, Ellis V. The chronic effects of whey proteins on blood pressure, vascular function, and inflammatory markers in overweight individuals. *Obesity* (Silver Spring). 2010 Jul;18(7):1354-9

[243] Pal S, Ellis V, Dhaliwal S. Effects of whey protein isolate on body composition, lipids, insulin and glucose in overweight and obese individuals. *Br J Nutr*. 2010 Sep;104(5):716-23

appetite suppression and weight loss in overweight or obese individuals.[244] This is a very interesting study showing that even though whey protein acutely elevates insulin levels postprandially, the reduced appetite and calorie intake induced by whey protein consumption may actually help patients lose weight.

o Review: Lactokinins are whey protein-derived ACE inhibitory peptides (*Nahrung*, Jun 1999): Whey protein contains lactokinins, peptides that function as ACE-inhibitors. "Peptides derived from the major whey proteins, i.e. alpha-lactalbumin (alpha-la) and beta-lactoglobulin (beta-lg) in addition to bovine serum albumin (BSA), inhibit ACE. ... While they do not have the inhibitory potency of synthetic drugs commonly used in the treatment of hypertension, these naturally occurring peptides may represent nutraceutical/functional food ingredients for the prevention/treatment of high blood pressure."[245]

o Review: Milk protein-derived peptide inhibitors of angiotensin-I-converting enzyme (*British Journal of Nutrition*, Nov 2000): "Numerous casein and whey protein-derived angiotensin-I-converting enzyme (ACE) inhibitory peptides/hydrolysates have been identified. Clinical trials in hypertensive animals and humans show that these peptides/hydrolysates can bring about a significant reduction in hypertension. These peptides/hydrolysates may be classified as functional food ingredients and nutraceuticals due to their ability to provide health benefits i.e. as functional food ingredients in reducing the risk of developing a disease and as nutraceuticals in the prevention/treatment of disease."[246]

o Review: Hypotensive peptides from milk proteins (*Journal of Nutrition*, Apr 2004): "Milk proteins, both caseins and whey proteins, are a rich source of ACE inhibitory peptides. Several studies in spontaneously hypertensive rats show that these casokinins and lactokinins can significantly reduce blood pressure. Furthermore, a limited number of human studies have associated milk protein-derived peptides with statistically significant hypotensive effects (i.e., lower systolic and diastolic pressures)."[247]

• **Probiotics**: The term "probiotics" generally refers to beneficial microorganisms—most commonly bacteria but also including the probiotic yeast *Saccharomyces boulardii*—that are consumed either in the supplement/nutraceutical form of tablets, capsules, powders or as fermented foods such as yogurt, kefir, kombucha, miso, tempeh, cottage cheese (some types), and sauerkraut. Due to their numerous benefits, probiotics have been included as the fifth component of the 5-part nutritional protocol published by Vasquez[248] in 2005 and described in all subsequent editions of *Integrative Orthopedics*, *Integrative Rheumatology*, and especially *Chiropractic and Naturopathic Mastery of Common Clinical Disorders*. As science has continued to progress (both qualitatively and quantitatively), so has our knowledge of the diversity and mechanisms of the health-promoting benefits of probiotic supplementation. This section reviews several of the mechanisms behind the antihypertensive (and also cardioprotective, antidiabetes, antidyslipidemic, and anti-inflammatory) benefits of probiotic supplementation.

---

[244] Pal S, Ellis V. The acute effects of four protein meals on insulin, glucose, appetite and energy intake in lean men. *Br J Nutr*. 2010 Oct;104(8):1241-8

[245] FitzGerald RJ, Meisel H. Lactokinins: whey protein-derived ACE inhibitory peptides. *Nahrung*. 1999 Jun;43(3):165-7

[246] FitzGerald RJ, Meisel H. Milk protein-derived peptide inhibitors of angiotensin-I-converting enzyme. *Br J Nutr*. 2000 Nov;84 Suppl 1:S33-

[247] FitzGerald RJ, Murray BA, Walsh DJ. Hypotensive peptides from milk proteins. *J Nutr*. 2004 Apr;134(4):980S-8S

[248] **Vasquez A**. A Five-Part Nutritional Protocol that Produces Consistently Positive Results. *Nutritional Wellness* 2005 September Available in the printed version and on-line at http://optimalhealthresearch.com/protocol This essay was also republished in "Chiropractic and Naturopathic Mastery of Common Clinical Disorders" in 2009 http://optimalhealthresearch.com/clinical_mastery.html

Starting with and strongly relying upon a review article by Lye et al[249] named "The improvement of hypertension by probiotics: effects on cholesterol, diabetes, renin, and phytoestrogens", this section will concisely review the more prominent antihypertensive benefits and mechanisms of probiotic supplementation. Lye et al emphasize the role of dyslipidemia in the genesis of HTN by stating, "…lipid metabolism disorders are often the causes of hypertension." Relevant to this paradigm, they review data from controlled studies in humans, rats, and/or pigs showing that antidyslipidemic benefits (reduction in total serum cholesterol, very low density lipoprotein, intermediate density lipoprotein, and LDL cholesterol and increase in HDL cholesterol) have been documented due to the use of *Lactobacillus acidophilus*, *Lactobacillus casei*, *Bifidobacterium longum*, and *Saccharomyces boulardii* (when used with bacterial probiotics). The antidyslipidemic benefit of supplementation with *L. acidophilus*, *B. breve*, *Lactococcus lactis* and other probiotics is mediated in part or in whole part via ❶ cholesterol assimilation during growth (i.e., the bacteria actively take up cholesterol for their own use), ❷ binding of cholesterol to the cellular surface, in part via exopolysaccharides (EPS) which adhere to the cell surface and absorb cholesterol, and ❸ probiotic elaboration of the enzyme bile salt hydrolase (BSH; cholyglycine hydrolase) which catalyzes the hydrolysis of glycine- and/or taurine-conjugated bile salts into amino acid residues and free bile acids, the latter of which contain cholesterol and are preferentially excreted in the feces rather than being reabsorbed in the intestines. Thus, probiotics function in part (mechanisms 1 and 2) similarly to the anticholesteremic drug cholestyramine, which exerts its cholesterol-lowering effect via enhanced fecal excretion of cholesterol. Also, the authors note the correlation between diabetes mellitus, insulin resistance, and HTN, and that probiotics may also mediate an antihypertensive benefit by ❹ ameliorating diabetes and insulin resistance; in their words, "The consumption of probiotics is a new therapeutic strategy in preventing or delaying the onset of diabetes and subsequently reducing the incident of hypertension." With regard to this fourth mechanism, the postulated mechanism of the antihypertensive and antidiabetes benefit is worthy of appreciation both as a mechanism and as an independent benefit. The authors state that the antidiabetes benefit of probiotics is due to the reduction in systemic inflammation mediated via improvements in intestinal microecology which effect a reduction in systemic absorption of intestinally-derived bacterial lipopolysaccharides [LPS], which are inherently proinflammatory; the authors write, "…the composition of natural intestinal gut microflora often determine the degree of inflammation contributing to the onset of diabetes and obesity. The concentration of plasma lipopolysaccharides, the proinflammatory factor, is inversely correlated with the population of *Bifidobacterium* spp. … Several studies have also shown that bifidobacteria can reduce the intestinal endotoxin levels and improve mucosal barrier thus reducing systemic inflammation and subsequently reduced the incidence of diabetes." This **systemic anti-inflammatory benefit derived from the (re)establishment of eubiosis** is wholly consistent with the model of dysbiosis-induced systemic inflammation and autoimmunity detailed in both the 2006 and 2007 editions of *Integrative Rheumatology*.[250] In summarizing this mechanism, we must (again) conclude that probiotics are antidysbiotic and anti-inflammatory (dependent on and independent from LPS reduction) and that ❺ the

---

[249] Lye HS, Kuan CY, Ewe JA, Fung WY, Liong MT. The improvement of hypertension by probiotics: effects on cholesterol, diabetes, renin, and phytoestrogens. *Int J Mol Sci*. 2009 Aug 27;10(9):3755-75. http://www.ncbi.nlm.nih.gov/pmc/articles/PMC2769158/
[250] **Vasquez A**. Integrative Rheumatology. IBMRC 2006, 2007 and all future editions. http://optimalhealthresearch.com/rheumatology.html

antihypertensive benefit of probiotic supplementation is mediated at least in part via reducing systemic LPS-induced inflammation and thus subsequent insulin resistance and endothelial dysfunction, which independently and synergistically promote HTN. In either *in vitro*, animal, or human studies, the beneficial effects of probiotic supplementation have been demonstrated (in descending order of efficacy) from the use of living and growing probiotic populations, non-growing probiotics, and dead cells. Finally but not exhaustively, we should appreciate as mentioned previously that ❻ probiotic bacteria interact with dietary components—especially proteins from cow's milk—to produce antihypertensive peptides which, in particular, have ACE-inhibiting functions. As summed by Lye et al, "Probiotics are able to grow in milk products because they posses a proteolytic system that degrades casein along with lactose hydrolyzing enzymes. **Upon fermentation, the proteinases of various probiotics are capable of releasing ACE inhibitory peptides and thus a blood-pressure lowering effect can be derived from the milk proteins.** Several studies have demonstrated that *Lactobacillus helveticus* are capable of releasing antihypertensive peptides which are ACE inhibitory tripeptides Val-Pro-Pro (VPP) and Ile-Pro-Pro (IPP) from milk protein casein."

o Randomized, placebo-controlled, double-blind study: Effect of powdered fermented milk with *Lactobacillus helveticus* on subjects with high-normal blood pressure or mild hypertension (*Journal of the American College of Nutrition*, Aug 2005): This study used a randomized, placebo-controlled, double-blind design in 40 subjects with high-normal blood pressure (HN group: SBP 130–139 mm Hg and DBP 85–89 mm Hg) and 40 subjects with mild hypertension (MH group: SBP 140–159 mm Hg and DBP 90–99 mm Hg).[251] Each subject ingested 12 g of powdered fermented milk (in tablet form) with *L. helveticus* CM4 daily for 4 weeks (test group) or the same amount of placebo tablets for 4 weeks (placebo group). The authors noted that **among the patients with high-normal blood pressure, the change in SBP in the test group was 3.2 mm Hg lower than that in the placebo group, and DBP decreased more in the test group than in the placebo group during treatment, by 5.0 mm Hg** at the end of week 4. Further, they write, "**In the [Mild Hypertension] group, SBP decreased by 11.2 mm Hg and there was a statistically non-significant decrease in DBP of 6.5 mm Hg** compared with the placebo group." Their conclusions read, "Daily ingestion of the tablets containing powdered fermented milk with *L. helveticus* CM4 in subjects with high-normal blood pressure or mild hypertension reduces elevated blood pressure without any adverse effects." Readers should appreciate that this group with mild hypertension (SBP 140–159 mm Hg and DBP 90–99 mm Hg) represents the largest group of HTN patients and that this benefit of peptides from fermented milk—a reduction in blood pressure of -11.2/-6.5—is on par with the antihypertensive effect derived from many commonly used FDA-approved pharmaceutical drugs.

• **Cocoa & Dark Chocolate (*Theobroma cacao*)**: Cacao has been cultivated for thousands of years in South and Central America; currently most production comes from Africa as well as various other countries such as Belize. The word chocolate came into English from Spanish and entered Spanish either from the Aztecs ("chocolatl" or "chicolatl") or the Maya ("chokol"). Among its numerous constituents, alkaloids such as theobromine and phenethylamine and

---

[251] Aihara K, Kajimoto O, Hirata H, Takahashi R, Nakamura Y. Effect of powdered fermented milk with Lactobacillus helveticus on subjects with high-normal blood pressure or mild hypertension. *J Am Coll Nutr.* 2005 Aug;24(4):257-65

various antioxidants such as epicatechin and procyanidins have received the most attention. Dark chocolate *without added sugar* and *without the addition of excess fat or cow's milk* provides antioxidant, cardioprotective, neuroprotective, and anticancer benefits. **People who regularly consume higher levels of cocoa (suggested range 10-30 grams up to 100 grams daily) have lower BP and a -50% relative reduction in cardiovascular and all-cause mortality**; regarding the mechanism of action for the BP-lowering effect of chocolate: **flavonoids in cacao upregulate nitric oxide synthase in endothelial cells, and thus chocolate improves endothelial function.**[252] The cocoa content should be at least 65% and preferably 85%-90%. In December 2009, MD Anderson Cancer Center endorsed dark chocolate for its probable cancer-preventive benefits.[253] Because of its stimulating effects, cocoa should be consumed in the earlier part of the day in order to avoid sleep disturbance.

- o Systematic review and meta-analysis: Benefits of cocoa products on blood pressure (*American Journal of Hypertension*, Jan 2010): For this systematic review, the authors performed a meta-analysis of randomized controlled trials assessing the antihypertensive effects of flavanol-rich cocoa products. They found that among 10 randomized controlled trials with a total of 297 individuals (either healthy normotensive adults or patients with prehypertension/stage 1 hypertension), **systolic BP dropped -4.5 mm Hg while diastolic BP dropped -2.5 mm Hg following cocoa consumption** for durations of 2-18 weeks. The authors concluded that "The meta-analysis confirms the BP-lowering capacity of flavanol-rich cocoa products...."[254] Rather than rendering the typical cautionary note ("...questions such as the most appropriate dose and the long-term side effect profile warrant further investigation before cocoa products can be recommended as a treatment option in hypertension."), the authors might have been more wise to suggest increased consumption of chocolate for its antihypertensive and cardioprotective benefits and its greater safety profile compared to pharmaceutical drugs.

- o Randomized controlled trial: Effects of habitual cocoa intake on blood pressure and bioactive nitric oxide (*JAMA—Journal of the American Medical Association*, Jul 2007): The authors of this clinical trial review previously published research and note that regular intake of cocoa-containing foods is linked to lower cardiovascular mortality and that short-term interventions show that **high doses of cocoa can improve endothelial function and reduce BP due to the action of the cocoa polyphenols**. Their clinical trial design was a randomized, controlled, investigator-blinded, parallel-group trial involving 44 adults aged 56 through 73 years (24 women, 20 men) with untreated upper-range prehypertension or stage 1 hypertension without comorbidity; the treatment was 6.3 g (30 kcal) per day of dark chocolate containing 30 mg of polyphenols or a placebo of polyphenol-free white chocolate. Main outcome measures were ❶ BP, ❷ plasma markers of vasodilative nitric oxide (S-nitrosoglutathione), ❸ oxidative stress (8-isoprostane), and ❹ bioavailability of cocoa polyphenols. "RESULTS: From baseline to 18 weeks, **dark chocolate reduced mean systolic BP by -2.9 mm Hg and diastolic BP by -1.9 mm Hg** without changes in body weight, plasma levels of lipids, glucose, and 8-isoprostane.

---

[252] Nahas R. Complementary and alternative medicine approaches to blood pressure reduction: An evidence-based review. *Can Fam Physician*. 2008 Nov;54(11):1529-33 http://www.cfp.ca/cgi/content/full/54/11/1529

[253] "In addition to being delicious, moderate amounts of dark chocolate may play a role in cancer prevention. ... To get those cancer prevention benefits, the chocolate should contain at least 65% cocoa. Winters R. Focused on Health - December 2009. http://www.mdanderson.org/publications/focused-on-health/issues/2009-december/share-the-health.html Accessed January 15, 2010

[254] Desch S, Schmidt J, Kobler D, Sonnabend M, Eitel I, Sareban M, Rahimi K, Schuler G, Thiele H. Effect of cocoa products on blood pressure: systematic review and meta-analysis. *Am J Hypertens*. 2010 Jan;23(1):97-103

Hypertension prevalence declined from 86% to 68%. The BP decrease was accompanied by a sustained increase of S-nitrosoglutathione by 0.23 nmol/L, and a dark chocolate dose resulted in the appearance of cocoa phenols in plasma. White chocolate intake caused no changes in BP or plasma biomarkers. CONCLUSIONS: Data in this relatively small sample of otherwise healthy individuals with above-optimal BP indicate that **inclusion of small amounts of polyphenol-rich dark chocolate as part of a usual diet efficiently reduced BP and improved formation of vasodilative nitric oxide.**"[255]

o Randomized controlled single-blind crossover trial: Benefits of acute dark chocolate and cocoa ingestion on endothelial function (*American Journal of Clinical Nutrition*, Jul 2008): The purpose of this clinical trial (n = 45, BMI = 30, age = 53y) was to assess the acute effects of solid dark chocolate and liquid cocoa intake on endothelial function and blood pressure in overweight adults. First, subjects were randomly assigned to consume a **solid dark chocolate bar (containing 22 g cocoa powder)** or a cocoa-free placebo bar (containing 0 g cocoa powder). In the second part of the trial, subjects were randomly assigned to consume **sugar-free cocoa** (containing 22 g cocoa powder), **sugared cocoa** (containing 22 g cocoa powder), or a **placebo** (containing 0 g cocoa powder). "RESULTS: **Solid dark chocolate and liquid cocoa** ingestion improved endothelial function (measured as [ultrasound-visualized] flow-mediated dilatation) compared with placebo (**dark chocolate: 4.3%** compared with -1.8% [for placebo]; **sugar-free** and sugared cocoa: **5.7%** and 2.0% compared with -1.5%). **Blood pressure decreased after the ingestion of dark chocolate and sugar-free cocoa** compared with *placebo* (**dark chocolate: systolic, -3.2 mm Hg** compared with 2.7 mm Hg; and **diastolic -1.4 mm Hg** compared with 2.7 mm Hg; **sugar-free cocoa: systolic, -2.1 mm Hg** compared with 3.2 mm Hg; and **diastolic: -1.2** mm Hg compared with 2.8 mm Hg. **Endothelial function improved significantly more with sugar-free than with regular cocoa** (5.7 % compared with 2.0%). CONCLUSIONS: The acute ingestion of both solid dark chocolate and liquid cocoa improved endothelial function and lowered blood pressure in overweight adults. Sugar content may attenuate these effects, and sugar-free preparations may augment them."[256] The practical application of this research is important to communicate to patients: to obtain the cardioprotective benefits of chocolate, the chocolate must be consumed without added sugar, i.e., it must be **dark chocolate**, *not* sugar-sweetened milk chocolate.

o Population-based inception cohort study with 8-year follow-up: Chocolate consumption and mortality following a first acute myocardial infarction: the Stockholm Heart Epidemiology Program (*Journal of Internal Medicine*, Sep 2009): Authors of this study[257] followed 1,169 non-diabetic patients hospitalized with a confirmed first acute myocardial infarction (AMI) between 1992 and 1994. Participants self-reported usual chocolate consumption over the preceding 12 months with a standardized questionnaire distributed during hospitalization. Participants were followed for 8 years. "RESULTS: **Chocolate consumption had a strong inverse association with cardiac mortality.** When

---

[255] Taubert D, Roesen R, Lehmann C, Jung N, Schömig E. Effects of low habitual cocoa intake on blood pressure and bioactive nitric oxide: a randomized controlled trial. *JAMA*. 2007 Jul 4;298(1):49-60

[256] Faridi Z, Njike VY, Dutta S, Ali A, Katz DL. Acute dark chocolate and cocoa ingestion and endothelial function: a randomized controlled crossover trial. *Am J Clin Nutr*. 2008 Jul;88(1):58-63 http://www.ajcn.org/cgi/content/full/88/1/58

[257] Janszky I, Mukamal KJ, Ljung R, Ahnve S, Ahlbom A, Hallqvist J. Chocolate consumption and mortality following a first acute myocardial infarction: the Stockholm Heart Epidemiology Program. *J Intern Med*. 2009 Sep;266(3):248-57

compared with those never eating chocolate, the multivariable-adjusted hazard ratios were 0.73 (95% confidence interval, 0.41-1.31) for those consuming chocolate less than once per month, 0.56 (0.32-0.99) for up to once per week, and **0.34 (0.17-0.70) and twice or more per week respectively**. [Note: dose-response relationships suggest causality.] Chocolate consumption generally had an inverse but weak association with total mortality and nonfatal outcomes. In contrast, intake of other sweets was not associated with cardiac or total mortality. CONCLUSIONS: Chocolate consumption was associated with lower cardiac mortality in a dose dependent manner in patients free of diabetes surviving their first AMI. Although our findings support increasing evidence that chocolate is a rich source of beneficial bioactive compounds, confirmation of this strong inverse relationship from other observational studies or large-scale, long-term, controlled randomized trials is needed." The importance of this study is that it suggests that the cardioprotective benefits of cocoa are not limited to short-term alleviation of hypertension but extend to a more generalized cardioprotective benefit; beyond this, the reduction in all-cause mortality is what we would expect from a functional food rich in bioactive health-promoting constituents. Limitations to this study include the self-selected nature of the intervention and lack of randomization; however, the large number of subjects (n = 1,169) serves to mitigate these methodological limitations.

- **Melatonin**: Melatonin is an endogenously produced hormone from the pineal gland that plays numerous physiologic roles beyond its sedative effect for sleep promotion. Trace amounts of melatonin are found in food; when taken as a dietary supplement, melatonin demonstrates chronobiologic, sedative, antioxidant, antitumor, and immunomodulatory benefits.
  - Double-blind placebo-controlled clinical trial: Melatonin reduces night blood pressure in patients with nocturnal hypertension (*American Journal of Medicine*, Oct 2006): The authors begin by noting that "Nocturnal hypertension is associated with a high risk of morbidity and mortality." In this study, 38 adult patients medicated for HTN were randomized to receive melatonin 2 mg or placebo for 4 weeks. The results read as follows, "Melatonin treatment reduced nocturnal systolic BP significantly from 136 to 130 mm Hg (P=.011), and diastolic BP from 72 to 69 mm Hg (P=.002), whereas placebo had no effect on nocturnal BP." Thus, the authors concluded, "**Thus, an addition of melatonin 2 mg at night to stable antihypertensive treatment may improve nocturnal BP control in treated patients with nocturnal hypertension**."[258] This study showed that the addition of melatonin to standard drug treatment for HTN resulted in a **decrease in nighttime blood pressure of -6/-3 mm Hg** among patients with nocturnal HTN.
  - Randomized placebo-controlled double-blind crossover study: Blood pressure response to melatonin in type 1 diabetes (*Pediatric Diabetes*, Mar 2004): Eleven normotensive adolescent patients with type 1 diabetes of average 7-year duration and 10 healthy controls aged 14-18y participated in a randomized placebo-controlled double-blind crossover study of 5 mg melatonin for 1 week followed by a 1-week washout. Results showed that, "In the patients with type 1 diabetes, the decline in **diastolic blood pressure** during sleep was significantly greater on melatonin (17.8 mmHg) than on placebo (16.0

---

[258] Grossman E, Laudon M, Yalcin R, Zengil H, Peleg E, Sharabi Y, Kamari Y, Shen-Orr Z, Zisapel N. Melatonin reduces night blood pressure in patients with nocturnal hypertension. *Am J Med*. 2006 Oct;119(10):898-902

mmHg, p < 0.01)."[259] This study showed use of melatonin 5 mg resulted in a **decrease in nighttime diastolic pressure of -1.6 mm Hg** among type-1 diabetic patients. Longer duration of treatment would be expected to provide more robust results.

o Randomized, double-blind, placebo-controlled, crossover trial: Daily nighttime melatonin reduces blood pressure in male patients with essential hypertension (*Hypertension*, Feb 2004): The authors of this study show uncommon insight in their introduction which reads: "Patients with essential hypertension have disturbed autonomic cardiovascular regulation and circadian pacemaker function. ... Our objective was to determine whether enhancement of the functioning of the biological clock by repeated nighttime melatonin intake might reduce ambulatory blood pressure in patients with essential hypertension." Sixteen men with untreated essential HTN were given oral melatonin 2.5 mg at 1 hour before sleep, while 24-hour ambulatory blood pressure and actigraphic estimates of sleep quality were measured. Results showed that **repeated melatonin intake reduced systolic and diastolic blood pressure during sleep by -6 and -4 mm Hg, respectively**, with no effect on heart rate.[260]

- **Treatment of hypothyroidism**: Obviously, HTN caused by primary, secondary, or peripheral/metabolic hypothyroidism is not primary/essential HTN because it is due to the thyroid hormone disorder/dysfunction. Clinicians can choose any of several—or a combination thereof—methods to correct thyroid dysfunction, not the least of which are gluten avoidance in gluten-intolerant patients[261], zinc[262] and selenium supplementation[263,264,265,266], administration of *inactive* T4 (levothyroxine) and/or T3 (liothyronine, the most active thyroid hormone[267,268]), or the use of bovine/porcine-sourced glandular thyroid products—the latter should be avoided in patients with antibody-positive thyroid autoimmunity.

---

[259] Cavallo A, Daniels SR, Dolan LM, Khoury JC, Bean JA. Blood pressure response to melatonin in type 1 diabetes. *Pediatr Diabetes*. 2004 Mar;5(1):26-31

[260] Scheer FA, Van Montfrans GA, van Someren EJ, Mairuhu G, Buijs RM. Daily nighttime melatonin reduces blood pressure in male patients with essential hypertension. *Hypertension*. 2004 Feb;43(2):192-7

[261] "In most patients who strictly followed a 1-yr gluten withdrawal (as confirmed by intestinal mucosa recovery), there was a normalization of subclinical hypothyroidism. ... CONCLUSIONS: The greater frequency of thyroid disease among celiac disease patients justifies a thyroid functional assessment. In distinct cases, gluten withdrawal may single-handedly reverse the abnormality." Sategna-Guidetti C, Volta U, Ciacci C, Usai P, Carlino A, De Franceschi L, Camera A, Pelli A, Brossa C. Prevalence of thyroid disorders in untreated adult celiac disease patients and effect of gluten withdrawal: an Italian multicenter study. *Am J Gastroenterol*. 2001 Mar;96(3):751-7

[262] "RESULTS: Thirteen had low levels of serum free T3 and normal T4. ... After oral supplementation of Zn sulphate (4-10 mg/kg body weight) for 12 months, levels of serum free T3 and T3 normalized, serum rT3 decreased, and the TRH-induced TSH reaction normalized. ... CONCLUSION: Zn may play a role in thyroid hormone metabolism in low T3 patients and may in part contribute to conversion of T4 to T3 in humans." Nishiyama S, Futagoishi-Suginohara Y, Matsukura M, Nakamura T, Higashi A, Shinohara M, Matsuda I. Zinc supplementation alters thyroid hormone metabolism in disabled patients with zinc deficiency. *J Am Coll Nutr*. 1994 Feb;13(1):62-7

[263] Duntas LH, Mantzou E, Koutras DA. Effects of a six month treatment with selenomethionine in patients with autoimmune thyroiditis. *Eur J Endocrinol*. 2003 Apr;148(4):389-93 http://eje-online.org/cgi/reprint/148/4/389

[264] Gartner R, Gasnier BC, Dietrich JW, Krebs B, Angstwurm MW. Selenium supplementation in patients with autoimmune thyroiditis decreases thyroid peroxidase antibodies concentrations. *J Clin Endocrinol Metab*. 2002 Apr;87(4):1687-91 http://jcem.endojournals.org/cgi/content/full/87/4/1687

[265] "We recently conducted a prospective, placebo-controlled clinical study, where we could demonstrate, that a substitution of 200 wg sodium selenite for three months in patients with autoimmune thyroiditis reduced thyroid peroxidase antibody (TPO-Ab) concentrations significantly." Gartner R, Gasnier BC. Selenium in the treatment of autoimmune thyroiditis. *Biofactors*. 2003;19(3-4):165-70

[266] "A highly significant linear correlation between the T3/T4 ratio and indices of Se status was observed in the older group of subjects. Indices of Zn status did not correlate with thyroid hormones, ... We concluded that reduced peripheral T4 conversion is related to impaired Se status in the elderly." Olivieri O, Girelli D, Stanzial AM, Rossi L, Bassi A, Corrocher R. Selenium, zinc, and thyroid hormones in healthy subjects: low T3/T4 ratio in the elderly is related to impaired selenium status. *Biol Trace Elem Res*. 1996 Jan;51(1):31-41

[267] McDaniel AB. Thyroid Assessment: Controversies and Conundrums. Institute for Functional Medicine Fourteenth International Symposium. Tuscon, Arizona. May 23-26, 2007. Reviewed in more detail in: **Vasquez A**. Integrative Rheumatology. IBMRC 2006, 2007 and all future editions. http://optimalhealthresearch.com/rheumatology.html and **Vasquez A**. Musculoskeletal Pain: Expanded Clinical Strategies. Institute for Functional Medicine. May 2008

[268] Friedman M, Miranda-Massari JR, Gonzalez MJ. Supraphysiological cyclic dosing of sustained release T3 in order to reset low basal body temperature. *P R Health Sci J*. 2006 Mar;25(1):23-9

- **Berberine**: Used for it's health-promoting properties for thousands of years, berberine is a naturally-occurring plant alkaloid present in *Hydrastis canadensis* (goldenseal), *Coptis chinensis* (goldenthread), *Berberis aquifolium* (Oregon grape), *Berberis vulgaris* (barberry), and *Berberis aristata* (tree turmeric). Naturopathic physicians have commonly employed berberine-containing treatments for anti-infective benefits, particularly against gastrointestinal dysbiosis and respiratory tract infections. Within the past few years, numerous experimental studies in animals and clinical trials in humans have clearly demonstrated that berberine possesses many cardioprotective benefits, only one of which is its ability to promote normalization of elevated blood pressure. Given its well-documented antimicrobial effects, berberine quite likely improves overall health by reducing microbe-induced total inflammatory load (TIL) in addition to its direct benefits on metabolic and genomic processes. The current author appreciates berberine's numerous benefits demonstrated in clinical practice and in recent research, but prefers to limit its high-dose (1,000 mg/d) use to 3-6 months.
  - Clinical trial: Treatment of type 2 diabetes and dyslipidemia with the natural plant alkaloid berberine (*Journal of Clinical Endocrinology and Metabolism*, Jul 2008): In this randomized placebo-controlled trial, 116 patients with diabetes mellitus type-2 and dyslipidemia were randomly allocated to receive berberine (1,000 mg/d) or placebo for 3 months. Significant benefits were shown by berberine in insulin sensitivity, glucose homeostasis, and plasma lipids; except for mild to moderate constipation in five subjects in the berberine group, no major adverse effects were observed. With regard to blood pressure, results showed that systolic blood pressure decreased from 124 to 117 mm Hg and diastolic blood pressure decreased from 81 to 77 mm Hg in subjects treated with berberine (i.e., total reduction of -7/-4 mm Hg); this effect was superior to that shown in patients treated with placebo, who showed reduction of -3/-3 mm Hg. Note that these patients—even though they were diabetic—were not hypertensive. The authors concluded the text of their article by stating, "Given the benefits of berberine in lowering blood glucose, lipids, body weight, and blood pressures, we speculate that berberine may be used for patients with type-2 diabetes and metabolic syndrome."[269]
- **Garlic, *Allium sativum***: As both food and medicine, garlic has a long history of use dating back thousands of years. Cardioprotective mechanisms are reported to include alleviation of hypertension, reduction in serum lipids, platelet aggregation, and improvements in insulin sensitivity and endothelial function; obviously these vasculoprotective effects would be expected to produce additive and perhaps synergistic clinical benefits. Accordingly, epidemiologic studies have shown inverse relationships between garlic consumption and cardiovascular disease prevalence; while various mechanisms are in effect, a recent *in vitro* study showed that human RBCs convert garlic-derived organic polysulfides (allyl-substituted sulfur compounds) into hydrogen sulfide (H2S), an endogenous cell signaling molecule that exerts vasculoprotective effects in endothelial cells.[270] Per *in vitro* studies, extracts from garlic leaf and bulbs have shown ability to inhibit 5-lipoxygenase,

---

[269] Zhang Y, Li X, Zou D, Liu W, Yang J, Zhu N, Huo L, Wang M, Hong J, Wu P, Ren G, Ning G. Treatment of type 2 diabetes and dyslipidemia with the natural plant alkaloid berberine. *J Clin Endocrinol Metab*. 2008 Jul;93(7):2559-65
[270] Benavides GA, Squadrito GL, Mills RW, Patel HD, Isbell TS, Patel RP, Darley-Usmar VM, Doeller JE, Kraus DW. Hydrogen sulfide mediates the vasoactivity of garlic. *Proc Natl Acad Sci* U S A. 2007 Nov 13;104(46):17977-82 http://www.pnas.org/content/104/46/17977.full.pdf

cyclooxygenase, thrombocyte aggregation, and angiotensin-converting enzyme (ACE).[271] Garlic's antimicrobial properties and its numerous immune-enhancing effects might also be included in its spectrum of cardioprotective properties, since occult infections in general (i.e., multifocal polydysbiosis, particularly the orodental and gastrointestinal subtypes[272,273]) and bacterial lipopolysaccharide (LPS) in particular are correlated in humans with HTN, diabetes mellitus, and cardiovascular disease; additionally, garlic's ability to modulate cytokine expression and inhibit activation of NF-kappaB could further mitigate the cardiovasculotoxic effects of inflammation and dysbiosis.

- Critical review: Garlic and cardiovascular disease (*Journal of Nutrition*, Mar 2006): The authors note that epidemiologic studies show an inverse correlation between garlic consumption and progression of cardiovascular disease and that garlic has many cardioprotective properties:
  - Garlic inhibits enzymes involved in lipid synthesis, most notably beta-hydroxy-beta-methylglutaryl-CoA (HMG-CoA) reductase, the rate limiting enzyme in cholesterol biosynthesis,
  - Garlic decreases platelet aggregation,
  - Garlic prevents lipid peroxidation of erythrocytes and LDL,
  - Garlic improves antioxidant status,
  - Garlic inhibits angiotensin-converting enzyme (ACE).

  Garlic's inconsistent results on BP, the authors suggest, is due ❶ to a combination of usage of different garlic preparations, ❷ uncertainty about which active constituents should be provided, and their respective bioavailability, ❸ inadequate randomization, ❹ selection of inappropriate subjects, and ❺ insufficient duration of trials.[274] However, the gestalt of garlic's cardioprotective benefits strongly suggest its value in dietary utilization for patient's with elevated cardiovascular risk, which obviously includes patients with hypertension.

- Double-blind, placebo-controlled trial: Time-released garlic powder tablets lower systolic and diastolic blood pressure in men with mild and moderate arterial hypertension (*Hypertension Research*, Jun 2009): This double-blind placebo-controlled trial with 84 hypertensive men employed either ❶ time-released garlic powder tablets (600-2400 mg Allicor) or ❷ "regular garlic pills" (900 mg Kwai). Allicor (600 mg daily) resulted in a reduction of both systolic and diastolic blood pressures by 7.0 mm Hg and 3.8 mm, respectively, with no advantage noted at the higher 2400 mg/d dose. Use of Kwai resulted in a similar decrease in systolic blood pressure (-5.4 mm Hg), but no decrease in diastolic blood pressure was observed with Kwai. Noting that both garlic preparations provided an antihypertensive benefit, the authors concluded, "The results of this study show that time-released garlic powder tablets are more effective for the treatment of mild

[271] "The inhibition rates as IC50 values of both extracts for 5-LO, CO, and TA showed a good correlation with the %-content of the major S-containing compounds (thiosulfinates and ajoenes) of the various extracts. … In the ACE test the water extract of the leaves of wild garlic containing glutamyl-peptides showed the highest inhibitory activity followed by that of the garlic leaf and the bulbs of both drugs." Sendl A, Elbl G, Steinke B, Redl K, Breu W, Wagner H. Comparative pharmacological investigations of Allium ursinum and Allium sativum. *Planta Med*. 1992 Feb;58(1):1-7
[272] **Vasquez A**. Integrative Rheumatology. IBMRC 2006, 2007 and all future editions. http://optimalhealthresearch.com/rheumatology.html
[273] **Vasquez A**. Reducing Pain and Inflammation Naturally. Part 6: Nutritional and Botanical Treatments Against "Silent Infections" and Gastrointestinal Dysbiosis, Commonly Overlooked Causes of Neuromusculoskeletal Inflammation and Chronic Health Problems. *Nutritional Perspectives* 2006; January
[274] Rahman K, Lowe GM. Garlic and cardiovascular disease: a critical review. *J Nutr*. 2006 Mar;136(3 Suppl):736S-740S

and moderate arterial hypertension than are regular garlic supplements."[275] Of note, a different study by the same primary author (Igor Sobenin) also demonstrated lipid-modifying effects of time-released garlic powder tablets, (Allicor 600 mg daily) in a double-blinded placebo-controlled randomized study among 42 men: total cholesterol reduced by >7%, LDL cholesterol reduced by approximately 12%, and HDL cholesterol increased by 11.5%.[276]

o Systematic review and meta-analysis: Effect of garlic on blood pressure (*BioMed Central - Cardiovascular Disorders*, Jun 2008): The authors reviewed eleven criteria-selected studies published between 1955 and October 2007 identified from Medline and Embase databases. Results showed, "...the mean decrease in the hypertensive subgroup was 8.4 mm Hg for SBP (n = 4; $p < 0.001$), and 7.3 mm Hg for DBP (n = 3; $p < 0.001$). Regression analysis revealed a significant association between blood pressure at the start of the intervention and the level of blood pressure reduction (SBP: $R = 0.057$; $p = 0.03$; DBP: $R = -0.315$; $p = 0.02$). CONCLUSION: Our meta-analysis suggests that garlic preparations are superior to placebo in reducing blood pressure in individuals with hypertension."[277]

o Meta-analysis: Effects of garlic on blood pressure in patients with and without systolic hypertension (*Annals of Pharmacotherapy*, Dec 2008): For this meta-analysis, the authors performed a systematic search of MEDLINE, CINAHL, and the Cochrane Central Register of Controlled Trials to identify randomized controlled trials in humans evaluating garlic's effect on blood pressure; to this was added a manual search of published literature, and the complete search yielded 10 trials for review. The authors write, "Garlic reduced SBP by **16.3 mm Hg** (95% CI 6.2 to 26.5) and DBP by **9.3 mm Hg** (95% CI 5.3 to 13.3) compared with placebo in patients with elevated SBP. ... This meta-analysis suggests that garlic is associated with blood pressure reductions in patients with an elevated SBP although not in those without elevated SBP. Future research should focus on the impact of garlic on clinical events and the assessment of the long-term risk of harm."[278] While the authors' cautionary note is reasonable given the potential for adverse effects from nearly any agent, the risk-benefit scales appear to tip in favor of garlic's overall cardioprotective, antihypertensive, eulipidemic benefits in addition to its wide availability and low cost; indeed, given these results, an argument could be made that withholding garlic—like CoQ10 and fish oil and vitamin D3—could be unethical in patients at elevated CVD risk.

o Beyond mechanics and into the Functional Medicine Matrix: Garlic (*Allium sativum* L.) modulates cytokine expression in lipopolysaccharide-activated human blood thereby inhibiting NF-kappaB activity (*Journal of Nutrition*, Jul 2003): Given the well established role of inflammation in CVD initiation and progression, and the potential role of occult infections (i.e., various types and locations of dysbiosis), an anti-inflammatory mechanism to garlic's cardioprotective benefits is intriguing. The authors write, "This paper shows that garlic powder extracts (GPE) and single garlic metabolites modulate

---

[275] Sobenin IA, Andrianova IV, Fomchenkov IV, Gorchakova TV, Orekhov AN. Time-released garlic powder tablets lower systolic and diastolic blood pressure in men with mild and moderate arterial hypertension. *Hypertens Res*. 2009 Jun;32(6):433-7

[276] Sobenin IA, Andrianova IV, Demidova ON, Gorchakova T, Orekhov AN. Lipid-lowering effects of time-released garlic powder tablets in double-blinded placebo-controlled randomized study. *J Atheroscler Thromb*. 2008 Dec;15(6):334-8 http://www.jstage.jst.go.jp/article/jat/15/6/334/_pdf

[277] Ried K, Frank OR, Stocks NP, Fakler P, Sullivan T. Effect of garlic on blood pressure: a systematic review and meta-analysis. *BMC Cardiovasc Disord*. 2008 Jun 16;8:13 http://www.biomedcentral.com/1471-2261/8/13

[278] Reinhart KM, Coleman CI, Teevan C, Vachhani P, White CM. Effects of garlic on blood pressure in patients with and without systolic hypertension: a meta-analysis. *Ann Pharmacother*. 2008 Dec;42(12):1766-71

lipopolysaccharide (LPS)-induced cytokine levels in human whole blood" and that these favorable modifications in GPE-altered cytokine levels "reduced nuclear factor (NF)-kappaB [NFkB] activity in human cells exposed to these samples." Pretreatment with garlic extracts reduced LPS-induced production of proinflammatory cytokines interleukin (IL)-1beta from 15.7 to 6.2 micro g/L (greater than 50% reduction) and tumor necrosis factor (TNF)-alpha from 8.8 to 3.9 micro g/L (greater than 50% reduction). In an additional experiment, exposure of human embryonic kidney cell line (HEK293) cells to GPE-treated blood sample supernatants reduced NFkB activity by 25% (unfertilized garlic) and 41% (sulfur-fertilized garlic). The authors conclude, "In summary, garlic may indeed promote an anti-inflammatory environment by cytokine modulation in human blood that leads to an overall inhibition of NFkB activity in the surrounding tissue."[279] Beyond demonstrating an anti-inflammatory effect of garlic, this study also serves as a reminder that suppression of proinflammatory cytokines can favorably downregulate NFkB activity in a "retroactive" manner, since NFkB activation generally precedes elaboration of proinflammatory cytokines; thus, garlic extracts appear capable of breaking the proinflammatory vicious cycle, illustrated below from Vasquez.[280]

Activation of NF-kappaB leads to enhanced transcription of pro-inflammatory mediators, and the vicious cycle of inflammation-induced activation of NF-kappaB

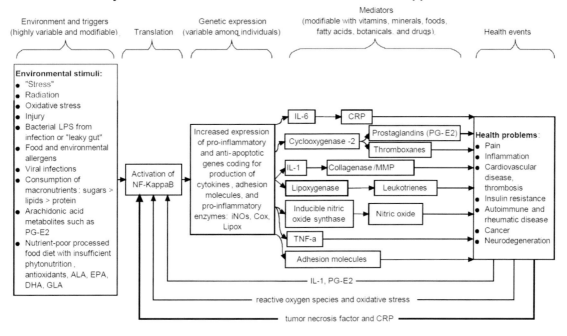

---

[279] Keiss HP, Dirsch VM, Hartung T, Haffner T, Trueman L, Auger J, Kahane R, Vollmar AM. Garlic (Allium sativum L.) modulates cytokine expression in lipopolysaccharide-activated human blood thereby inhibiting NF-kappaB activity. *J Nutr*. 2003 Jul;133(7):2171-5 http://jn.nutrition.org/cgi/content/full/133/7/2171
[280] **Vasquez A**. Integrative Orthopedics. IBMRC 2007; page 373. **Vasquez A**. Integrative Rheumatology. IBMRC 2006, 2007; page 433. **Vasquez A**. Chiropractic and Naturopathic Mastery of Common Clinical Disorders. IBMRC 2009; page 553.

- **Nattokinase**: Nattokinase is an enzyme extracted and purified from a Japanese food called Natto, a cheese-like food made from fermented soybeans.
  - Randomized, controlled trial: Effects of nattokinase on blood pressure (*Hypertension Research*, Aug 2008): 86 participants with pre-hypertension or stage-1 hypertension received nattokinase (2,000 FU/capsule) or a placebo capsule for 8 weeks. **Net changes in systolic and diastolic blood pressure were -5.55 mmHg and -2.84 mmHg, respectively, after the 8-week intervention**. Renin activity levels dropped by -1.17 ng/mL/h for the nattokinase group compared with the control group. The authors concluded, "...nattokinase supplementation resulted in a reduction in SBP and DBP. These findings suggest that increased intake of nattokinase may play an important role in preventing and treating hypertension."[281]
- **Treatment of "central neurogenic hypertension" with surgical techniques—focus on neurovascular (de)compression at the level of the left ventrolateral medulla oblongata**: Physical compression or mechanical irritation of neuronal structures can result in systemic hypertension through a variety of mechanisms; these mechanisms have been most thoroughly described in the biomedical research literature under the disciplines of Surgery as well as of Manipulative Medicine and Spinal Manipulation. Readers should appreciate the basic commonality between surgical intervention and physical manipulation: both interventions have the potential to change physiological relationships experienced between two or more anatomical components via either direct means (i.e., physical alteration) or indirect mechanisms (e.g., reflexive or adaptive changes). Several studies describing surgical alleviation of neurogenic hypertension will be reviewed and summarized here, while those focusing on manipulative treatments will be discussed in the subsection immediately following. Dr Peter Jannetta (MD) is generally attributed with the origination of the concept of medulla oblongata vascular compression by the vertebral artery as one of the causes of hypertension; he has demonstrated that neurovascular compression can be surgically treated by microvascular decompression (MVD) with resultant antihypertensive benefits.[282] Initially, patients selected for surgery (generally either left retromastoid craniectomy or lateral suboccipital craniectomy) were chosen for their cranial nerve deficits such as trigeminal neuralgia, hemifacial spasm, glossopharyngeal neuralgia, Bell's palsy, and spasmodic torticolis, and alleviation of HTN was a "side benefit" of the surgery. Later, severe recalcitrant HTN alone without overt CN deficits has become sufficient basis for surgery in carefully selected patients in appropriate treatment centers, perhaps within a prospective research protocol (per Geiger *et al* in 1998, reviewed below). Also, as stated in a previous section, the perspectives offered by Reis[283] is worthy of recall because of the two truths contained therein, namely that neurogenic contributors to HTN can be ❶ *omnipotent* (Reis: "A neural or neurochemical imbalance in brain **can produce** hypertension"), or ❷ *contributory/amplificatory* (Reis: "Impaired NTS [nucleus tract solitarius] function can produce an **amplification** of the action of the environmental stresses on blood pressure. Thus environmental stimuli or the expression of behaviors which normally result in trivial elevations of blood pressure will, after the NTS is perturbed, result in marked elevations [of

---

[281] Kim JY, Gum SN, Paik JK, Lim HH, Kim KC, Ogasawara K, Inoue K, Park S, Jang Y, Lee JH. Effects of nattokinase on blood pressure: a randomized, controlled trial. *Hypertens Res.* 2008 Aug;31(8):1583-8
[282] See "Discussion": http://www.ncbi.nlm.nih.gov/pmc/articles/PMC1346999/pdf/annsurg00224-0102.pdf
[283] Reis DJ. The nucleus tractus solitarius and experimental neurogenic hypertension: evidence for a central neural imbalance hypothesis of hypertensive disease. *Adv Biochem Psychopharmacol.* 1981;28:409-20

blood pressure])." Per descriptions in the literature, central neurogenic hypertension is typically difficult to control, chronic, and progressive.

o   <u>Review and case series: Neurogenic hypertension etiology and surgical treatment: observations in 53 patients (*Annals of Surgery*, Mar 1985)</u>: Among 53 patients with simultaneous cranial nerve (CN) dysfunctions and systemic hypertension, 51 of these 53 patients were noted to have arterial compression of the **left lateral medulla oblongata** by looping arteries at the base of the brain (note: neurovascular compression was *not* noted in *normotensive* patients); all 53 patients underwent left retromastoid craniectomy and microvascular decompression (MVD) for treatment of the cranial nerve dysfunctions. More specifically, treatment by vascular decompression of the medulla was performed in 42 of the 53 patients. Relief in the hypertension was seen in 32 of 42 (76% of total) patients and improvement in four; "improvement" was defined in this article as "more than a 20-mm drop in both systolic and diastolic pressures", and thus the total number of patients with a highly meaningful antihypertensive response was 36 of 42 (85% of total). Generally, the problem appears localized to the left vagal nerve and the left lateral medulla oblongata (more specifically between the inferior olive anteriorly and the root entry zone (REZ) or CN 9 and CN 10 posteriorly) and is most commonly caused by arteriosclerosis and arterial ectasia which contribute to arterial elongation and looping, which can eventually lead to pulsatile compression of the left lateral medulla; hypertension can then develop from compromise of the balance in the neural control systems that regulate blood pressure. Because systemic HTN can further contribute to arterial elongation, a vicious cycle of HTN followed by progressive arterial ectasia followed by additional neuronal compromise which results in additional HTN may be established. Specific arteries that can contribute to medulla and/or cranial nerve neurocompression include the left vertebral artery (due to normal anatomy, ectasia, or severe atherosclerosis), posterior inferior cerebellar artery, superior cerebellar artery, basilar artery, and anterior inferior cerebellar artery. Neural pathways involved in BP control relevant to this discussion as reviewed by Jannetta *et al* include ❶ carotid baroreceptors with afferents traveling in CN 9 to the nucleus tractus solitarius, ❷ aortic baroreceptors with afferents traveling in CN 10 (i.e., aortic vagal afferents), ❸ cardiac vagal afferents, ❹ descending sympathetic output to vascular smooth muscle; of these, *vasodepressive* cardiac vagal afferent fibers are unmyelinated and are thus most susceptible to compression (per Jannetta *et al*, 1985) thus neurovascular compressive compromise at the REZ of the medulla likely causes HTN (at least in large part) by disinhibition, i.e., impairment of vasodepressive cardiac vagal afferent input. Furthermore, the pulsatile nature of arterial compression may cause greater damage than constant pressure and may desynchronize neural cardiac-pressor control centers. Following surgical displacement of the offending artery away from the brainstem by use of an implant of plastic sponge, muscle, or synthetic felt, many of these patients with chronic systemic HTN who had been taking "large doses of strong medications" were able to reduce or altogether discontinue their drug dependency over the course of days to months following the surgical microvascular decompression. Thus, neurovascular decompression of the left medulla oblongata is a treatment option worth considering in affected and appropriately selected patients with chronic hypertension.[284]

o Exemplary case report: Decreases in blood pressure and sympathetic nerve activity by microvascular decompression of the rostral ventrolateral medulla in essential hypertension (*Stroke*, Aug 1999): The authors of this report begin by noting that neurovascular compression of the rostral ventrolateral medulla, a major center regulating sympathetic nerve activity, may be causally related to essential hypertension, and that microvascular decompression of the rostral ventrolateral medulla decreases elevated blood pressure in some patients. A 47-year-old male with "essential hypertension" and hemifacial nerve spasms was found to have neurovascular compression of the rostral ventrolateral medulla and facial nerve; **microvascular decompression of the rostral ventrolateral medulla successfully reduced blood pressure from 152/110 mm/Hg** while on amlodipine, quinapril, and doxazosin **to 108/74** with only low-dose quinapril (the authors note that quinapril was being tapered to discontinuation at time of publication). Microvascular decompression of the rostral ventrolateral medulla also reduced plasma and urine norepinephrine levels, and reduced other markers of excessive sympathetic nerve activity.[285] Reductions in plasma and urine epinephrine and norepinephrine following MVD in their case report were listed previously in this chapter and are included here again in context to show that post-intervention reduction in sympathetic nerve activity can be documented objectively, and that clinical antihypertensive benefits (BP reductions of 10–30% at 48h postsurgery) can be associated with *relative* reductions in catecholamine levels that may be *within* or *outside of* the normal reference range:

- plasma epinephrine (range <0.93 nmol/L) dropped from 0.22 to <0.05,
- plasma norepinephrine (range 0.89 - 3.37 nmol/L) dropped from 0.95 to 0.30,
- urine epinephrine (range 5.5 – 76.4 nmol/d) dropped from 83.5 to 26.2,
- urine norepinephrine (range 0.06 – 0.024 mmol/d) dropped from 0.52 to 0.39.

o Prospective study (n=14) with long-term follow-up: Temporary reduction of blood pressure and sympathetic nerve activity in hypertensive patients after microvascular decompression (*Stroke*, Jan 2009): Fourteen patients with essential hypertension underwent microvascular decompression of the brain stem. Vasoconstrictor muscle sympathetic nerve activity (recorded by microneurography: burst frequency, bursts/min) and blood pressure (24-hour profiles) were measured before surgery and 7 days, 3 months, and every 6 months postoperatively. **Muscle sympathetic nerve activity** decreased from preoperative levels (35 bursts/min) a nadir of 19 bursts/min before spontaneously rising again to 34 bursts/min; in more detail, the sympatholytic benefits were noted as follows: a reduction from preoperative levels of 35 bursts/min to 19 bursts/min (at 3 months postoperatively), 19 bursts/min (at 6 months), and 23 bursts/min (at 12 months) but were minimized to statistical and clinical insignificance to 28 bursts/min (at 18 months) and 34 bursts/min (at 24 months). **Systolic and diastolic blood pressure** decreased from 162/98 mm Hg preoperatively to 133/85 mm Hg (at 7 days postoperatively), 136/86 mm Hg (at 3 months), 132/85 mm Hg (at 6 months), 132/85 mm Hg (at 12 months), and then increased to 158/96 mm Hg at 24 months; thus both

---

[284] Jannetta PJ, Segal R, Wolfson SK Jr. Neurogenic hypertension: etiology and surgical treatment. I. Observations in 53 patients. *Ann Surg.* 1985 Mar;201(3):391-8 http://www.ncbi.nlm.nih.gov/pmc/articles/PMC1250685/pdf/annsurg00109-0147.pdf

[285] Morimoto S, Sasaki S, Takeda K, Furuya S, Naruse S, Matsumoto K, Higuchi T, Saito M, Nakagawa M. Decreases in blood pressure and sympathetic nerve activity by microvascular decompression of the rostral ventrolateral medulla in essential hypertension. *Stroke.* 1999 Aug;30(8):1707-10

blood pressure and hypersympathotonia were reduced by MVD surgery but both returned many months thereafter. The fact that hypersympathotonia returned before HTN would appear to indicate that the former caused the latter despite the fact that the latter can cause the former as discussed in a preceding section. (For review: hypersympathotonia causes HTN via vasoconstriction and activation of the renin-angiotensin system, while HTN causes activation of the sympathetic nervous system when chronic HTN induces elongation and tortuosity of the arteries [left vertebral artery, posterior inferior cerebellar artery, superior cerebellar artery, basilar artery, and anterior inferior cerebellar artery] that are in close proximity to the nucleus tract solitarius and related pressure-controlling neurologic structures.) The authors of the study[286] conclude that, "The data are a hint for sympathetic overactivity as a pathomechanism in this subgroup of patients" while also noting that in the patients selected for this study, the life-threatening severity of their hypertension was probably of such an extent that end-organ damage and various neurohormonal vicious cycles had probably already been established so as to make long-term suppression of HTN particularly challenging. The authors of this paper, published in 2009 in the American Heart Association's journal *Stroke*, close with the following four main conclusions:

- Neurovascular compression of the RVLM causes neurogenic hypertension mediated by a central sympathetic hyperactivity.
- Surgical microvascular decompression reduces central sympathetic outflow and reduces blood pressure, at least temporarily.
- In this study, neither blood pressure improvement nor sympathetic deactivation was sustained effectively for the long-term.
- Until more conclusions are established regarding appropriate imaging and patient selection, MVD is not recommended as cure for HTN and should be performed only in prospective study protocols.

o <u>Case series (n=8) using microvascular decompression as therapy for severe chronic HTN: Decrease of blood pressure by ventrolateral medullary decompression in essential hypertension (*The Lancet*, Aug 1998)</u>: Previously, this group of authors showed that 83% of patients with primary HTN, 24% of patients with secondary HTN, and 7% of normotensive controls showed evidence of looping vessels at the left ventrolateral medulla consistent with neurovascular compression as seen on magnetic resonance imaging. In this study, the authors investigated whether neurosurgical microvascular decompression substantially decreases blood pressure long-term in patients with severe essential hypertension. Eight patients—all of whom had experienced one or more life-threatening hypertensive crises—who had received *three or more* antihypertensive drugs without adequate control of blood pressure, intolerable side-effects, or both, underwent microvascular decompression at the root-entry zone (REZ) of cranial nerves 9 and 10 after neurovascular compression of the ventrolateral medulla oblongata was seen with magnetic resonance angiography (MRA). Three months after surgery, blood pressure and antihypertensive drug regimens had decreased substantially in 7 of 8 patients. Four patients who were followed up for more than 1 year became normotensive. No

---

[286] Frank H, Heusser K, Geiger H, Fahlbusch R, Naraghi R, Schobel HP. Temporary reduction of blood pressure and sympathetic nerve activity in hypertensive patients after microvascular decompression. *Stroke*. 2009 Jan;40(1):47-51 http://stroke.ahajournals.org/cgi/content/full/40/1/47

complications associated with decompression occurred except that one patient experienced a transient vocal-cord paresis after the laryngeal part of the vagus nerve was maneuvered during surgery. The authors concluded, "We showed a direct causal relation between raised blood pressure and irritation of cranial nerves 9 and 10. A subgroup of patients with essential hypertension may exist who have secondary forms of hypertension related to neurovascular compression at the ventrolateral medulla and who may be successfully treated with decompression."[287]

- **Treatment of "central and peripheral neurogenic hypertension" with chiropractic and osteopathic manipulative techniques**: Spinal manipulative therapy has proven safe and effective for musculoskeletal spinal pain as well as some extra-spinal disorders, notably asthma.[288] Chiropractic manipulation differs from the types of manipulation provided by other professions (e.g., osteopathic, naturopathic) and thus research substantiating the effectiveness of chiropractic manipulation may not be applicable to different manipulative approaches. Based on the material reviewed in the previous section, readers should already have some appreciation of the rationale, potential benefits, and potential limitations of upper cervical spinal manipulation for the treatment of HTN via reduction of **central neurogenic hypertension** (i.e., potentially via reduction in medullary compression and NTS irritation) as well as via reduction of **peripheral neurogenic hypertension** insofar as upper cervical and cranial/occipital manipulation has been suggested—mainly by theory, extrapolation of anatomy, and less so by strong clinical trials—to potentially decompress, de-facilitate, or otherwise generally relieve from mechanical (and thus physiologic) irritation CN 9, CN 10, and the cervical sympathetic ganglia, all of which are involved in regulation of blood pressure, heart rate, and/or peripheral resistance.

  o Double-blind, placebo-controlled pilot study of chiropractic upper cervical manipulation for treatment of hypertension: Atlas vertebra realignment and achievement of arterial pressure goal in 50 *pain-free* hypertensive patients (*Journal of Human Hypertension*, May 2007): The authors introduce this study by writing, "Anatomical abnormalities of the cervical spine at the level of the Atlas

> **Cervical spine manipulation for chronic hypertension**
>
> "At week 8, there were differences in **systolic BP (-17 mm Hg, NUCCA [chiropractic]** versus -3 mm Hg, placebo) and **diastolic BP (-10 mm Hg, NUCCA [chiropractic]** versus -2 mm Hg). … No adverse effects were recorded. We conclude that restoration of Atlas alignment is associated with marked and sustained reductions in BP similar to the use of two-drug combination therapy.
>
> … most single agent antihypertensive [drugs] yield an 8 mm Hg drop in pressure in people with Stage 1 hypertension…"
>
> Bakris G, Dickholtz M Sr, Meyer PM, et al. Atlas vertebra realignment and achievement of arterial pressure goal in hypertensive patients: a pilot study. *J Hum Hypertens*. 2007 May;21(5):347-52. For video footage, see the official NUCCA website at http://www.nucca.org/ and: http://www.youtube.com/watch?v=aXfIlp5KBT0, http://www.youtube.com/watch?v=3z-LQvs_BXo

---

[287] Geiger H, Naraghi R, Schobel HP, Frank H, Sterzel RB, Fahlbusch R. Decrease of blood pressure by ventrolateral medullary decompression in essential hypertension. *Lancet*. 1998 Aug 8;352(9126):446-9

[288] For review, see Vasquez A. *Chiropractic and Naturopathic Mastery of Common Clinical Disorders*. 2009, especially pages 347-386. http://optimalhealthresearch.com/clinical_mastery For another intriguing and insightful brief review discussing manipulation and asthma, see also: Mein EA, Greenman PE, McMillin DL, Richards DG, Nelson CD. Manual medicine diversity: research pitfalls and the emerging medical paradigm. *J Am Osteopath Assoc*. 2001 Aug;101(8):441-4 http://www.jaoa.org/cgi/reprint/101/8/441

vertebra are associated with relative ischemia of the brainstem circulation and increased blood pressure (BP). Manual correction of this mal-alignment has been associated with reduced arterial pressure." The authors used a double-blind, placebo-controlled design at a single center among 50 *pain-free* drug-naïve (n=26) or washed-out (n=24) patients with Stage 1 hypertension; patients were randomized (n=25 in each treatment or placebo group) to receive a National Upper Cervical Chiropractic (NUCCA) procedure or a sham procedure. Significant findings included the following, "At week 8, there were differences in **systolic BP (-17 mm Hg, NUCCA** versus -3 mm Hg, placebo) and **diastolic BP (-10 mm Hg, NUCCA** versus -2 mm Hg [placebo]). … No adverse effects were recorded. We conclude that restoration of Atlas alignment is associated with marked and sustained reductions in BP similar to the use of two-drug combination therapy."[289] Because the patients were pain-free at the start of the study, relief of neck pain due to treatment with chiropractic manipulation does not explain antihypertensive benefit. Pretreatment patient assessment for NUCCA-specific chiropractic treatment (rather than all forms of chiropractic treatment, of which exist many different techniques) includes ❶ assessment for dynamic functional leg-length discrepancy in the supine position while the patient actively rotates the neck left and right in the transverse/horizontal plane, ❷ paracervical skin temperature measurement, ❸ postural analysis with a proprietary device named Anatometer[290] for precise static biomechanical measurements, and ❹ craniocervical radiographs which are then assessed with NUCCA-specific roentgenometric techniques. As with any procedure involving exposure to ionizing radiation, long-term risk-to-benefit ratios need to be determined and compared to the risk-to-benefit ratios of other treatments; if radiographic evaluation could be eliminated from the assessment protocol without compromising treatment safety efficacy then both costs and risks would be reduced. Impressively, **85% of patients in the chiropractic-treated group required only one treatment to maintain the antihypertensive benefit during the study's duration of two months**. NUCCA treatment of the atlas vertebra resulted in significant measurable changes in atlas lateral and rotational positioning (measured by the pre- and post-treatment radiographs), lateral displacement of C-7 vertebra, frontal-plane pelvic distortion, and lateral-plane pelvic distortion which correlated with the reductions in blood pressure. Lastly for this discussion, readers should appreciate that the NUCCA chiropractic technique uses a gentle direct technique of spinal manipulation which is not the typical, more forceful, high-velocity low-amplitude (HVLA) type which is more commonly used by the majority of chiropractic and (to a lesser extent) osteopathic clinicians; in the current article, NUCCA treatment was described as "A series of precise, subtle, external nudges causes Atlas to recoil into normalized alignment, reseating occipital condyles into Atlas' lateral masses", and the technique's delivery can be observed in the video hyperlinks provided and specifically at http://www.nucca.org/. Readers of this section may have—hopefully—seen beyond the "data" of this study to appreciate the paradigm shifts implied, which are built upon and/or include but are not limited to the following: ❶ a single gentle musculoskeletal

---

[289] Bakris G, Dickholtz M Sr, Meyer PM, Kravitz G, Avery E, Miller M, Brown J, Woodfield C, Bell B. Atlas vertebra realignment and achievement of arterial pressure goal in hypertensive patients: a pilot study. *J Hum Hypertens*. 2007 May;21(5):347-52
[290] Anatometer is manufactured by Benesh Corporation: http://www.anatometer.com

manipulation delivered to the atlas vertebra can lower blood pressure just as effectively as the use of two-drug antihypertensive treatment; ❷ a single gentle musculoskeletal manipulation delivered to the atlas vertebra can affect the positioning of the C-7 vertebra as well as pelvic positioning in the frontal and lateral planes; ❸ subtle changes (invisible to the naked eye) in the positioning of the atlas vertebra, the C-7 vertebra, and pelvis correspond to clinically and statistically significant changes in arterial pressure that can be sustained for at least two months; ❹ individually and collectively, these findings present us with paradigm shifts regarding the local effects of spinal manipulation, body-wide musculoskeletal effects of spinal manipulation, and the systemic nonmusculoskeletal effects of spinal manipulation.

- o Case report: Chiropractic management of a hypertensive patient (*Journal of Manipulative and Physiological Therapeutics*, Oct 1993): In this single illustrative case report, the clinician authors describe their experience with a 38-year-old male previously diagnosed with and medicated for chronic essential HTN; the patient's presenting complaints were HTN, drug-related side effects, and low back pain. Chiropractic treatment emphasized specific contact, short lever arm spinal adjustments as the primary mode of chiropractic care. The authors noted, "**During the course of chiropractic treatment, the patient's need for hypertensive medication was reduced**. The patient's medical physician gradually withdrew the medication over 2 months." Appreciating the BP-normalizing benefits of chiropractic manipulation and how these benefits may—paradoxically—lead to iatrogenic complications in patients whose physiologic homeostasis is restored, the authors caution that "specific contact short lever arm spinal adjustments may cause a hypotensive effect in a medicated hypertensive patient that may lead to complications (e.g., hypotension). Since a medicated hypertensive patient's blood pressure may fall below normal while he or she is undergoing chiropractic care, it is advised that the blood pressure be closely monitored and medications adjusted, if necessary, by the patient's medical physician."[291] This point about the very real potential of drug-induced iatrogenic hypotension is analogous to the drug-induced iatrogenic hypoglycemia that can occur when patients' utilization of non-drug integrative treatments overlaps with their previously prescribed drug treatments. When working with medicated and particularly *polymedicated* HTN patients, clinicians have the responsibility to implement treatment in such a way as to minimize the risk for hypotension (and other complications, such as hypoglycemia, respectively)—for example, by starting with lower doses of nutritional supplements, implementing treatment in a step-wise manner, coordinating modifications/reductions in drug doses, and having the patient use more frequent self-monitoring (of blood pressure, blood glucose [etc], respectively); patient education and documentation of informed consent are standards of care for all interventions.

- o Randomized, controlled trial (active treatment, placebo treatment, or no treatment): Effects of chiropractic treatment on blood pressure and anxiety (*Journal of Manipulative and Physiological Therapeutics*, Dec 1988): This study (n=21) differs from the previously cited article "Atlas vertebra realignment and achievement of arterial pressure goal in hypertensive patients"[292] in that ❶ the thoracic spine (T1-T5) rather than the upper

[291] Plaugher G, Bachman TR. Chiropractic management of a hypertensive patient. *J Manipulative Physiol Ther*. 1993 Oct;16(8):544-9
[292] Bakris G, Dickholtz M Sr, Meyer PM, Kravitz G, Avery E, Miller M, Brown J, Woodfield C, Bell B. Atlas vertebra realignment and achievement of arterial pressure goal in hypertensive patients: a pilot study. *J Hum Hypertens*. 2007 May;21(5):347-52

cervical spine was the area of treatment, ❷ the treatment used a mechanical chiropractic adjusting device rather than manual manipulation, and ❸ the study included assessment for anxiety as well as for changes in BP, rather than BP alone. The mechanical chiropractic adjusting device used in this study is the Activator Adjusting Instrument[293], which delivers a highly-localized 28-pound thrust within 1/300 of a second. The authors concluded, "**Results indicated that systolic and diastolic blood pressure decreased significantly in the active treatment condition**, whereas no significant changes occurred in the placebo and control conditions. State anxiety significantly decreased in the active and control conditions. **Results provide support for the hypothesis that blood pressure is reduced following chiropractic treatment.**"[294]

o   Pilot study to determine the feasibility of a practice-based randomized controlled clinical trial with three parallel groups: Chiropractic adjustments and brief massage treatment at sites of subluxation in subjects with essential hypertension (*Journal of Manipulative and Physiological Therapeutics*, May 2002): Treatment groups in this study consisted of ❶ chiropractic manipulation, ❷ brief soft tissue massage, or ❸ nontreatment control group.[295] The patient group consisted of 23 subjects, 24-50 years of age, with systolic or diastolic primary HTN. In the active chiropractic treatment group, the intervention consisted of 2 months of full-spine chiropractic care using Gonstead technique, described as specific-contact, short-lever-arm adjustments delivered at motion segments exhibiting signs of subluxation. The massage group received brief effleurage at localized regions of the spine believed to be exhibiting signs of subluxation. The nontreatment control group rested alone for a period of approximately 5 minutes in a treatment room. In both the chiropractic and massage therapy groups, all subjects were classified as either overweight or obese; in the control group, only 2 subjects were overweight—these baseline differences in the study groups are important as they suggest that more patients in the chiropractic treatment group probably had HTN as a component of the metabolic syndrome rather than HTN due specifically and solely to a musculoskeletal lesion. The authors report that at the end of the study period, the BP change was -6.3 mm Hg in the chiropractic group, -1.0 mm Hg in the massage group, and -7.2 mm Hg in the relaxation "control" group. The authors of this pilot feasibility study noted several methodological shortcomings and logistical complications of their study, most notably the limited subject pool of patients who have hypertensive disease but who are not taking medications for its control. A larger study group would have allowed improved randomization and thus equilibration of baseline patient characteristics such as body mass index, which shows a strong correlation with severity of HTN.

o   Review: Spinal manipulation and the efficacy of conservative therapeusis for the treatment of hypertension (*Journal of Manipulative and Physiological Therapeutics*, Mar 1986): These authors review relevant chiropractic and osteopathic literature of the day (published in 1986) and conclude that manipulative therapy has a rational basis in the

---

[293] http://www.activator.com. Activator Methods International, Ltd. (AMI) produces the Activator Method Chiropractic Technique and the associated Activator Adjusting Instrument. See also http://www.activatoronline.com/

[294] Yates RG, Lamping DL, Abram NL, Wright C. Effects of chiropractic treatment on blood pressure and anxiety: a randomized, controlled trial. *J Manipulative Physiol Ther.* 1988 Dec;11(6):484-8

[295] Plaugher G, Long CR, Alcantara J, Silveus AD, Wood H, Lotun K, Menke JM, Meeker WC, Rowe SH. Practice-based randomized controlled-comparison clinical trial of chiropractic adjustments and brief massage treatment at sites of subluxation in subjects with essential hypertension: pilot study. *J Manipulative Physiol Ther.* 2002 May;25(4):221-39

treatment of HTN based on the potential for spinal manipulation to promote restoration of homeostasis via reducing excess sympathetic tone and effecting a relative increase in parasympathetic tone. Spinal regions that are emphasized are ❶ the upper cervical spine (occiput-atlas) which correlates anatomically with the superior cervical sympathetic ganglia, ❷ the upper thoracic spine (T1-T6, especially T2-T3) which correlates with the thoracic sympathetic ganglia, and ❸ the lower thoracic spine (T11-T12) which correlates with sympathetic innervation via the renal ganglia/plexus that services the kidney. Clinicians should recall that sympathetic activation of the kidney increases production of renin (the enzyme), angiotensin-2 (the product of renin acting upon angiotensin-1), and aldosterone (produced by the adrenal cortex in response to stimulation by angiotensin-2) to effect systemic vasoconstriction and retention of sodium and water to increase blood volume and blood pressure. Comprehensive chiropractic treatment should include (but not be limited to) manipulation of spinal segments, massage and manipulation of regional soft tissues, mobilization of the ribs, and the implementation of dietary, nutritional, exercise/lifestyle, sleep pattern, and psychoemotional interventions. The authors conclude that alleviating HTN via resolution of musculoskeletal dysfunction and restoration of homeostasis is a more logical and ethical approach than is the suppression of HTN with the use of drugs that commonly have iatrogenic consequences.[296]

o Review: Effect of osteopathic manipulative therapy on autonomic tone as evidenced by blood pressure changes and activity of the fibrinolytic system (JAOA—Journal of the American Osteopathic Association, May 1968): The authors[297] describe their prior research experience with humans and animals in the investigation of the effects of osteopathic manipulation on blood pressure and activation of the sympathetic nervous system as evaluated by changes in the fibrinogen/fibrinolytic system; they wrote, "In research which has been conducted in this laboratory to date, the relationship between changes in blood pressure and the manipulative therapeutic approach not only has been validated in human beings with hypertension, but has also been demonstrated in normal persons as well as in experimental dogs. **Soft tissue manipulation of the upper thoracic and cervical vertebrae leads in almost every case to a decrease in blood pressure.**" These authors go on to note that "…a cumulative effect does occur, four or five treatments accomplishing a greater effect than a single treatment…" and that a reduction in pro-coagulative tendency occurs as evidenced by reductions in fibrinogen and other serum levels of coagulation factors.

o Clinical trial: Effect of osteopathic manipulative therapy on autonomic tone as evidenced by blood pressure changes and activity of the fibrinolytic system (JAOA—Journal of the American Osteopathic Association, Jun 1969): The authors[298] describe the use of an interventional protocol consisting of ❶ 15 minutes of rest in the supine position during measurement of blood pressure and laboratory indices, ❷ 5 minutes of soft tissue manipulation in the prone position ("The patient then assumes the prone position for 5 minutes. During this time soft tissue manipulation is applied equally to the left and right

[296] Crawford JP, Hickson GS, Wiles MR. The management of hypertensive disease: a review of spinal manipulation and the efficacy of conservative therapeusis. J Manipulative Physiol Ther 1986 Mar ;9(1):27-32

[297] Celander E, Koenig AJ, Celander DR. Effect of osteopathic manipulative therapy on autonomic tone as evidenced by blood pressure changes and activity of the fibrinolytic system. J Am Osteopath Assoc. 1968 May;67(9):1037-8

[298] Fichera AP, Celander DR. Effect of osteopathic manipulative therapy on autonomic tone as evidenced by blood pressure changes and activity of the fibrinolytic system. J Am Osteopath Assoc. 1969 Jun;68(10):1036-8

posterior cervical and thoracic areas. In the control experiment, no soft tissue manipulation is performed during this time interval.", and ❸ 15 minutes of rest in the supine position during measurement of blood pressure and laboratory indices. The authors wrote, "In our study after an initial rest period followed by manipulation there was a significant decrease (p<0.01) in both diastolic and systolic pressure in the hypertensive group." Furthermore, they noted laboratory evidence of reduced hemoconcentration, erythrocyte sedimentation rate, and a reduction in fibrinogen levels in 96% of patients with hypertension; among normotensive patients, fibrinogen levels decreased in 32% and increased in 51%.

o Blinded randomized clinical trial using chiropractic and diet to treat hypertension: Treatment of Hypertension with Alternative Therapies (THAT) Study (*Journal of Hypertension*, Oct 2002): Given the potential implications of the use of "chiropractic spinal manipulation and diet" for the treatment of HTN, this study[299] is potentially important and therefore worthy of detailed analysis; this is even more true when we appreciate that the authors titled this study "Treatment of Hypertension with Alternative Therapies" and thus broadened the implications of this article to all modes, genres, professions, and interventions that might fall under the rubric of "alternative medicine." The authors begin their abstract by stating that the objective of the study is to "To examine the effect of spinal manipulation on blood pressure" and then go on to describe the design of the study to be "This randomized clinical trial compared the effects of chiropractic spinal manipulation and diet with diet alone for lowering blood pressure in participants with high-normal blood pressure or stage I hypertension."; thus, from the outset, the study was not designed to truly investigate "alternative therapies" *per se* as the term should be applied (if it is to be used at all[300]) but rather only "chiropractic spinal manipulation" (within which many techniques exist) and "diet" (which can mean different things to different clinicians and can be variously applied to and implemented by diverse groups of patients). Per the study description, "One hundred and forty men and women, aged 25-60 years, with high-normal blood pressure or stage I hypertension, were enrolled. One hundred and twenty-eight participants completed the study. INTERVENTIONS: (i) A dietary intervention program administered by a dietitian [Diet] or (ii) a dietary intervention program administered by a doctor of chiropractic in conjunction with chiropractic spinal manipulation [DC+diet]. The frequency of treatment for both groups was three times per week for 4 weeks, for a total of 12 visits"; this might appear to be a reasonable study design insofar as it distinguishes the effectiveness of Diet from the effectiveness of DC+diet however the comparison is not balanced insofar as the Diet group was seen by a full-time dietician (who focuses only on nutrition) versus the diet advice administered by a full-time clinician with a broader range of responsibilities and daily actions who then by definition has less time to dedicate to dietary advice. Results of the study showed that "Average decreases in systolic/diastolic blood pressure were -4.9/5.6 mmHg for diet group and -3.5/4.0 mmHg for the chiropractic group. Between

---

[299] Goertz CH, Grimm RH, Svendsen K, Grandits G. Treatment of Hypertension with Alternative Therapies (THAT) Study: a randomized clinical trial. *J Hypertens*. 2002 Oct;20(10):2063-8

[300] MacIntosh A. "Understanding the Differences Between Conventional, Alternative, Complementary, Integrative and Natural Medicine" *Townsend Letter* 1999 July http://www.tldp.com/medicine.htm This is a brilliant -- if not obvious -- explanation that was powerful for the time it was written, and beyond. This article should be required reading for politicians, clinicians, and policy-makers and others with a stake in so-called "CAM."

group changes were not statistically significant. CONCLUSIONS: For patients with high normal blood pressure or stage I hypertension, chiropractic spinal manipulation in conjunction with a dietary modification program offered no advantage in lowering either diastolic or systolic blood pressure compared to diet alone." This conclusion could easily be interpreted to imply that chiropractic manipulation is inefficacious and/or that the dietary advice given by the chiropractic doctors in this study was of poor quality or that it even negated the potential benefits of spinal manipulation (or vice versa). For many clinicians and policy-makers, this is probably as far as they might go with this study, with the take-away message being that both diet and spinal manipulation are essentially inefficacious for the treatment of hypertension. However, detailed reading of the article reveals several study characteristics that may have contributed to the report of inefficacy, which is suspiciously noteworthy for its severity in both groups treated with diet therapy. Critique of the article follows:

> | Respect for truth |
> | --- |
> | "…I think that respect for the truth and a concern for the truth—these are among the foundations of civilization. And I was for a long time disturbed by the lack of truth and lack of concern for the truth that I seemed to observe in much of the speech and writing that was being produced." |
> | Professor Emeritus Harry G. Frankfurt PhD. *On Bullshit*, Princeton University Press. http://press.princeton.edu/video/frankfurt/ |

❶ Participants in this study did not have hypertension to begin with. Participants for this study were relatively healthy with systolic pressures below 160 mmHg and diastolic pressures of 85–99 mmHg. Since patients with less severe degrees of hypertension would be expected to show less numerical improvement, this study's use of subjects with average blood pressure of 135/88 mm Hg—a level which is considered nonhypertensive—slanted the scales toward a conclusion of inefficacy because the subjects had no disease. In a very real sense therefore, the title of this article "Treatment of Hypertension with Alternative Therapies" is doubly misleading; first, the subjects did not have hypertension to begin with, and second, among the hundreds of "alternative therapies" available, only two were chosen for this study. A more accurate title of this article (as will become more clear in the following discussion) would have been "Treatment of nonhypertensive patients with weak dietary advice and nonspecific chiropractic manipulation lowers blood pressure by approximately 4/5 mm Hg."

❷ The diet advice given was standardized rather than customized. The study reads "DC/Diet patients received all of the written diet information received by the Diet group, but from the chiropractor. In addition, DC/Diet participants received chiropractic spinal manipulation." Regardless of whether the information was delivered by a chiropractic doctor or an experienced registered dietitian, the information was "prefabricated" rather than customized per patient. Better results are obtained when treatments are customized per patient; thus, this study failed to offer optimal diet therapy and not surprisingly found lackluster results.

❸ The study prohibited the use of several of the most effective "alternative therapies" for hypertension despite being titled "Treatment of Hypertension with Alternative Therapies". The requirement that "All treating clinicians agreed not to offer dietary advice other than that included in the standard diet instructions (e.g.

supplements), aerobic exercise advice, acupuncture or activator treatment to participants" was good for the standardization of the study but it eliminates the possibility of implementing some of the most valuable "alternative therapies" that exist for the treatment of HTN, such as vitamin D3, CoQ-10, exercise, and weight loss. Again, the study was given a misleading title.

❹ The "specific diet intervention instructions" used in this study were suspiciously inefficacious and were not disclosed in the materials and methods. The authors fail to disclose the details of their diet intervention, thus ensuring that their study can never be subjected to scientific scrutiny by replication. Further, the only details provided are that subjects were given "written instructions on how to modify their current diet and were also given diet sheets, which included low-fat, low-salt recipes. The nutritionist explained the diet and covered a pre-set list of topics." The low-fat aspect of the diet strongly suggests that the diet was low in the health-promoting cardioprotective fatty acids previously reviewed, namely ALA, GLA, EPA, DHA, and oleic acid; the diet pattern suggested was probably neither Paleo nor Mediterranean. Diets that are relatively lower in fat tend to be by default relatively higher in carbohydrates, which leads to insulin release, retention of sodium and water, systemic inflammation, endothelial dysfunction, and the perpetuation of hypertension. That the diet was highly inefficacious is made obvious by the results provided in Table @ of their study, which shows that participants in both groups lost essentially zero weight (-0.8 lbs) during the 4-week study duration; this proves the inappropriate design of the intervention diet provided to both groups because clinical experience and clinical trials have repeatedly demonstrated that patients on effective optimized diets generally lose 4-8 lbs per month. Failure of the diet intervention to effect weight loss in both therapeutic groups having an average BMI of 30.5 *which clearly shows that most patients in this study met objective criteria for obesity* provides objective proof that the interventional diet was of faulty design; again, these patients should have lost 4-8 lbs during the study period had the diet been appropriately designed, delivered, and implemented.

❺ The subjects in the chiropractic group were healthier than those in the diet group. "The diet group overall weighed more than the chiropractic group at 200 versus 187 lbs, and this difference was borderline significant (P = 0.06)." Regardless of statistical significance, the clinical significance of a 13-pound weight difference is noteworthy. Because the DC+diet group was healthier from the start of the study, less improvement would have been expected. The DC+diet group also had fewer smokers and fewer patients taking medications; these differences between groups were not mathematically significant, but they may have been additively or synergistically clinically significant.

❻ Exclusion of patients with pain negates the recognition of chiropractic's probable antihypertension-via-analgesia benefit from spinal manipulation. The authors acknowledge, "Because spinal manipulation has been reported to lower pain levels for individuals with back pain, and there is a correlation between pain levels and blood pressure, participants reporting average pain levels of five or above on a 0–10 point visual analog type scale were also excluded." In the real world, if a patient with pain and hypertension has both conditions relieved via spinal manipulation's antinociceptive benefits, then this would be documented as a dual benefit from a single therapy. This study's design eliminated the possibility of detecting and documenting this benefit.

❼ <u>Positive selection of subjects likely confused the findings of the study</u>. Recruitment methods quite likely selected patients already using "alternative therapies" and who may have already been "maximally improved" from their former baseline of hypertension severity. "All methods [of subject recruitment] incorporated the same message and highlighted the alternative therapy aspect of the study."; this would have resulted in positive selection of patients interested in and perhaps already using CAM treatments including nutritional supplements and exercise. Since the authors did not include use of nutritional supplements, exercise, acupuncture, diet therapy (etc) in their exclusion criteria, some of the test subjects may have already been maximally treated with self-selected or professionally-directed treatments. The exclusion criteria failed to control for this important variable.

❽ <u>With all of these problems invalidating the design, implementation, and conclusions of the study, its publication calls into question either the intent or the wakefulness of the journal's editorial board</u>. Supposedly, the purpose of having an Editor and an Editorial Board is to create what is called the "peer-review" process by which an article undergoes at least some modicum of scientific *or perhaps even intellectual* scrutiny prior to publication so that drivel is not incorporated into our collective body of knowledge that we use to direct patient care. Bad research is bad enough, but when it becomes codified by publication in a journal such as *Journal of Hypertension* and then indexed into Medline by the US National Library of Medicine, then it has the power to influence the healthcare received by thousands of patients, nationally and internationally. The publication of articles such as this calls into question the value and reliability of the peer-review process, the quality and intent of journal editors and editorial boards, and the value of doctorate-level training *prima facie* if its results are such as these. In sum, this study had numerous flaws—the three most important are ❶ the patients were nonhypertensive from the start, ❷ the dietary intervention was standardized (rather than individualized) and was clearly inefficacious as demonstrated by its inability to effect weight loss in a group of obese patients, and ❸ the interventional diet was prefabricated rather than reflecting the type of dietary intervention that a chiropractic doctor might actually use in real clinical practice. Thus, this study completely failed to offer any legitimate insight into the "treatment of hypertension with alternative therapies" and it unscientifically and inaccurately slanders both chiropractic manipulation and dietary intervention for the treatment of hypertension.

Musculoskeletal Manipulation and Manual Medicine: Samples of Commonly Used Chiropractic and Osteopathic Techniques

Manual medicine in general and spinal manipulation in particular are mentioned in nearly every section of **Integrative Orthopedics**, and select techniques are described with accompanying text and photographs. Manipulative techniques are included in this textbook to remind practitioners of a few of the more useful and commonly applied maneuvers and to provide descriptions and citations for refinement of their application. However, the level of detail provided here is insufficient unless the reader has received hands-on professionally-supervised training in an accredited institution wherein other important concepts have been taught and implemented under experienced guidance. Competence and proficiency in the art and skill of manipulation cannot be learned from a textbook; these can only be approached with personal mentoring and in-person coursework amply provided in colleges and post-graduate trainings specializing in manipulative technique. **Manipulative medicine** is a *time-space* objective-subjective-intuitive **kinesthetic phenomenon** which might be described as occurring in four dimensions—*anteroposterior, transverse/horizontal, vertical*, and *chronological* due to variations in speed and power; all the while, the doctor is monitoring subjective and objective responses of the what might be considered the fifth dimension—the doctor's dynamic *perception of, influence upon*, and *interaction with* the patient's affect, posture, muscle tension, dynamic joint positioning, tissue response, and compressive tension. As the doctor assesses and provides force to the spinal lesion, the patient's response changes the quality of the lesion, and so the doctor must adapt to a moving target—the lesion being treated. These sections presume professional training by the reader has already been begun or completed and that the reader is familiar with manipulative concepts, technique, terminology, and commonly used abbreviations. Again, the intention here is to remind clinicians of manipulation in general and these specific techniques in particular; only a few *subjectively chosen* techniques are included from the several hundred vertebral, myofascial, visceral, and extravertebral/extremity maneuvers that are available.

General Layout and Description of Manipulative Techniques
- **Patient position**: Patient position may be prone, supine, lateral recumbent or "side-posture", standing, or seated.
- **Doctor position**: Usually standing, either upright, forward flexed, or using an oblique fencer's stance; knees are almost always bent in order to bring doctor's torso near treatment area to increase mechanical force from the upper limbs.
- **Assessment**: *Subjective*: Patient's experience, sensations, and effect on daily living. *Motion palpation*: Intersegmental motion analysis generally used for assessing the presence of vertebral (and extravertebral) motion restrictions or aberrant motion. The patient is relaxed and passive while the doctor takes the joint that is being assessed through its normal range of motion in various directions while palpating near adjacent joint surfaces for nuance of pattern and end-feel. Motion lesions are generally described as **restrictions** and/or **hypermobility.** *Static palpation*: Boney and other landmarks are compared symmetrically and to the practitioner's experience for the detection of abnormality consistent with subjective, motion, and soft tissue findings; static palpations are usually described in terms of prominence or relative superiority/inferiority when compared symmetrically. *Soft tissue palpation*: Subcutaneous tissues, tendons, ligaments, muscles, and joint spaces can be palpated to assess myofascial status and function. Soft tissue findings commonly include edema, joint swelling, bogginess, "ropiness" of muscles, tenderness, restricted motion of soft tissues, hypertonicity, spasm, and adhesions.

- **Treatment contact, directive hand**: Generally the doctor provides therapeutic contact with one of the contact surfaces of the hands—digital, hypothenar, pisiform, index, thumb, thenar, or "calcaneal" (when using the "heel" of the hand)[301]; other contacts such as the elbow or chest might be used for deep myofascial or compressive manipulative procedures, respectively. The treatment contact is provided by the directive hand—the hand that is delivering the therapeutic thrust or direction; the treatment contact of the directive hand works in cooperation with the supporting contact of the supporting hand.
- **Supporting contact**: This generally refers to the supportive hand, the one that is either holding or stabilizing the patient in contrast to the hand that is delivering the manipulative force. The indirect hand can provide at least three different types of support.
- **Neutral/stabilizing support**: The supportive hand plays a relatively neutral role with regard to the manipulative force.
- **Synergistic/cooperative/assistive support**: In this situation, the supportive hand moves with the therapeutic force in the same direction. An example of this would be the head-holding hand moving in the same direction as the directive/treatment hand when performing manipulation of the upper cervical spine.
- **Counterthrust/resistive support**: In this situation, the supportive hand moves counter/against the direction of the directive force. A common example is the force applied to the upper torso when performing a side-posture manipulation of the lumbar spine or pelvis.
- **Pretreatment positioning**: Joints are generally—but not always—taken to the end range of motion before the manipulative thrust is applied because the general purpose of high-velocity low-amplitude manipulation is to break myofascial restrictions and/or forcefully activate joint proprioceptors. In chiropractic terms, this is described as taking the joint into the **paraphysiologic space** because the physiologic range of motion is temporarily though safely exceeded[302]; in osteopathic terms, this part of the range of motion is described as being within the range of **passive motion** but still within the **anatomic barrier.**[303]
- **Therapeutic action**: For joint manipulation, this is usually the **chiropractic adjustment** or the **osteopathic HVLA** (high-velocity low-amplitude thrust); **thrust vectors** can be straight, curvilinear, or rotary into **segmental directions** of rotation, extension, flexion, side-bending, traction, and combinations of those directions. Other common manual techniques include stretching, post-isometric stretching, massage, compression, percussion, joint springing, mobilization, articulation, traction.
- **Resources**: The most commonly cited works here include: *States Manual, Second Edition* by Constance Kirk DC, Dana Lawrence DC, Nila Valvo DC; *Kimberly Manual, 2006 Edition* by Paul Kimberly DO; *Chiropractic Technique* by Thomas Bergmann DC, David Peterson DC, Dana Lawrence DC; *Chiropractic Management of Spine-Related Disorders* edited by Meridel Gatterman DC.
- **Context**: The following samples are an obvious underrepresentation of the diversity of manipulative techniques available, which easily numbers into the hundreds. Various techniques are—of course—described with greater range and depth in textbooks wholly dedicated to the topic of manipulation, which by itself is not the subject of this text. Rather, **use these samples as reminders to include *or at least consider* manipulative therapy** when composing your treatment plan; oftentimes, the manipulative therapy is the fastest and shortest route between *pain* and *relief from pain* and also from *dysfunction* toward *homeostasis*.

---

[301] Kirk CR, Lawrence DJ, Valvo NL. States Manual of Spinal, Pelvic, and Extravertebral Technics. Second Edition. Lombard, Illinois: National College of Chiropractic; 1985, page 20

[302] Leach RA. (ed). The Chiropractic Theories: A Textbook of Scientific Research, 4th Edition. Baltimore:Lippincott,Williams,Wilkins,2004,page 32-33

[303] Kimberly PE. Outline of Osteopathic Manipulative Procedures. The Kimberly Manual 2006. Kirksville College of Osteopathic Medicine. Walsworth Publishing , Marceline, Mo, page 7

Cervical Spine: Rotation Emphasis for Treatment of Rotational Restriction

- **Patient position**: Supine, neck slightly flexed.
- **Doctor position**: At 45° angle from head of table; may also be in a more lateral position aside the patient's head and neck; while it is acceptable to assess and set-up with straight legs, at the time of impulse, doctor's legs should be bent to provide the doctor with greater power, stability, and biomechanical safety.
- **Assessment**: <u>Subjective</u>: neck pain, headaches. <u>Motion palpation</u>: rotation restriction; primary or compensatory hypermobile segments may be detected above or below the restricted segment. <u>Static palpation</u>: vertebra may feel relatively posterior on the side opposite the rotational restriction, e.g., a right rotational restriction may present with a relative left rotational malposition that brings the vertebral lamina and articular pillars posterior on the left. <u>Soft tissue</u>: tenderness, may also have muscle spasm.
- **Treatment contact**: Doctor uses either an index or proximal phalange contact on the posterior aspect of the transverse process and/or articular pillar. The doctor's vector and hence the positioning of the forearm of the contact hand must change depending on the level of the cervical spine that is being treated. Notice in this photograph that the thumb of the doctor's contact hand is placed on the angle of the mandible, this is more to help anchor the contact and stabilize the doctor's wrist than to assist with the manipulation; very little pressure and zero thrust are applied to the mandible.
- **Supporting contact**: Head is held into rotation and slight flexion; as with all techniques, nuanced adjustments in flexion-extension, rotation, and side-bending are made until the premanipulative tension is localized to the specific direction/tissue of restriction.
- **Pretreatment positioning**: Slight flexion and extension may be used below and above the treatment contact to create motion restriction at the adjacent motion segments; this helps to focus the motion and therapeutic force at the specific; importantly the support hand is largely responsible for proper positioning with the correct amount of nuanced flexion-extension and side-bending so that the rotational force is accurately delivered.

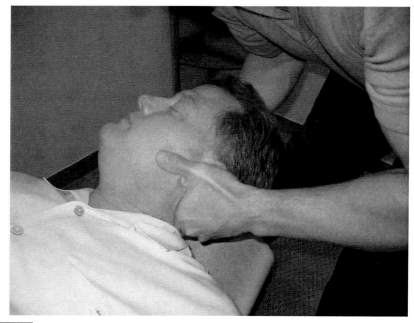

- **Therapeutic action**: Rotational thrust with contact hand; support hand keeps head off table so that rotational motion can occur.
- **Resources**: *States Manual, Second Edition*[304] page 47

---

[304] Kirk CR, Lawrence DJ, Valvo NL. <u>States Manual of Spinal, Pelvic, and Extravertebral Technics. Second Edition</u>. Lombard, Illinois: National College of Chiropractic; 1985

Cervical Spine: Lateral Flexion (Side-Bending) Emphasis; Treatment of Lateral Malposition or Lateral Flexion Restriction

- **Patient position**: Supine, head is neutrally placed—neither flexed nor extended; slight flexion is allowed; this technique can also be adapted for use in a seated position.
- **Doctor position**: At 45° angle from head of table; may also be in a more lateral position aside the patient's head and neck.
- **Assessment**: Subjective: neck pain, headaches. Motion palpation: lateral flexion restriction. Static palpation: vertebra may feel laterally displaced. Soft tissue: tenderness, may also have muscle spasm.
- **Treatment contact**: Using an index (metacarpal-phalangeal) contact at the tip of the transverse process or slightly posterior to the transverse process; an index phalangeal contact can also be used on the articular pillars as long as doctor is careful not to thrust in a rotational direction; notice in this picture how Dr Harris has the forearm of his contact hand perfectly aligned in the treatment vector, which is almost purely in the patient's transverse/horizontal plane; notice also that Dr Harris has his knees bent and is forward flexed to bring his torso closer to his contact and thereby minimize stress and strain on his own shoulders; with slight modifications in vector direction, this technique can be applied throughout the cervical spine from C0-C7.
- **Supporting contact**: Lateral aspect of head, opposite contact; generally the supporting hand is neutral, however it can supply some traction and can help induce lateral flexion at impulse; with more aggressive adjustments, the supporting hand can supply a counterforce to minimize motion following the application of a faster and more powerful thrust.
- **Pretreatment positioning**: Lateral flexion at the targeted cervical segment; the slightest amount of contralateral rotation is applied. The doctor establishes an "index" contact on the posterolateral aspect of the cervical vertebrae (i.e., the "paravertebral gutter"[305]).

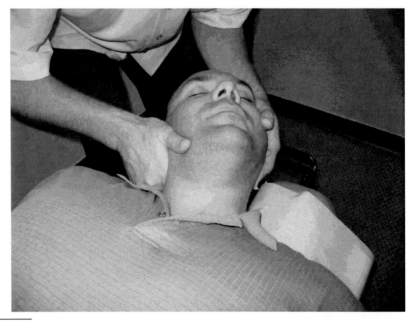

- **Therapeutic action**: Establish minimal premanipulative tension once the end range of motion has been reached, then use quick and very shallow trust to induce lateral flexion.
- **Resources**:[306, 307, 308]

---

[305] "There are eleven pairs of thoracic zygapophysial joints, with one pair located between each vertebral level. These joints contribute to the floor of the 'paravertebral gutter', the region between the spinous and transverse processes. In the cervical and lumbar regions this gutter is shallow, formed mainly by the laminae and articular pillars, whereas in the thoracic region the gutter is deeper and broader, being formed by the laminae, articular pillars and transverse processes." Cornwall J, Mercer s. Thoracic Zygapophysial joint palpation. *New Zealand Journal of Physiotherapy* 2006: 34(2); 56-59
[306] Kirk CR, Lawrence DJ, Valvo NL. States Manual of Spinal, Pelvic, and Extravertebral Technics. Second Edition. Lombard, Illinois: National College of Chiropractic; 1985
[307] Kimberly PE. Outline of Osteopathic Manipulative Procedures. The Kimberly Manual 2006. Kirksville College of Osteopathic Medicine. Walsworth Publishing , Marceline, Mo
[308] Bergmann TF, Peterson DH, Lawrence DJ. Chiropractic Technique. New York; Churchill Livingstone: 1993

Thoracic Spine: Supine Thoracic Flexion, "Anterior Thoracic"

- **Patient position**: Supine on table; to facilitate positioning, patient's leg opposite doctor may be flexed at hip and knee with foot flat on table. Patient is instructed to place right hand on right trapezius and left hand on left trapezius; the patient is instructed, "Place your hands behind your neck and do not interlace your fingers."
- **Doctor position**: Facing table at 45° angle in fencer stance with feet apart and knees bent. Doctor must be midline and balanced at time of impulse in order to provide symmetric force.
- **Assessment**: <u>Subjective</u>: mechanical midback pain. <u>Motion palpation</u>: flexion restriction. <u>Static palpation</u>: extension malposition; focal loss of thoracic kyphosis; focal approximation of spinous processes consistent with extension malposition; vertebra may feel anteriorly displaced. <u>Soft tissue</u>: local paravertebral myohypertonicity is common; local paresthesia is very common, and patients are often exquisitely sensitive to the lightest touch.
- **Treatment contact**: Closed fist contact with spinous processes between doctor's distal interphalangeal joints and thenar eminence; the trust is delivered from the doctor's chest through the patient's arms which compress the patient's chest; Dr Harris (pictured as patient) prefers to use a forearm contact to reduce wear-and-tear on his hands and wrists.
- **Supporting contact**: The supporting contact is the hand-arm that supports the patient's upper torso; the supporting contact pulls toward the doctor and superiorly at time of impulse.
- **Pretreatment positioning**: Patient lifts head from table; doctor uses supporting hand and arm to lift patient off table to allow placement of contact hand and to facilitate spinal flexion.
- **Therapeutic action**: Doctor uses **body drop thrust** technique at 45° toward ground and toward the head of the table; the trust should simultaneously generate compression and long-axis traction; the contact hand remains tense to provide solid leverage inferior to the targeted motion segment; the supporting hand and arm pull toward doctor at time of impulse to accentuate traction and spinal flexion; patient is instructed to breath deeply then relax and exhale; upon exhalation, the doctor establishes and maintains premanipulative tension to achieve joint flexion, then applies HVLA thrust; the thrust must be fast and shallow; slow and deep impulses can sprain the interspinous ligaments.

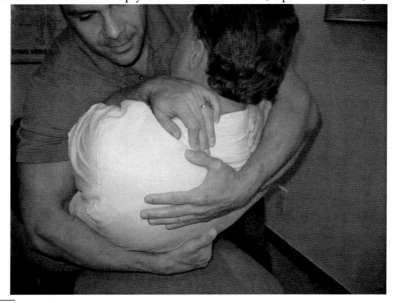

- **Resources**: *States Manual*[309] page 67, *Kimberly Manual, 2006 Edition*[310] page 93-94, *Chiropractic Technique*[311] page 349

[309] Kirk CR, Lawrence DJ, Valvo NL. <u>States Manual of Spinal, Pelvic, and Extravertebral Technics. Second Edition</u>. Lombard, Illinois: National College of Chiropractic; 1985
[310] Kimberly PE. <u>Outline of Osteopathic Manipulative Procedures. The Kimberly Manual 2006</u>. Kirksville College of Osteopathic Medicine. Walsworth Publishing , Marceline, Mo
[311] Bergmann TF, Peterson DH, Lawrence DJ. <u>Chiropractic Technique</u>. New York; Churchill Livingstone: 1993

Posterior Ribs: Manipulation of the Costovertebral Junction

- **Patient position**: Supine on table; to facilitate positioning, patient's leg opposite doctor may be flexed at hip and knee with foot flat on table. Patient's arms are crossed over the front of their body; my preference is that the arm closest to the doctor (the arm opposite to the side of the thorax being treated) is atop.
- **Doctor position**: Modified fencer's stance facing cephalad.
- **Assessment**: <u>Subjective</u>: mechanical paraspinal pain; often discomfort with inhalation. <u>Motion palpation</u>: stiffness at the affected costo-transverse junction. <u>Static palpation</u>: prominence in the posterior direction of the rib near the costo-transverse junction. <u>Soft tissue</u>: local tenderness to palpation is very common.
- **Treatment contact**: Contact on the specific rib immediately lateral to the costo-transverse junction is made with the doctor's thenar eminence with the doctor's hand in a firm, pursed position. Initial contact is made superior and lateral to the final location of manipulative contact in order to attain proper premanipulative tissue tension.
- **Supporting contact**: The doctor's supporting (noncontact) hand along with the doctor's torso deliver the manipulative thrust through the patient's arm atop the patient's thorax.
- **Pretreatment positioning**: Patient is supine; after positioning the contact hand posteriorly, the doctor grasps the patient's upper arm, then pulls downward and then applies progressively compressive force (body weight, not muscular force) while raising the supporting contact and rolling the patient over atop the contact hand.
- **Therapeutic action**: Body-drop thrust generally superiorly and laterally in the direction of the patient's opposite shoulder; the angle of the thrust changes depending on the spinal-costal level being treated, with more superior segments requiring a more superiorly directed thrust, while lower segments require a progressively laterally-yet-sagittally directed thrust. Notably, the manipulative thrust is applied to the anterior thorax via contact with the patient's upper arm, yet the true manipulative force is from posterior to anterior via the doctor's thenar eminence positioned posteriorly.

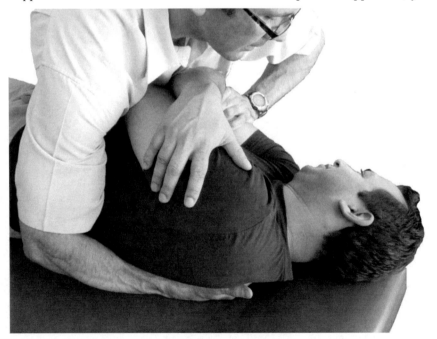

- **Resources**: See appropriate sections in previously listed textbooks, particularly *States Manual, Second Edition*[312], and *Chiropractic Technique*.[313]

---

[312] Kirk CR, Lawrence DJ, Valvo NL. <u>States Manual of Spinal, Pelvic, and Extravertebral Technics. Second Edition</u>. Lombard, Illinois: National College of Chiropractic; 1985
[313] Bergmann TF, Peterson DH, Lawrence DJ. <u>Chiropractic Technique</u>. New York; Churchill Livingstone: 1993

Lumbar Side-Posture Rotational Manipulation/Mobilization, "Lumbar Roll"

- **Patient position**: Side-posture, lateral recumbent; lower leg is straight; upper leg is flexed at hip and knee with foot behind calf of the leg that is straight on the table.
- **Doctor position**: Facing table at 45° angle in fencer stance with feet apart and knees bent. Notice in the photograph how Dr Harris approximates his center of gravity and biomechanical leverage directly over his therapeutic contact.
- **Assessment**: Subjective: asymptomatic or with lumbar pain; lumbar disc herniation[314], use a cautious and gentle technique if the patient has radicular symptoms, and as a rule of thumb the patient should be positioned with the symptomatic leg down on the table (e.g., "good leg *up*, bad leg *down*"). Motion palpation: focal restrictions with focal pain are perhaps better treated with a lesion-specific technique such as the "push-pull" maneuver; this is an excellent technique if the patient has general discomfort without localization, or has pain and will benefit from rotational manipulation for its muscle stretching and afferent-stimulating analgesic benefits. Static palpation: minor displacements and malpositions may be noted; if specific biomechanical lesions are found, use a more specific technique such as the "push-pull" maneuver. Soft tissue: palpate for hypertonicity/spasm with or without relative muscle atrophy; patients with chronic low-back pain tend to have weaker extensor muscles than the general population; however, during an acutely painful episode, their otherwise weakened muscles will be hypertonic thus leading to a paradoxical **atrophic hypertonicity.**
- **Treatment contact**: Doctor uses a palmar/calcaneal ("heel of the hand") contact over the lumbar facet joints. Rotation and traction are provided at the time of impulse with the doctor's thigh which is compressed and providing long-axis traction against the patient's upper leg, which is flexed at the hip and knee.
- **Support**: Doctor's cephalad hand applies rotational resistance to patient's shoulder as shown.
- **Pretreatment positioning**: Premanipulative tension is attained and maintained prior to **body drop impulse**. The premanipulative tension and the therapeutic impulse are established and delivered through the contact hand and the doctor's caudad leg which has compressive contact with the patient's flexed leg.
- **Therapeutic action**: Body drop thrust impulse with rotational emphasis. Notice how Dr Harris has the forearm of his contact hand perpendicular to the patient's coronal plane to direct his impulse in a posterior-to-anterior direction.
- **Resources**: *States Manual, Second Edition*[315] pages 95, 105, 106

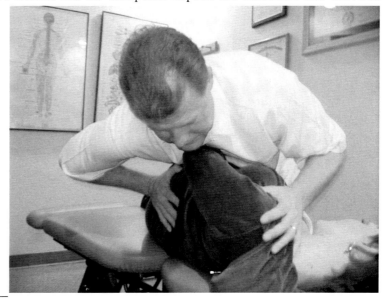

---

[314] Quon JA, Cassidy JD, O'Connor SM, Kirkaldy-Willis WH. Lumbar intervertebral disc herniation: treatment by rotational manipulation. *J Manipulative Physiol Ther*. 1989 Jun;12(3):220-7
[315] Kirk CR, Lawrence DJ, Valvo NL. States Manual of Spinal, Pelvic, and Extravertebral Technics. Second Edition. Lombard, Illinois: National College of Chiropractic; 1985

Lumbar Spine: Side-Posture Segmental Rotation (Lumbar "Push-Pull")

- **Patient position**: Lateral recumbent (side-posture) with no/minimal lateral flexion and minimal thoracic rotation; upper leg is flexed at hip and knee, with foot placed/locked behind the calf that is on the table; the patient grasps his/her own forearms and maintains modest tension to provide anchoring for the doctor's caudad arm, which is placed under the patient's superior arm; the patient's lower leg is straight.
- **Doctor position**: Doctor is facing the table standing on the cephalad leg while the caudad leg is flexed at the hip and knee and placed atop the patient's flexed upper leg to provide additional leverage at the time of manipulative thrust. Regarding the doctor's cephalad arm, the humerus is directed toward the patient's shoulder, and the elbow is bent allowing the forearm to push into the sulcus formed by the pectoralis major and deltoid; doctors forearm emerges under patient's elbow, so that fingertips are on the superior/lateral aspect of the lumbar spinous process of the superior vertebra of the targeted motion segment. Regarding the doctor's caudad arm, the elbow is flexed and the forearm is placed along the posterior aspect of the patient's superior ilium; fingers hook the inferior/lateral aspect of the lumbar spinous process of the inferior vertebra of the targeted motion segment.
- **Assessment**: <u>Subjective</u>: asymptomatic or lumbar pain, which may not be at the affected segment. <u>Motion palpation</u>: rotational restriction. <u>Static palpation</u>: may have rotational malposition. <u>Soft tissue</u>: may have muscle spasm at nearby area of hypermobility.
- **Treatment contact**: The doctor's cephalad contacts are at the patient's deltopectoral sulcus and directly on the superior/lateral aspect of the lumbar spinous process of the superior vertebra of the targeted motion segment. This maneuver has three caudad contacts: 1) doctor's fingertips pull directly on the inferior/lateral aspect of the lumbar spinous process of the inferior vertebra of the targeted motion segment; 2) doctor's forearm on patient's ilium; 3) doctors caudad lower leg is atop patient's flexed leg.
- **Support**: All contacts are active.
- **Pretreatment positioning**: Rotational tension is applied and focused at the lumbar spinal segment being treated. Thoracic rotation and lateral flexion are minimized to the extent possible. Modest lumbar lateral flexion toward the table helps to gap the inferior articular process of the superior segment from the superior articular process of the inferior segment.
- **Therapeutic action**: 1) Doctor's cephalad elbow thrusts toward patient's shoulder to create simultaneous rotation and long-axis traction; 2) cephalad fingertips push toward the ground while atop the superior/lateral aspect of the lumbar spinous process of the superior vertebra of the targeted motion segment; 3) doctor's caudad fingertips hook and pull the inferior vertebra; 4) forearm pushes patient's ilium into rotation; 5) extension "kick" of doctor's knee quickly creates rotational force. All five actions must occur simultaneously.

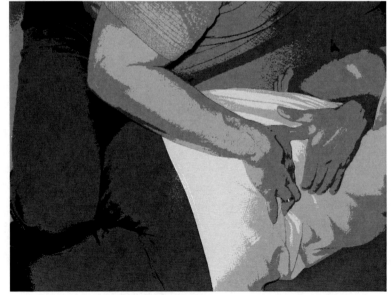

- **Resources**: *Chiropractic Technique*[316] page 428

---

[316] Bergmann TF, Peterson DH, Lawrence DJ. <u>Chiropractic Technique</u>. New York; Churchill Livingstone: 1993

- **<u>Approaching an integrated model for the understanding of "essential" hypertension</u>**: This diagram provides a reasonable representation of several of the key factors that generate and perpetuate the common clinical syndromes of overweight-obesity, hypertension, insulin resistance and diabetes mellitus type-2. Clinicians can use this single page for patient education so that patients will have access to a more complete understanding of their condition and how the integration of various interventions such as dietary improvement, exercise, nutritional supplementation, and spinal manipulation can work together to provide additive and synergistic health benefits.

<u>Integrated Model of So-called Primary Hypertension</u>: A sample of interconnected lifestyle-physiologic mechanisms contributing to the hyperinsulinemia-inflammation-hypertension syndrome commonly known as "idiopathic hypertension", "type-2 diabetes", and metabolic syndrome.

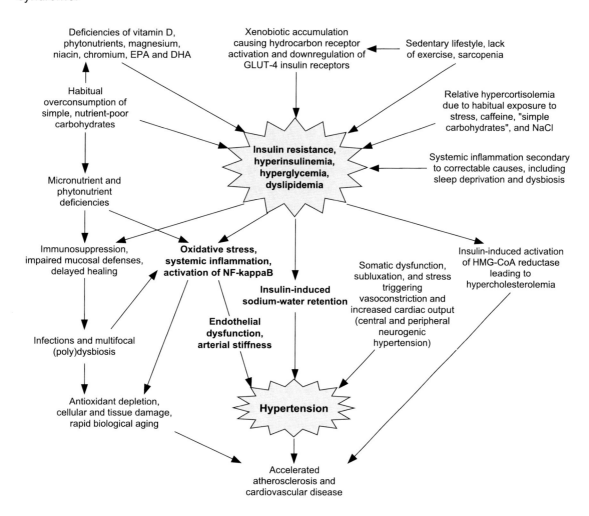

- **<u>Using the Functional Medicine Matrix to understand chronic hypertension</u>**: This diagram provides a representation of the Functional Medicine Matrix as applied to chronic hypertension. Note that Functional Medicine as a specific paradigm and discipline differs importantly from integrative medicine, which is mostly defined by its quantitative compilation of drug and nondrug treatments rather than by a specific model and clinical approach. The Functional Medicine serves as a clinician's learning and teaching tool to help clinicians understand and appreciate the complex interconnected aspects of disease and then to teach patients about their illnesses and thereby provide reassurance and enhanced opportunities for improved compliance.

Unofficial Functional Medicine Matrix Model of High Blood Pressure (Hypertension): Modified from the original diagram by Vasquez in 2003 for the Institute for Functional Medicine (IFM). The Functional Medicine Matrix is owned by the Institute for Functional Medicine. See www.FunctionalMedicine.org for updated information and additional training.

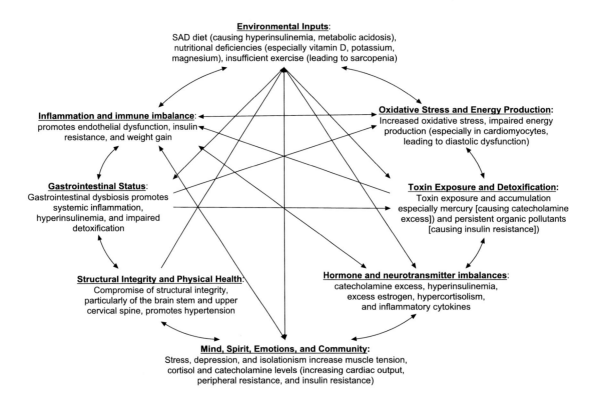

- **HTN—a singular etiology, multiple etiologies, or both?**: The following diagram shows how the simple act of what is referred to here as "living out of accord with nature" sets the stage for numerous biochemical and physiologic factors which contribute to HTN. Thus, this singular etiology or cause leads to numerous secondary etiologies or causes which all culminate in volume overload, sympathetic activation, systemic inflammation, and vasoconstriction. "Living out of accord with nature" has been a theme of so-called modernized/ Westernized/ industrialized societies since their subtle and progressive development. Dr Price's *Nutrition and Physical Degeneration: A Comparison of Primitive and Modern Diets and Their Effects*[317] documented in 1945 the effects that this "progress" was

---

[317] Price WA. <u>Nutrition and Physical Degeneration: A Comparison of Primitive and Modern Diets and Their Effects</u>. Price-Pottinger Nutr Foundtn: 1945

having on the health of societies that became "modernized"—their health status and social structures fell into decline, often complete ruin. More recently, O'Keefe and Cordain[318] wrote in their review article entitled *Cardiovascular disease resulting from a diet and lifestyle at odds with our Paleolithic genome: how to become a 21st-century hunter-gatherer* that,

> "Accumulating evidence suggests that this mismatch between our modern diet and lifestyle and our Paleolithic genome is playing a substantial role in the ongoing epidemics of obesity, hypertension, diabetes, and atherosclerotic cardiovascular disease. … Although the human genome has remained largely unchanged (DNA evidence documents relatively little change in the genome during the past 10,000 years), our diet and lifestyle have become progressively more divergent from those of our ancient ancestors."

Whether we call the problem "living out of accord with nature" or "the mismatch between our modern diet and lifestyle and our Paleolithic genome" the concept is the same, and the biophysiologic and social results are obviously negative. America's social fabric has deteriorated to the point that most Americans have only 2-3 friends and no confidants[319], and the progressively larger epidemics of obesity, depression, cancer, diabetes mellitus, and cardiovascular disease are well publicized and known to all.

Failure to meet nature-based physiologic expectations is a major cause of different secondary causes of hypertension

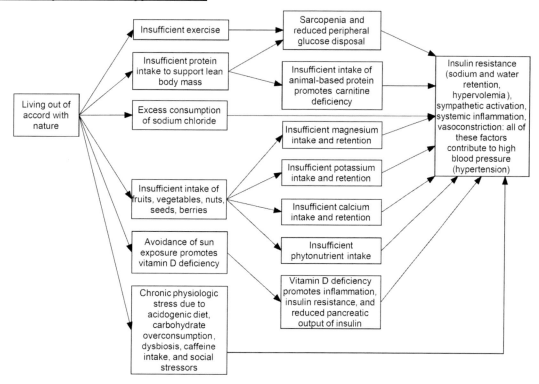

---

[318] O'Keefe JH Jr, Cordain L. Cardiovascular disease resulting from a diet and lifestyle at odds with our Paleolithic genome: how to become a 21st-century hunter-gatherer. *Mayo Clin Proc.* 2004 Jan;79(1):101-8

[319] McPherson M, Smith-Lovin L, Brashears ME. Social Isolation in America: Changes in Core Discussion Networks over Two Decades. *American Sociological Review* 2006; 71: 353-75 http://www.asanet.org/galleries/default-file/June06ASRFeature.pdf

Clinical pearls: Easy methods for objectively assessing treatment involvement

1. **Vitamin D levels**: Serum 25-OH-cholecalciferol can be tested as a surrogate marker for compliance with nutritional supplementation (detailed later); levels should rise within one month and plateau at the optimal range within 2-3 months if dose and compliance are appropriate. Since most patients will have low levels of 25-OH-D at initial assessment, retesting serum levels after 1-2 months of supplementation is an easy way to assess compliance with and effectiveness of this aspect of the treatment plan.

2. **Recall**: Patients should be able to recite their daily regimen of nutritional supplementation, pharmaceutical drugs, dietary prescriptions/proscriptions, and exercise-lifestyle habits. *If the patient cannot recall their daily health-promoting activities, then compliance is likely either low or nonexistent.*

3. **Consciousness**: Ideally, patients should be able to recite their personal values and goals, as these are the driving forces that either *support* or *subvert* their daily health-related behaviors. Conscious physicians should encourage consciousness-raising in their patients.

4. **Weight optimization**: Often, the "scale of truth" can be used for objective determination of compliance with the Paleo-Mediterranean Diet and particularly its low-carbohydrate and ketogenic variants. Overweight patients who comply with dietary optimization and lifestyle modification can generally achieve weight loss of 4-8 lbs (13-18 kg) per month. Certainly not all benefits of diet optimization are mediated through weight loss; however, the fact remains that weight loss is an important goal for the majority of hypertensive patients. Failure of weight loss can also be used to assess compliance and effectiveness of clinical trials involving dietary intervention; obviously, those trials that fail to effect weight loss were affected by inadequate compliance on behalf of the group of subjects (unlikely) or failure to design an appropriate dietary intervention on behalf of the researchers (more likely).

5. **Urinary sodium and potassium**: With a decided and consistent shift away from the Standard American-type diet (SAD) and toward the health-promoting Paleo-Mediterranean Diet (PMD) and particularly with its supplemented version (sPMD), the urinary sodium:creatinine ratio will decrease, as will the urinary sodium:potassium ratio.

- **Drug treatments for chronic HTN**: From a practical standpoint, the many drugs used for the suppression of HTN can be placed in one of five categories; the mnemonic offered in the *Saint-Frances Guide*[320] is "A.B.C.D.E." which stands for ❶ ACEis (angiotensin converting enzyme inhibitors) and ARBs (angiotensin II Receptor Blockers), ❷ BBs (beta-blockers), ❸ CCBs (calcium channel blockers), ❹ diuretics, and ❺ everything else (e.g., central alpha-agonists, alpha-blockers, vasodilators). For uncomplicated HTN, the initial treatment is a diuretic, generally hydrochlorothiazide (HCTZ), since the thiazide diuretics have the best cost-effectiveness of various drug classes; as noted by Howland and Mycek[321], "Current treatment recommendations are to **initiate therapy with a thiazide diuretic unless there are compelling reasons to employ other drug classes**. … Recent data suggest that diuretics are superior to beta-blockers in older adults." For complicated HTN (resistant to treatment or with concomitant illness), a different first-line or additive second drug is chosen from a different class based on patient characteristics, as outlined below. While clinicians might choose a higher initial dose based on HTN severity or the doctor's experience and preference, as a general rule the most reasonable course is to start with a single drug at a low dose in order to minimize risk for adverse effects and to readily determine the offending agent in the event of an expected or idiosyncratic side effect. In the outline below, patient profiles are matched to drug classes; when specific drugs are listed, they are chosen based on general

[320] Bent S, Gensler LS, Frances C. Saint-Frances Guide: Clinical Clerkship in Outpatient Medicine. 2nd Edition. Philadelphia; Wolters Kluwer: 2008, 90
[321] Howland RD, Mycek MJ. Lippincott's Illustrated Reviews: Pharmacology, Third Edition. Baltimore: Lippincott Williams and Wilkins; 2006, 213-226

frequency of use with preference for those administered once daily due to improved compliance. If drug treatment is well tolerated but insufficient to achieve BP goal, then *treatment compliance is verified* before increasing the dose and eventually adding a second drug from a different class. For the patient-centered and drug-centered tables that follow, primary sources of information are Lippincott's Illustrated Reviews: Pharmacology, Third Edition[322] for pharmacology and The 5-Minute Clinical Consult, 18th Edition[323] for more clinical information and doses; Ebell's review and clinical worksheet ("Hypertension Encounter Guide") published in "Initial evaluation of hypertension" in *American Family Physician* (March 2004)[324] was also used as a very practical point-of-care guide. The tables that follow were originally written by Alex Vasquez and reviewed by Robert Richard DO[325] in January

---

Suggested Practical HTN Drug Protocol
(Always check for drug allergies/intolerances)

1. **Thiazide diuretic: Hydrochlorothiazide 12.5-25 mg/d po** initially for most patients, not with renal insufficiency. For patients with DM or proteinuria, start with ACEi. Add **spironolactone 25-50 mg/d** if hypokalemia develops.
2. **ACEi: Lisinopril 10-40 mg/d po**, give the first dose in the office to monitor for hypotensive syncope or angioedema. If cough or angioedema develop, switch to ARB, particularly **losartan 25-100 mg/d** due to modest uricosuric effect. ACEi and ARB are contraindicated in pregnancy.
3. **CCB: Amlodipine 2.5-10 mg/d po**, particularly for patients with migraine, COPD, asthma.
4. **BB: Metoprolol 50-100 mg/d po** (up to bid), especially with angina or MI; not with bradycardia, insulin-requiring DM, depression, or sexual dysfunction.
5. **Loop diuretic: Furosemide 20-320 mg/d po** if patient has severe volume overload; effective with renal insufficiency.

Ebell MH. Initial evaluation of hypertension. *Am Fam Physician*. 2004 Mar 15;69:1485-7
http://www.aafp.org/afp/2004/0315/p1485.html
Domino FJ (editor-in-chief). The 5-Minute Clinical Consult. 2010. 18th Edition. Philadel.; WoltersKluwer: 2009, 656-7

2010 for the publication of *Chiropractic Management of Chronic Hypertension* (from which this more current text is derived); later editions of this publication have undergone additional professional and peer review.

- The medical profession's near-exclusive reliance upon drug treatments for HTN is fraught with problems, particularly including adverse drug effects, failure to address the underling primary cause(s) of the metabolic disturbance(s), of which, HTN is only the tip of the proverbial iceberg, and patient noncompliance. According to a 2001 editorial published in the *New England Journal of Medicine*, "Approximately one-half of patients who are prescribed antihypertensive medications discontinue therapy by the end of the first year."[326]
- In representative medical pharmacology textbooks[327] the primary variables considered for the support of antihypertensive pharmacotherapy are ❶ cardiac output (controlled with beta-blockers), ❷ peripheral resistance (treated with vasodilators such as ACEi and CCB), and ❸ blood volume (reduced by the first-line use of diuretics). One interconnecting theme in this

[322] Howland RD, Mycek MJ. Lippincott's Illustrated Reviews: Pharmacology, Third Edition. Baltimore: Lippincott Williams and Wilkins; 2006, 213-226
[323] Domino FJ (editor in chief). The 5-Minute Clinical Consult. 2010. 18th Edition. Philadelphia; Wolters Kluwer: 2009, 656-7
[324] Ebell MH. Initial evaluation of hypertension. *Am Fam Physician*. 2004 Mar 15;69(6):1485-7 http://www.aafp.org/afp/2004/0315/p1485.html
[325] Robert Richard DO is Medical Director of the John Peter Smith Polytechnic Clinic and Chair of Community Medicine at Texas College of Osteopathic Medicine. Dr Richard's review of these tables does not imply his endorsement of their content nor of the content of this document as a whole. Furthermore, Dr Richard's review does not imply endorsement by JPS Health Network or Texas College of Osteopathic Medicine.
[326] Chobanian AV. Control of hypertension--an important national priority. *N Engl J Med*. 2001 Aug 16;345(7):534-5
[327] Harvey RA, Champe PC (eds). Lippincott's Illustrated Reviews: Pharmacology, Third Edition. Philadelphia, Lippincott Williams and Wilkins; 1997

paradigm is that of activation of the sympathetic nervous system by some unknown insult or combination thereof. Whether due to "stress", faulty disinhibition of baroreceptors in the aortic arch, carotid sinuses, or renal juxtaglomerular cells, sympathetic activation increases cardiac output via increased rate and contractility, increases peripheral resistance via vasoconstriction, and increases blood volume via aldosterone-enhanced sodium (and thus water) retention. The enzyme renin converts angiotensinogen into angiotensin-1, which is converted via angiotensin converting enzyme (ACE) into the vasoconstrictor and trigger for aldosterone release angiotensin-2.

- Suggested doses of course need to be tailored to individual patient needs; doses suggested are for adults of average adult size and are administered by mouth (per os, p.o.) unless otherwise indicated. Note that IV and IM doses are generally much smaller than oral doses.

> **Analogy**
> **"Treating hypertension" simply by using drugs to lower blood pressure is like turning off a smoke alarm and then letting the fire continue to blaze.**
> High blood pressure is a manifestation of dysfunction. Rather than directing treatment toward the manifestation (i.e., the blood pressure elevation), clinicians would be more wise to address the nature and cause of the imbalance that is causing the elevation in blood pressure.
> If the metabolic-physiologic fire is extinguished, then the smoke alarm will silence itself though autoregulation, and spending billions of dollars and work-hours on alarm silencers (i.e., drugs) and alarm specialists will thereby become largely unnecessary. The results will include enhanced health via collateral benefits of natural treatments, reductions in costly and dangerous adverse drug effects, patient liberation from drug dependency, authentic patient empowerment, and improved fulfillment of medicine's purported tenets of beneficence, autonomy, and nonmalfesence.

Comorbidity profile suggesting specific first- or second-line treatment of hypertension

- **Tailoring drug selection per comorbidities:** Although the first choice for an antihypertensive drug is generally hydrochlorothiazide, the second drug and occasionally the first-line drug are selected based on patient tolerance and co-morbidities. The following quote by Chobanian[328] summarizes the general approach: "...for those who have had a heart attack, beta blockers and ACE inhibitors are preferred; for those at high risk for coronary heart disease, ACE inhibitors, beta blockers, calcium channel blockers, as well as diuretics are recommended; and for chronic kidney disease, ACE inhibitors and angiotensin receptor blockers are drugs of first choice." Additional details are provided below:
  - **Uncomplicated**: Thiazide diuretics (especially **HCTZ**) are first choice (can worsen gout and dyslipidemia); BB have historically been a common second choice, but recently atenolol has fallen out of favor[329] and with the increasing prevalence of DM which indicates ACEi and ARB treatment, these medications may become the preferred second line; the ARB **losartan** would seem particularly favorable in patients with metabolic syndrome and type-2 DM due to its uricosuric effect.
  - **Diabetes mellitus**: ACEis are renoprotective (but not used with renovascular disease), ARB's are second choice due to cost and less historical use; beta-blockers are generally

---

[328] Chobanian AV. Press Conference Remarks: The Seventh Report of the Joint National Committee on Prevention, Detection, Evaluation, and Treatment of High Blood Pressure (JNC 7). May 14, 2003. http://www.nhlbi.nih.gov/guidelines/hypertension/speaker2.htm Accessed November 2010
[329] Domino FJ (editor in chief). The 5-Minute Clinical Consult. 2010. 18th Edition. Philadelphia; Wolters Kluwer: 2009, 656-7

avoided in insulin-requiring DM due to blunting of protective responses to hypoglycemia.

o **Renal disease**: ACEis are renoprotective (but not used with renovascular disease), ARBs are second choice. Nondihydropyridine CCBs reduce intrarenal filtration pressure thus reducing proteinuria. Thiazides require renal function and are generally not useful if creatinine is >2 mg/dl.

o **African American**: African-Americans tend to respond better to diuretics and CCB than to BB or ACEi.[330]

o **Asthma and COPD**: Use a CCB. Generally avoid beta-blockers with any airway disease, B1-selective metoprolol might be considered

o **Angina**: BB and CCB improve outcomes independent of BP-lowering; when BB and CCB are combined, the CCB should be a dihydropyridine (i.e., from the class of "-pyridines" or "-pines"). Do not combine a BB with a negative inotropic non-dihydropyridine CCB so as to avoid inducing heart block.

o **Erectile dysfunction**: Avoid beta-blockers; thiazides may exacerbate. Consider concomitant administration of arginine and/or a phosphodiesterase-5 inhibitor; also consider treatment for excess estrogen in men with a serum estradiol greater than 30 picogram/mL (for details see the anti-estrogen protocol outlined in chapter 4 of *Integrative Rheumatology*[331]). Implement diet and lifestyle modification for weight optimization; optimize endothelial health.

o **Systolic HTN**: Dihydropyridine CCB ("-pyridines" or "-*pines*") are preferred because of their relative selectivity for the peripheral vasculature—the vascular *tree*.

o **CAD or prior MI**: BB are top choice if not contraindicated by problematic asthma, COPD, or DM.

o **Pregnancy**: Use methyldopa, hydralazine, magnesium; pregnancy contraindicates ACEi and ARB due to teratogenic effects.

o **CHF**: BB are particularly useful for diastolic CHF to slow heart rate and allow greater filling time: Carvedilol is BB of choice in this situation. Monitor for signs of excessive cardiosupresion such as edema, SOB, rales, bradycardia. Carvedilol is a non-selective beta blocker/alpha-1 blocker indicated in the treatment of mild to moderate CHF. Do not use BB or CCB with bradycardia; generally do not use verapamil (negative inotrope CCB) with CHF. Diuretics such as Lasix are mainstays of CHF treatment, particularly for exacerbations. ACEi and ARB drugs are also routinely used in CHF.

o **Bradycardia**: Do not use BB or CCB with bradycardia.

o **Edema**: Sodium and water restriction along with use of loop diuretics (e.g., furosemide/Lasix) is common treatment. Lasix is generally dosed "to effect."

The next several pages provide a review of each drug class per page. When available and to maintain the drug-per-page formatting, space is provided at the bottom of the page for clinicians to write their own notes on drug usage and preferences. Preferred/representative drugs are listed based on the author's experience, training (especially observed prescribing patterns by attending physicians) and research; following the so-called preferred drug is optional at the discretion of the clinician.

---

[330] Howland RD, Mycek MJ. Lippincott's Illustrated Reviews: Pharmacology, Third Edition. Baltimore: Lippincott Williams and Wilkins; 2006, 213-226
[331] **Vasquez A**. Integrative Rheumatology. IBMRC 2006, 2007 and all future editions. http://optimalhealthresearch.com/rheumatology.html

ACEi: angiotensin-2 converting enzyme inhibitors

- Pharmacology and introduction: Blocking formation of angiotensin-2 reduces peripheral vascular resistance and aldosterone secretion; vasodilation is effected by reduced breakdown of bradykinin; sympathetic tone may be reduced. For best safety, the initial dose of an ACEi can be given in the office under supervision due to risks for first-dose syncope and life-threatening angioedema; this advised practice is rarely followed.

- Unique benefits of class: ACE inhibitors provide renoprotection, hence their routine use in patients with DM, with or without HTN. Thiazide, BB, and ACEi can be safely used together. As summarized by Domino (ed), "ACE inhibitors should be used in patients with diabetes, proteinuria, atrial fibrillation, or CHF but not in pregnancy."

- Unique adverse effects and contraindications: Not used with **renal artery stenosis** (can cause acute renal failure) or **pregnancy** (teratogenic); may cause **cough (10%) and angioedema** due to reduced breakdown of bradykinin. Reduced aldosterone secretion promotes hypotension and **hyperkalemia—potassium levels should be monitored** *especially in diabetic* **patients and those with renal insufficiency and/or renal vascular stenosis; coadministration of ACEi and spironolactone is generally contraindicated** due to risk of hyperkalemia.

- Representative drug of class (dose range):

Drug, starting dose, comments	*Benefits*	*Risks*
Lisinopril 10 mg/d (up to 80 mg/d; max dose in renal failure is 40 mg/d) po; available as 2.5 mg, 5 mg, 10 mg, 20 mg, 30 mg and 40 mg tablets: Lisinopril is an orally administered long-acting angiotensin converting enzyme inhibitor. This is a very commonly used medication in medical practice and hospitals. Half-life is approximately 12 hours; absorption of Lisinopril is approximately 25%, with large intersubject variability (6% to 60%) at all doses tested (5 mg to 80 mg).	☑ Antihypertensive, vasodilatory, anti-aldosterone effect, ☑ Beneficial in CHF, ☑ Beneficial after MI, ☑ Benefits within 1 hour, peak at 6 hours, duration 24 hours; full benefit takes weeks, ☑ Concomitant administration of Lisinopril and hydrochlorothiazide further reduces blood pressure in Black and non-Black patients.	☒ Contraindicated in **pregnancy**—black box warning. Do not use during lactation. ☒ Not to be used in patients with ACEi hypersensitivity, higher risk for **life-threatening angioedema** in African-American patients, ☒ Benefit blunted by NSAIDs, ☒ Can reduce renal filtration of potassium, **lithium**—especially use caution in patients with sCr >2mg/dL. ☒ Removal of angiotensin II negative feedback on renin secretion leads to increased plasma renin activity.

Clinician notes:

ARB: angiotensin-2 receptor blocker/antagonist

- <u>Pharmacology and introduction</u>: ARBs block reception of angiotensin-2 and thus reduce vasoconstriction and aldosterone secretion; risk-benefit profile is similar to ACEi except that bradykinin-mediated benefits (vasodilation) and risks (cough, angioedema) are not seen. ARBs improve endothelial dysfunction in patients with HTN and/or CAD, reduce cardiovascular mortality and morbidity, and have anti-inflammatory benefits.
- <u>Unique benefits of class</u>: Hypotensive and renoprotective benefits without the risks of cough and angioedema compared with ACEi.
- <u>Unique adverse effects and contraindications</u>: Fetotoxicity contraindicates ARB use in pregnancy—this is a black box warning.
- <u>Representative drug of class (dose range)</u>:

Drug, starting dose, comments	*Benefits*	*Risks*
Losartan 50 mg/d (up to 100 mg/d), available as 25 mg, 50 mg and 100 mg; among the ARBs, this drug provides the additional benefit of reducing uric acid levels, which is relevant for fructose-induced urate-mediated metabolic syndrome; however, a recent clinical trial showed no differences between ramipril and losartan in lowering BP and both drugs showed a trend to improve metabolic parameters such as serum glucose, serum triglycerides, and uric acid equally.[332]	☑ Half-life is 6-9 hours with no plasma accumulation after repeated daily dosing. ☑ Food slows and reduces absorption but this is not clinically significant.	☒ Contraindicated in **pregnancy**—black box warning. Do not use during lactation. ☒ Less effective in African-American patients. ☒ Most of the anti-HTN benefits of Losartan are due to its active carboxylic acid metabolite formed via the action of cytochrome P450 2C9 and 3A4. Generally, 14% of Losartan is converted into the active metabolite; in 1% of patients, they only convert 1% of Losartan to the active metabolite and therefore the drug is inefficacious for them. ☒ Consider caution and lower doses in patients with renal disease: plasma concentrations are increased by 50 to 90% in patients with mild (creatinine clearance of 50 to 74 mL/min) or moderate (creatinine clearance 30 to 49 mL/min) renal insufficiency.

---

[332] Spinar J, Vítovec J, Soucek M, Dusek L, Pavlík T; CORD Invesigators. CORD: COmparsion of Recommended Doses of ACE inhibitors and angiotensin II receptor blockers. *Vnitr Lek*. 2009 May;55(5):481-8

BB: beta-adrenergic receptor blockers, "beta blockers"

- Pharmacology and introduction: Primary mechanism of drug action is via blockade of B1 receptors; this reduces cardiac output, sympathetic tone, and renin secretion. Major adverse effects include bradycardia, fatigue, depression, sexual dysfunction, exacerbation of asthma and COPD, and **rebound hypertension with rapid discontinuation of drug**.
- Unique benefits of class: Thiazide, BB, and ACEi can be safely used together. BB considered more effective in Caucasians than Africans, more effective in young than elderly. BB are particularly used in HTN patients who also have **supraventricular tachyarrhythmia, previous MI, angina, migraine, and anxiety**.
- Unique adverse effects and contraindications: Do not use BB or CCB with **bradycardia** due to potential for inducing **heart block or hypotension**. Nonselective BB such as propranolol which target B1 (heart) and B2 (lungs) have potential to **exacerbate asthma and COPD**; however, **propranolol's B1 blockade helps reduce renin levels**. Patients with PVD may have a worsening of limb ischemia secondary to reduced perfusion. **Hypotension, fatigue, depression, sexual dysfunction,** and **rebound hypertension** are common adverse BB effects; lowering of HDL and elevation of TRIGs has also been noted. Sudden discontinuation of BB can result in **rebound hypertension** (presumably due to upregulation of beta-adrenergic receptors under prolonged suppression). Of note, **atenolol** is no longer considered first-line treatment due to recent evidence of **inefficacy** in preventing HTN complications.[333]
- Representative drug of class (dose range):

Drug, starting dose, comments	*Benefits*	*Risks*
Metoprolol in extended release (Toprol-XL) 25 mg/d; available as 25 mg, 50 mg, 100 mg, 200 mg: This drug is preferred in patients with angina or MI.	☑ Benefits HTN, supraventricular tachyarrhythmia, previous MI, angina, migraine, and anxiety.	☒ Patients must not discontinue drug without tapering dose; sudden discontinuation can cause severe rebound HTN, angina, and MI. ☒ Do not use in patients with bradycardia or heart block. Fatigue, depression, sexual dysfunction, and weight gain can be caused by beta-blockers. ☒ Beta-blockers blunt the physiologic responses to hypoglycemia and are thus associated with hypoglycemic risk in diabetic patients taking glucose-lowering drugs such as insulin.

---

[333] Domino FJ (editor in chief). The 5-Minute Clinical Consult. 2010. 18th Edition. Philadelphia; Wolters Kluwer: 2009, 656-7

CCB: calcium channel blockers (dihydropyridine class)

- <u>Pharmacology and introduction</u>: The "-pyrines" block calcium entry into vascular smooth muscle and thus cause relative arterial dilation and thus a reduction in peripheral resistance. *Memory tool*: Remember that *pyridines* sounds like *pines* and that these drugs work on the *vascular tree* to lower blood pressure via systemic arterial dilation.
  - Not detailed here are the non-dihydropyridine class of CCB (i.e., including diltiazem/Cardizem and Verapamil) which are not used for HTN but rather are used for their cardioselective effects. *Memory tool*: Remember that the *non*-dihydropyridine CCBs are cardiosuppressive via a *negative* inotropic effect.
- <u>Unique benefits of class</u>: Generally safe in HTN patients with asthma, DM, angina, and PVD.
- <u>Unique adverse effects and contraindications</u>: Do not use BB or non-dihydropyridine CCB with bradycardia. Adverse effects include constipation (10%, especially with nifedipine), headache, and fatigue.
- <u>Representative drug of class (dose range)</u>:

Drug, starting dose, comments	*Benefits*	*Risks*
Amlodipine 5 mg/d, or start with 2.5 mg/d if being used as a secondary drug or if patient has liver disease; available as 2.5 mg, 5 mg, 10 mg:	☑ Amlodipine is indicated for HTN, chronic stable angina, vasospastic angina, and CAD if the ejection fraction is >40%. ☑ Generally safe in HTN patients with asthma, DM, angina, and PVD.	☒ Generally do not use this drug if patient has aortic stenosis, hypersensitivity, severe CAD or severe CHF. ☒ CCB are generally fourth-line drugs after thiazide diuretics, followed by either ACI/ARB and then BB. ☒ Numerous drug interactions, including barbiturates, phenytoin, rifampin, antipsychotics, amiodarone, erythromycin, fluconazole, and the related drugs sildenafil (Viagra) and tadalafil (Cialis).

<u>*Clinician notes*</u>:

_____

_____

_____

Diuretic—loop class: furosemide /Lasix

- <u>Pharmacology and introduction</u>: A key mechanism of action of most diuretics is enhanced excretion of sodium. Sodium (Na) retention promotes water retention and subsequent volume expansion, while also contributing to vasoconstriction and arterial stiffness via enhanced adrenergic reactivity and via promotion of intracellular hypercalcinosis (possibly due to enhanced sodium-calcium exchange).[334]
- <u>Unique benefits of class</u>: Fast action even in patients with renal insufficiency; efficacy of Lasix is via diuresis and venodilation.
- <u>Unique adverse effects and contraindications</u>: Chronic use promotes depletion of potassium, magnesium, and thiamine. Diuretic effect is potent and acute.
- <u>Representative drug of class (dose range)</u>:

Drug, starting dose, comments	*Benefits*	*Risks*
Furosemide 20 mg/d po is reasonable starting dose; may increase up to 600 mg/d as needed; available as 20 mg, 40 mg, 80 mg: Dose must be step-wise increased to find patient-specific threshold dose and frequency for individual patient, works for **6** hours (hence the name La**six**); higher doses not better than threshold dose.	☑ This is a very commonly used drug; commonly used PRN for outpatients with edema, including idiopathic edema. ☑ Used for systemic edema, pulmonary edema, CHF, hypercalcemia, and – rarely—HTN. ☑ This drug can be used in patients with renal insufficiency, but not with anuria or urethral obstruction	☒ This is a potent diuretic that can cause volume depletion and secondary syncope and hypoperfusion. This is a potent diuretic that can cause electrolyte depletion, including hyponatremia. Scheduled follow-up and laboratory tests for electrolytes are required. ☒ Avoid nighttime use to avoid nocturia.

<u>*Clinician notes*</u>:

_____

_____

_____

_____

_____

Loop diuretics cause electrolyte and thiamine loss

Loop diuretics such as furosemide/Lasix are commonly used in the treatment of heart failure and other edematous states in elderly patients, but the depletion of thiamine, magnesium, potassium, and calcium can exacerbate heart failure and contribute to co-morbidity such as depression, delirium, and dementia.

Felípez L, Sentongo TA. Drug-induced nutrient deficiencies. *Pediatr Clin North Am.* 2009;56:1211-24

---

[334] Benowitz NL. "Antihypertensive Agents." In Katzung BG (editor). <u>Basic and Clinical Pharmacology. Tenth Edition</u>. New York: McGraw Hill Medical; 2007, 163

Diuretic—thiazide class: hydrochlorothiazide (HCTZ)

- Pharmacology and introduction: Drug of choice for initial treatment of HTN. Sulfa sensitivity does not necessarily contraindicate thiazide use, even though thiazides are sulfa derivatives; use with caution. Thiazide diuretics are ineffective in patients with renal insufficiency; the loop diuretic furosemide is effective in patients with renal insufficiency.
- Unique benefits of class: Thiazide, BB, and ACEi can be safely used together. Particularly beneficial in elderly (as long as renal function is intact) and Africans. Promotion of calcium retention may benefit osteoporosis and reduce calcium nephrolithiasis. Thiazide diuretics reduce peripheral vascular resistance, perhaps via sodium elimination.
- **Unique adverse effects and contraindications**: Not useful in patients with renal insufficiency (creatinine clearance < 50 mL/min).
  - Thiazide diuretics can worsen **hyperuricemia** (70% of patients) and **gout** due to competition for renal excretion (organic acids).
  - **Hypokalemia** (70%)—potassium levels should be monitored in patients predisposed to cardiac arrhythmia and those treated with digitalis. Coadministration with ACEi/lisinopril helps negate the tendency toward hypokalemia.
  - **Hyperglycemia (10%), dyslipidemia, hypomagnesemia**
  - Promotion of calcium retention can promote **hypercalcemia** when HCTZ is combined with vitamin D3, even with the use of modest doses of vitamin D (e.g., 2,000 IU/d).[335]
  - Exacerbation of (fructose-induced) metabolic syndrome was recently proven experimentally [animal study] and published in a peer-reviewed journal[336]; this effect is mediated at least in part due to potassium depletion.
- Representative drug of class (dose range):

Drug, starting dose, comments	*Benefits*	*Risks*
Hydrochlorothiazide started at 12.5-25 mg/d; may use up to 50 mg/d for HTN: When used for the treatment of peripheral edema (rare), the dose is as high as 200 mg/d po qd.	☑ HCTZ is the first-line drug of choice for the routine outpatient management of chronic hypertension. Other drugs such as ACEi/ARB and BB are commonly added as second line agents after the initiation of HCTZ.	☒ HCTZ exacerbates many of the pathophysiologic components of the metabolic syndrome, such as hyperuricemia, potassium insufficiency, hyperglycemia, dyslipidemia, hypomagnesemia and magnesium insufficiency.

Clinician notes:

---

[335] **Vasquez A**, Manso G, Cannell J. The clinical importance of vitamin D (cholecalciferol): a paradigm shift with implications for all healthcare providers. *Altern Ther Health Med*. 2004 Sep-Oct;10(5):28-36 http://optimalhealthresearch.com/cholecalciferol.html
[336] Reungjui S, Roncal CA, Mu W, Srinivas TR, Sirivongs D, Johnson RJ, Nakagawa T. Thiazide diuretics exacerbate fructose-induced metabolic syndrome. *J Am Soc Nephrol*. 2007 Oct;18(10):2724-31 http://jasn.asnjournals.org/content/18/10/2724.full.pdf

Diuretic—potassium-sparing: spironolatone

- <u>Pharmacology and introduction</u>: Potassium-sparing diuretics are weak diuretics; **spironolactone** is the prototype and also has anti-androgen action and is therefore used in hirsutism.
- <u>Unique benefits of class</u>: Spironolactone is commonly used with HCTZ; it beneficially diminishes cardiac remodeling seen in CHF. Spironolactone reduces incidence of spontaneous bacterial peritonitis (SBP) in patients with cirrhosis.
- <u>Unique adverse effects and contraindications</u>: Spironolactone has antiandrogen effects, can promote sexual dysfunction in men and gynecomastia; can precipitate hyperkalemia and hypermagnesemia.
- <u>Representative drug of class (dose range)</u>:

Drug, starting dose, comments	*Benefits*	*Risks*
Spironolactone: start HTN dose at 12.5 mg/d; available as 25 mg, 50 mg, 100 mg; dosed as high as 200 mg/d for edema and 400 mg po qd x21-28 days for the diagnosis of hyperaldosteronism	☑ Useful as a second line or third line drug in the treatment of HTN following the use of HCTZ; also used as second line agent with Lasix. ☑ Used in the treatment of hypokalemia, hyperaldosteronism, ascities, hirsutism, CHF, and edema due to CHF, renal failure, and cirrhosis.	☒ Tumorigenic effect noted in animals suggests that spironolactone may exacerbate cancer and should therefore be used sparingly. ☒ Hyperkalemia is a real clinical concern associated with potassium-sparing diuretics such as spironolactone.

Clinician notes:

_____

_____

_____

_____

_____

_____

_____

_____

Alpha-1-blocker: alpha-adrenergic receptor type-1 antagonist

- Pharmacology and introduction: Reduce BP via relaxation of venous and arterial smooth muscle. These drugs are certainly not used as first-line treatments for HTN, generally speaking.
- Unique benefits of class: Can be used when other drugs have not been effective; can benefit men with prostatic hyperplasia.
- Unique adverse effects and contraindications: Sodium-water retention, hypotension, syncope, and reflex tachycardia are common; reflex tachycardia can be prevented with BB.
- Representative drug of class:

Drug, starting dose, comments	*Benefits*	*Risks*
Prazosin: start with 1 mg/d for the treatment of HTN; available as 1 mg, 2 mg, 5 mg; highest recommended dose for HTN is 15 mg/d.	☑ Used in the treatment of HTN, prostate enlargement (1 mg po bid)	☒ First-dose syncope and hypotension are common with prazosin.

Clinician notes:

_____

_____

_____

_____

_____

_____

_____

_____

_____

_____

_____

_____

_____

_____

Alpha-2 agonists: alpha-adrenergic receptor class-2 agonist

- Pharmacology and introduction: Centrally acting drugs reduce sympathetic output via central feedback inhibition. Rebound hypertension with clonidine withdrawal mandates tapering discontinuation.
- Unique benefits of class: Safe for use in renal disease; generally used with diuretic.
- Unique adverse effects and contraindications: Generally used with a diuretic to counteract the sodium-water retention. Sedation and dry nose may occur. Rebound hypertension mandates *tapering* discontinuation. **Alpha-2 agonists are best avoided due to high risk of rebound HTN following noncompliance or missed/skipped dose.**
- Representative drug of class:

Drug, starting dose, comments	Benefits	Risks
Clonidine: start at 0.1 mg bid for HTN; max dose is 2.4 mg; available as 0.1 mg, 0.2 mg, and 0.3 mg for oral administration, also available for injection: x.	☑ **Useful for acute and severe HTN; not routinely used for routine chronic HTN.** Can be administered orally or intravenously for the rapid reduction of severe hypertension. ☑ Epidural administration is used in the treatment of severe pain.	☒ **High risk of rebound HTN following noncompliance or missed/skipped dose.** Taper dose over 4 days to reduce risk of rebound HTN.

Clinician notes:

_____

_____

_____

_____

_____

_____

_____

_____

_____

_____

Vasodilators: Direct-acting smooth muscle relaxants: hydralazine

- <u>Pharmacology and introduction</u>: Vasodilators are used for treatment-resistant HTN, acute severe HTN, and pregnancy-related HTN. During my hospital training, we used these drugs commonly in emergency settings and in obstetrics; generally these drugs were administered intravenously at 10 mg per dose repeated as needed for HTN control. Hydralazine's mechanism of action includes limiting calcium release from the sarcoplasmic reticulum of smooth muscle thereby resulting in relaxation of arterioles and veins; hydralazine recently has been identified as a nitric oxide donor.
- <u>Unique benefits of class</u>: Rapid onset of action; safe for use during pregnancy.
- <u>Unique adverse effects and contraindications</u>: Sodium-water retention can be avoided with BB and diuretic. BB can be used to avoid vasodilator-induced tachycardia.
- <u>Representative drug of class</u>:

Drug, starting dose, comments	*Benefits*	*Risks*
Hydralazine: oral dose for moderate-severe HTN is 10-50 mg po starting with 10 mg po qid for 2-4 days then 25 mg po qid for 1 week; max dose is 300 mg po qd25-150 mg twice daily; available for oral administration 10 mg, 25 mg, 50 mg, 100 mg: For acute HTN, the parenteral dose is 10-20 mg IM or IV each 2-4 hours; switch to oral dosing as soon as possible.	☑ Monotherapy is generally only used in the treatment of pregnancy-induced HTN and moderate-severe treatment-resistant HTN. This drug is commonly used in hospitals for the treatment of pregnancy-induced HTN and pre-eclampsia.	☒ Side effects include headache due to vasodilation and drug-induced systemic lupus erythematosus (SLE). May also cause neutropenia and other blood disorders. ☒ **Warning**: Vasodilators cause reflex tachycardia that can precipitate MI and CHF.

<u>Clinician notes</u>:

_____

_____

_____

_____

_____

_____

_____

Selected Essays, Perspectives, and Previously Published Articles

Intracellular Hypercalcinosis: A Functional Nutritional Disorder with Implications Ranging from Myofascial Trigger Points to Affective Disorders, Hypertension, and Cancer

Alex Vasquez, D.C., N.D.

This article was originally published in *Naturopathy Digest*
http://www.naturopathydigest.com/archives/2006/sep/vasquez.php

Introduction:

Let's explore the possibility that elevated levels of calcium *within the cell* (intracellular hypercalcinosis) might predispose toward a wide range of clinical problems including migraine, hypertension, myofascial trigger points, inflammation, and cancer. Further, let's review the data showing that several commonly employed nutritional interventions can be used synergistically to counteract and correct this problem. By the time readers complete this article, they will have 1) an understanding of this problem, 2) a protocol for how to correct this problem, and 3) be able to explain the biochemical rationale for using these nutritional protocols in patients who might otherwise be treated with drugs in general and calcium-channel-blocking drugs in particular.

Although prescription drugs are often used by medical doctors in a "willy-nilly manner" (according to Harvard Medical School Professor Dr. Jerry Avorn[337]), let's assume for a moment that legitimate reasons exist for the widespread use of drugs that block calcium channels in cell membranes—the "calcium-channel-blocking drugs." Although it is counterintuitive to promote health by interfering with the body's natural function, calcium-channel-blocking drugs are routinely used in pharmaceutical medicine for a broad range of problems including hypertension, heart rhythm disturbances, bipolar disorder, and anxiety/panic disorders. Widespread medical use of calcium-channel-blocking drugs appears to validate the supposition that excess intracellular calcium is an important contributor to these and perhaps other problems. Therefore, if intracellular hypercalcinosis is the problem, then any safe and cost-effective treatment that can correct this problem should be met with the same widespread acceptance given to calcium-channel-blocking drugs, which are universally accepted and utilized in the allopathic "conventional medicine" society.

At the very least, we can generally state that all phenomena that contribute to calcium deficiency result in an increase in intracellular calcium levels (the "calcium paradox") due to the effect of parathyroid hormone, which specifically promotes calcium uptake in cells while mobilizing calcium from bone. Additionally, a few other nutritional influences (such as fatty acid imbalances) modulate cellular calcium balance, and these will be discussed in the section on clinical interventions.

The Problem of Excess Intracellular Calcium:

Although the current author is the first to coin the phrase "intracellular hypercalcinosis"[338], several other authors have pointed to the problem of the "calcium paradox" and the means by which *body-wide calcium deficiency* can result in *intracellular calcium overload*, which triggers a cascade of events leading to adverse health effects. Most notably, the work of Takuo Fujita[339,340]

---

[337] America The Medicated. http://www.cbsnews.com/stories/2005/04/21/health/main689997.shtml
[338] http://optimalhealthresearch.com/archives/intracellular-hypercalcinosis
[339] Fujita T. Calcium paradox: consequences of calcium deficiency manifested by a wide variety of diseases. *J Bone Miner Metab.* 2000;18(4):234-6

stands out in its clarity and specificity in linking intracellular hypercalcinosis with disorders such as hypertension, arteriosclerosis, diabetes mellitus, neurodegenerative diseases, malignancy, and degenerative joint disease.

Mechanisms by which intracellular hypercalcinosis contributes to disease have been defined, at least partially. However, we must remember that nutritional disorders never occur in isolation, and that the effects of intracellular hypercalcinosis observed clinically are overlaid with manifestations of the primary nutritional/metabolic disorder. Stated differently, contrary to what the pharmaceutical paradigm's monotherapeutic use of calcium-channel-blocking drugs would imply, intracellular hypercalcinosis never occurs by itself. For example, if intracellular hypercalcinosis is contributed to by vitamin D3 deficiency, then some of the observed clinical complications of that condition are due to and yet independent from the excess intracellular calcium since the primary problem (vitamin D3 deficiency) causes adverse effects and deficiency symptoms that are independent of its effect on intracellular calcium levels. To better understand the specific effects of excess intracellular calcium, a brief review of a few specific biochemical/physiologic mechanisms by which intracellular hypercalcinosis can contribute to disease is warranted. We must start by realizing that calcium is much more than a "bone nutrient" and that it functions as an electrolyte, intracellular messenger, and regulator of cell replication and metabolism. Let's talk about four pathways by which increased intracellular calcium promotes disease:

1. ***Adverse effects on membrane receptors and intracellular transduction***: The concentration of extracellular calcium exceeds the concentration of intracellular calcium by a ratio of 10,000 to one. When intracellular calcium levels rise even slightly, receptors and messaging systems in the cell membrane fail to function optimally. Thereby, increased intracellular calcium can predispose to insulin resistance (via interference with insulin receptors) and can promote neurodegeneration by amplifying the intracellular cascade of effects that follows activation of the brain's NMDA-receptors (excitoneurotoxicity). More specifically, we must note that the recently discovered "calcium-sensing receptor" (CaR, a G protein-coupled plasma membrane receptor) senses minute alterations in serum calcium levels and then ultimately translates these variations into changes in cellular function, notably alterations in cell replication (think cancer) and eicosanoid production (think inflammation).[341,342] Given that CaR are found in a wide range of cell types, including those found in bone, the kidneys, and immune system, we can see a pathway by which alterations in calcium balance could be implicated in a wide range of diseases. CaR-mediated alterations in cell function are likely to be complicated by disorders of vitamin D3 nutrition and metabolism (that commonly complicate disorders of calcium homeostasis), which affect an even wider range of cell types including those of the breast, prostate, ovary, lung, skin, lymph nodes, colon, pancreas, adrenal medulla, brain (pituitary, cerebellum, and cerebral cortex), aortic endothelium, and immune system, including monocytes, transformed B-cells, and activated T-cells. This is an example of the complexity involved in understanding nutrition in general and the effects of nutritional deficiency (always multifaceted) in particular.

2. ***Mitochondrial failure and cell death***: According to the most recent edition of the classic text Robbins Pathologic Basis of Disease (pages 15-16), increased intracellular calcium is a major cause of cell death. When calcium levels are increased within the cell, one adverse effect is the inhibition of mitochondrial function. Since calcium is pumped out of the cell in an energy-dependent process, and because dysfunctional mitochondria pour calcium into the intracellular space, calcium-induced mitochondrial failure results in an additional

---

[340] Fujita T, Palmieri GM. Calcium paradox disease: calcium deficiency prompting secondary hyperparathyroidism and cellular calcium overload. *J Bone Miner Metab*. 2000;18(3):109-25

[341] Peterlik M, Cross HS. Vitamin D and calcium deficits predispose for multiple chronic diseases. *Eur J Clin Invest*. 2005 May;35(5):290-304

[342] Heaney RP. Long-latency deficiency disease: insights from calcium and vitamin D. *Am J Clin Nutr*. 2003 Nov;78(5):912-9

increase in intracellular calcium. Further complicating this problem is the fact that the cell membrane becomes increasingly permeable to calcium as calcium levels increase. Elevated intracellular calcium levels activate enzymes such as ATPase, phospholipase, proteases, and endonucleases that synergistically promote cell death.

3. ***Pro-inflammatory effects of intracellular calcium***: The recent finding that intracellular calcium activates NF-kappaB[343] has obvious implications given the pivotal role of NF-kappaB in the promotion of systemic inflammation and diseases such as rheumatoid arthritis.[344] Thus, increased intracellular calcium appears to promote inflammation. This may explain in part how vitamin D3 supplementation (which lowers intracellular calcium levels) exerts its clinically impressive anti-inflammatory and immunomodulatory benefits.[345]

4. ***Enhanced production of lipid peroxides***: Fujita notes that lipid peroxides lead to an increase in cell membrane permeability to calcium, which results in increased intracellular calcium; this activates metabolic pathways that increase oxidative stress, thus leading to a vicious cycle stimulated by the production of additional lipid peroxides. Thus, intracellular hypercalcinosis promotes oxidative stress, which becomes self-perpetuating by this and other mechanisms. Of course, we all know by now that increased production of free radicals contributes to the development of many health problems, such as cancer, cardiovascular disease, arthritis, autoimmunity, diabetes, and other forms of rapid biological aging.

5. ***Myofascial trigger points, chronic muscle spasm, and increased vascular tone (hypertension)***: The release of calcium from the sarcoplasmic reticulum triggers muscle contraction and plays a role in hypertension (hence the use of calcium-channel-blocking drugs in the treatment of hypertension), chronic muscle spasm (especially when complicated by magnesium deficiency[346]), and the perpetuation of myofascial trigger points.[347] Reducing the levels of cytosolic and sarcoplasmic calcium promotes muscle relaxation.

Nutritional Interventions to Ameliorate Intracellular Hypercalcinosis:
Now that we've reviewed the data implicating intracellular hypercalcinosis as a legitimate contributor to a wide range of clinical disorders and diseases, let's explore some nutritional solutions.

1. ***Correction of vitamin D deficiency***: Vitamin D deficiency causes calcium deficiency which increases parathyroid hormone production resulting in increased intracellular calcium levels. Vitamin D deficiency is common (40-80% of most populations) and can be established via history and more objectively by measurement of serum 25-hydroxyl-vitamin D. Replacement doses are in the range of 1,000 IU per day for infants, 2,000 IU per day for children, and 4,000 IU per day for adults.[348] Vitamin D2 (ergocalciferol) should be avoided, and vitamin D3 (cholecalciferol) should be used, preferably in emulsified form to facilitate absorption, especially in older patients and those with impaired digestion and absorption.[349]

---

[343] "Furthermore, a calcium chelator, BAPTA-AM, attenuated the NF-kappaB activation... CONCLUSIONS: Induction of NF-kappaB within 30 min by TNF-alpha- and IL-1beta was mediated through intracellular calcium but not ROS." Chang JW, Kim CS, Kim SB, Park SK, Park JS, Lee SK. Proinflammatory cytokine-induced NF-kappaB activation in human mesangial cells is mediated through intracellular calcium but not ROS: effects of silymarin. *Nephron Exp Nephrol.* 2006;103:e156-65

[344] Tak PP, Firestein GS. NF-kappaB: a key role in inflammatory diseases. J Clin Invest. 2001 Jan;107(1):7-11. See also: **Vasquez A**. Reducing pain and inflammation naturally - Part 4: Nutritional and Botanical Inhibition of NF-kappaB, the Major Intracellular Amplifier of the Inflammatory Cascade. A Practical Clinical Strategy Exemplifying Anti-Inflammatory Nutrigenomics. *Nutritional Perspectives* 2005;July: 5-12 http://optimalhealthresearch.com/part4

[345] Timms PM, Mannan N, Hitman GA, et al. Circulating MMP9, vitamin D and variation in the TIMP-1 response with VDR genotype: mechanisms for inflammatory damage in chronic disorders? QJM. 2002 Dec;95(12):787-96. See also: **Vasquez A**, Manso G, Cannell J. The clinical importance of vitamin D (cholecalciferol): a paradigm shift with implications for all healthcare providers. *Altern Ther Health Med.* 2004 Sep-Oct;10(5):28-36 http://optimalhealthresearch.com/monograph04

[346] **Vasquez A**. Integrative Orthopedics. www.OptimalHealthResearch.com/orthopedics.html

[347] Simons DG. Cardiology and myofascial trigger points: Janet G. Travell's contribution. *Tex Heart Inst J.* 2003;30(1):3-7

[348] **Vasquez A**, Manso G, Cannell J. The clinical importance of vitamin D (cholecalciferol): a paradigm shift with implications for all healthcare providers. Altern Ther Health Med. 2004 Sep-Oct;10(5):28-36 http://optimalhealthresearch.com/monograph04

[349] **Vasquez A**. Subphysiologic Doses of Vitamin D are Subtherapeutic: Comment on the Study by The Record Trial Group. *The Lancet* 2005 Published on-line May 6 http://optimalhealthresearch.com/lancet

2. ***Reduction in dietary arachidonic acid intake***: Arachidonic acid promotes intracellular calcium uptake, as demonstrated in a recent study using human erythrocytes.[350] Rich sources of arachidonic acid include beef, liver, pork, lamb, and cow's milk.

3. ***Increase intake of eicosapentaenoic acid (EPA)***: EPA reduces intracellular calcium levels in experimental models[351] and anticancer, antihypertensive, and anti-inflammatory effects of EPA are seen clinically. One to three grams per day is reasonable for adults.

4. ***Urinary alkalinization***: Diet-induced chronic metabolic acidosis[352] promotes loss of calcium in urine[353] and thus indirectly contributes to calcium deficiency and the resultant rise in parathyroid hormone and intracellular calcium levels. An alkalinizing plant-based Paleo-Mediterranean diet should be the foundational treatment for numerous reasons[354]; however some patients may need to supplement with vegetable culture, potassium citrate, potassium bicarbonate, and/or sodium bicarbonate either chronically or on an "as needed" basis.

5. ***Ensuring adequate intake of calcium***: A healthy diet can supply upwards toward 1,000 mg of calcium per day, and some people may choose to supplement with an additional 500 to 1,500 mg daily. Calcium supplementation should be used with magnesium, vitamin D and other components of the supplemented Paleo-Mediterranean diet.[355]

6. ***Avoiding other dietary and lifestyle factors that promote calcium loss in urine***: Caffeine, sugar, alcohol/ethanol, and psychoemotional stress all increase calcium loss in urine and thus contribute to secondary hyperparathyroidism and intracellular hypercalcinosis.

Conclusions:

In this brief article, I have introduced and reviewed important concepts related to diet-induced alterations in cellular calcium balance. Notice that this discussion of calcium has transcended the usual conversation of simple "deficiency" and "excess." What I've done here is review data showing that we can indirectly modulate certain aspects of intracellular nutrition to promote optimal biochemical balance within the cell in order to optimize health and prevent and correct disease and dysfunction. Next time someone tells you that there is no scientific basis for interventional nutrition, sit them down and give them a lecture on causes and treatments for intracellular hypercalcinosis. Tell them it is only the tip of the iceberg, and that they'd be wise to take interventional nutrition seriously. Just because we buy groceries and nutritional supplements without a prescription (for now), this does not mean that these choices are not powerful or lacking in scientific merit. Amazing results can be achieved with diet modification and nutritional/botanical supplementation.

---

[350] "The Ca(2+) influx rate varied from 0.5 to 3 nM Ca(2+)/s in the presence of AA and from 0.9 to 1.7 nM Ca(2+)/s with EPA." Soldati L, Lombardi C, Adamo D, Terranegra A, Bianchin C, Bianchi G, Vezzoli G. Arachidonic acid increases intracellular calcium in erythrocytes. *Biochem Biophys Res Commun*. 2002 May 10;293(3):974-8

[351] "This is a consequence of the ability of EPA to release Ca2+ from intracellular stores while inhibiting their refilling via capacitative Ca2+ influx that results in partial emptying of intracellular Ca2+ stores and thereby activation of protein kinase R." Palakurthi SS, Fluckiger R, Aktas H, Changolkar AK, Shahsafaei A, Harneit S, Kilic E, Halperin JA. Inhibition of translation initiation mediates the anticancer effect of the n-3 polyunsaturated fatty acid eicosapentaenoic acid. *Cancer Res*. 2000 Jun 1;60(11):2919-25

[352] Maurer M, Riesen W, Muser J, Hulter HN, Krapf R. Neutralization of Western diet inhibits bone resorption independently of K intake and reduces cortisol secretion in humans. *Am J Physiol Renal Physiol*. 2003 Jan;284(1):F32-40

[353] Sellmeyer DE, Schloetter M, Sebastian A. Potassium citrate prevents increased urine calcium excretion and bone resorption induced by a high sodium chloride diet. *J Clin Endocrinol Metab*. 2002 May;87(5):2008-12

[354] **Vasquez A**. A Five-Part Nutritional Protocol that Produces Consistently Positive Results. *Nutritional Wellness* 2005 September http://optimalhealthresearch.com/protocol

[355] **Vasquez A**. Integrative Rheumatology. http://www.optimalhealthresearch.com/rheumatology.html

Nutritional Treatments for Hypertension

Alex Vasquez, D.C., N.D.

This article was originally published in *Naturopathy Digest*
http://www.naturopathydigest.com/archives/2006/nov/vasquez.php

Introduction:
Clinical problems associated with hypertension can be divided into two categories dependent upon the severity and duration of the elevated blood pressure. Mild elevations in blood pressure that are sustained over a period of many years and decades increases the risk of atherosclerosis, stroke, myocardial infarction, heart failure, and renal failure. Acute elevations in blood pressure, even if sustained for a relatively short time, can cause hypertensive encephalopathy, stroke, retinal hemorrhage, acute myocardial infarction, and acute left ventricular failure with pulmonary edema. Many different etiologies exist for hypertension, including but not limited to metabolic syndrome, hypothyroidism, renal failure, and adverse drug effects; the scope of this article is limited to uncomplicated prehypertension and Stage One Hypertension. Obviously, the goals of therapy are to bring the blood pressure down into the normal range and to prevent end-organ damage, especially to heart, brain, eyes, and kidneys.

Guidelines for the assessment and therefore management of hypertension change periodically based on new consensus and new research data. "Prehypertension" or early hypertension begins at 120 systolic over 80 diastolic, while "Stage One hypertension" is in the range of 140/90 - 160/100. Patients beyond Stage One Hypertension or those with a complex clinical presentation should generally be co-managed pharmaceutically (at least initially); a table describing hypertensive categories is provided below (Table 1). Doctors who choose to manage hypertension for their patients must include proper history, physical examination, laboratory assessment (e.g., chemistry/metabolic panel, urinalysis, thyroid and cardiovascular panels), and the treatment plan must include frequent follow-up (e.g., every 2-4 weeks) until the problem is resolved. If effectiveness cannot be obtained, sustained, or documented then the patient should receive both verbal and written referral to another physician, particularly an internist or cardiologist.

Table 1: Hypertension categorization*

Prehypertension:	>120/80
Stage One:	140/90 - 160/100
Stage Two:	160/100 - 210/120 without symptoms and without end-organ damage (i.e., no renal damage, headache, or edema). Clinicians should generally refer or co-manage these patients.
Urgent:	SBP ≥ 220 or DBP 125 - 129, or Stage 2 with symptoms or end-organ damage. Immediate referral for drug treatment is appropriate.
Emergency:	>220/130 is an emergency: 911 or ER

* Additional considerations that affect treatment and management: Insulin resistance / pre-diabetes / metabolic syndrome: dyslipidemia / high cholesterol, obesity, inactivity, personal and family medical history, other chief complaints and clinical and laboratory findings.

Nutritional treatments for hypertension:
Nutritional treatments for hypertension include the following considerations, which can generally be used in combination (rather than in isolation, as studied in the research). These will be listed and discussed in order of general effectiveness (see Table 2).

1. Short-term supervised fasting: Short-term inpatient supervised fasting appears to be the most effective treatment for chronic hypertension that has ever been documented. Working closely with his multidisciplinary team, **pioneering chiropractic physician Alan Goldhamer DC** documented reductions in hypertension of 60/17 in patients with severe

hypertension and reductions of 37/13 in patients with moderate hypertension.[356,357,358] Generally the program begins with 4-7 days of a raw vegetarian diet followed by 1-2 weeks of fasting and concluded with reintroduction of a vegetarian and health-promoting diet. Laboratory tests and professional supervision help ensure patient safety.

2. <u>Healthy diet and exercise</u>: Health-promoting diets such as either Paleo- and Mediterranean-style diets can lower blood pressure by as much as 17/13 according to some reports. Please see my previous articles in this magazine for description of the "supplemented Paleo-Mediterranean Diet."[359]

3. <u>CoQ10</u>: Coenzyme Q-10 in doses of 100-225 mg/day can lower blood pressure quite effectively, as documented in several clinical studies, some of which showed that CoQ-10 is more effective and safer than the use of antihypertensive drugs.[360,361,362] Reductions in blood pressure are generally in the range of 17/12 and are dose-dependent. A patient who does not respond to 100 mg per day may respond very well to 200 mg per day. Since it is a fat-soluble nutrient, CoQ-10 should be administered with dietary fat and/or consumed in a "pre-emulsified" form to enhance absorption which is a prerequisite for clinical effectiveness. Several trials have been reported showing enhanced absorption of CoQ-10 when administered in pre-emulsified form. CoQ-10 is very safe, and drug interactions are rare; caution should be used in patients taking coumadin.

4. <u>Sodium restriction</u>: Clinical responsiveness to low-sodium diets ranges from minimal to a maximal reduction in the range of 22/14 - 16/9.[363] Contraindications to low-sodium diet are uncommon (e.g., hyponatremia); low-sodium diets should generally be a component of all anti-hypertensive treatment plans.

5. <u>Vitamin D and calcium</u>: Vitamin D3 (cholecalciferol) and calcium supplementation can reduce blood pressure in hypertensive patients by approximately 13/7.[364] As I have discussed in extensive detail elsewhere, a reasonable dose of vitamin D3 for adults is in the range of 2,000 - 4,000 IU per day, and doctors new to vitamin D therapy should read my clinical monograph published in 2004 and available on-line.[365] The most important drug interaction with vitamin D is seen with hydrochlorothiazide, a commonly-used antihypertensive diuretic that promotes hypercalcemia; vitamin D therapy in patients taking hydrochlorothiazide must be implemented slowly, with professional supervision, and with weekly laboratory monitoring of serum calcium. Vitamin D probably corrects hypertension via several mechanisms, including but not limited to increased absorption of magnesium

---

[356] Goldhamer A, et al. Medically supervised water-only fasting in the treatment of hypertension. *J Manipulative Physiol Ther* 2001 Jun;24(5):335-9

[357] Goldhamer AC, et al. Medically supervised water-only fasting in the treatment of borderline hypertension. *J Altern Complement Med*. 2002 Oct;8(5):643-50

[358] Goldhamer AC. Initial cost of care results in medically supervised water-only fasting for treating high blood pressure and diabetes. *J Altern Complement Med*. 2002 Dec;8(6):696-7

[359] **Vasquez A**. Five-Part Nutritional Protocol that Produces Consistently Positive Results.*NutrWellness*2005 Sept http://optimalhealthresearch.com/protocol

[360] "RESULTS: The mean reduction in systolic blood pressure of the CoQ-treated group was 17.8 +/- 7.3 mm Hg (mean +/- SEM). None of the patients exhibited orthostatic blood pressure changes. CONCLUSIONS: Our results suggest CoQ may be safely offered to hypertensive patients as an alternative treatment option." Burke BE, Neuenschwander R, Olson RD. Randomized, double-blind, placebo-controlled trial of coenzyme Q10 in isolated systolic hypertension. *South Med J*. 2001 Nov;94(11):1112-7

[361] "These findings indicate that treatment with coenzyme Q10 decreases blood pressure possibly by decreasing oxidative stress and insulin response in patients with known hypertension receiving conventional antihypertensive drugs." Singh RB, Niaz MA, Rastogi SS, Shukla PK, Thakur AS. Effect of hydrosoluble coenzyme Q10 on blood pressures and insulin resistance in hypertensive patients with coronary artery disease. *J Hum Hypertens*. 1999 Mar;13(3):203-8

[362] "...51% of patients came completely off of between one and three antihypertensive drugs at an average of 4.4 months after starting CoQ10." Langsjoen P, Langsjoen P, Willis R, Folkers K. Treatment of essential hypertension with coenzyme Q10. *Mol Aspects Med*. 1994;15 Suppl:S265-72

[363] "The average fall in blood pressure from the highest to the lowest sodium intake was 16/9 mm Hg." MacGregor GA, Markandu ND, Sagnella GA, Singer DR, Cappuccio FP. Double-blind study of three sodium intakes and long-term effects of sodium restriction in essential hypertension. *Lancet*. 1989 Nov 25;2(8674):1244-7

[364] "A short-term supplementation with vitamin D(3) and calcium is more effective in reducing SBP than calcium alone. Inadequate vitamin D(3) and calcium intake could play a contributory role in the pathogenesis and progression of hypertension and cardiovascular disease in elderly women." Pfeifer M, Begerow B, Minne HW, Nachtigall D, Hansen C. Effects of a short-term vitamin D(3) and calcium supplementation on blood pressure and parathyroid hormone levels in elderly women. *J Clin Endocrinol Metab*. 2001 Apr;86(4):1633-7

[365] **Vasquez A**, Manso G, Cannell J. The clinical importance of vitamin D (cholecalciferol): a paradigm shift with implications for all healthcare providers. *Altern Ther Health Med*. 2004 Sep-Oct;10(5):28-36 http://optimalhealthresearch.com/monograph04

and reduction in intracellular calcium, as I described previously in this magazine.[366] Since vitamin D absorption decreases with age and in patients with intestinal disease (including dysbiosis[367]), absorption of fat-soluble vitamin D3 is enhanced when administered in pre-emulsified form.[368]

6. Prescription drugs: Use of the nutritional treatments described in this article can complement or replace antihypertensive drug therapy in many patients. When used singly, prescription antihypertensive drugs average a reduction in blood pressure of approximately 12/6. Initial reductions of 20/10 require combination therapy, according to a review article published in *American Family Physician* in 2003.[369]

7. Exercise: Moderate exercise can reduce blood pressure by approximately 7/7 in the short term. Longer-term exercise, particularly along with diet improvements and weight loss, can result in synergistic and curative benefits. Patients who have been sedentary for years and those with probable or documented cardiovascular disease should be evaluated by a physician and ECG before beginning an exercise program.

8. Fish oil: Fish oil supplementation had been shown to reduce blood pressure by approximately 3/2. For reasons that I have detailed elsewhere[370], fish oil should be co-administered with a source of GLA such as borage oil in order to maximize effectiveness and minimize subtle biochemical adverse effects. Importantly, fish oil is safer, less expensive, and more effective than "statin" antihypercholesterolemic drug treatment for reducing total and cardiovascular mortality.

9. Food allergy elimination: According to a clinical study of migraineurs published in *The Lancet*, identification and avoidance of food allergens can normalize blood pressure in hypertensive migraine patients.[371] The anti-hypertensive response to food allergy avoidance can be seen clinically even in patients who do not have migraine or other manifestations of allergy, but the more allergic symptoms that are seen and the more complete the response to allergy elimination, the more likely is a reduction in blood pressure.

Table 2: General effectiveness of therapies for chronic essential hypertension

	Therapy	Effectiveness
1.	Short-term supervised fasting:	-60/-17 for severe HTN and -37/-13 for moderate HTN*
2.	Healthy diet and exercise:	-17/-13
3.	CoQ10 100-225 mg/day:	-17/-12
4.	Sodium restriction:	22/14 - 16/-9
5.	Vitamin D and calcium:	-13/-7
6.	Prescription drugs:	-12/-6 * Reductions of 20/10 require combination therapy
7.	Exercise:	-7/-7
8.	Fish oil:	-3/-2
9.	Food allergy elimination:	variable response ranging from insignificant to curative

Conclusions: Many nutritional treatments for hypertension are documented in the research literature, and several of these treatments appear safer and more cost-effective than pharmaceutical antihypertensive drugs. Furthermore, the synergistic use of the nutritional and lifestyle interventions described above—e.g., supplemented Paleo-Mediterranean diet along with exercise, fish oil, vitamin D, CoQ-10, and sodium restriction-results in clinical benefits that far

[366] **Vasquez A**. Intracellular Hypercalcinosis. A Functional Nutritional Disorder With Implications Ranging From Myofascial Trigger Points to Affective Disorders, Hypertension and Cancer. Naturopathy *Digest* 2006, September http://www.naturopathydigest.com/archives/2006/sep/vasquez.php

[367] **Vasquez A**. Reducing Pain and Inflammation Naturally. Part 6: Nutritional and Botanical Treatments Against "Silent Infections" and Gastrointestinal Dysbiosis, Commonly Overlooked Causes of Neuromusculoskeletal Inflammation and Chronic Health Problems. *Nutritional Perspectives* 2006; January. http://optimalhealthresearch.com/dysbiosis

[368] **Vasquez A**. Subphysiologic Doses of Vitamin D are Subtherapeutic: Comment on the Study by The Record Trial Group. *Lancet* 2005 published online May 6 http://optimalhealthresearch.com/lancet

[369] Magill MK, Gunning K, Saffel-Shrier S, Gay C. New developments in the management of hypertension. *Am Fam Physician*. 2003 Sep 1;68(5):853-8 http://www.aafp.org/afp/20030901/853.html

[370] **Vasquez A**. Reducing Pain and Inflammation Naturally. Part 2: New Insights into Fatty Acid Supplementation and Its Effect on Eicosanoid Production and Genetic Expression. *Nutritional Perspectives* 2005; January: 5-16 http://optimalhealthresearch.com/part2.html

[371] Grant EC. Food allergies and migraine. *Lancet*. 1979 May 5;1(8123):966-9

exceed the results published in the single-intervention clinical trials that have documented the effectiveness of the individual components. The major drug interaction that one must look out for is the combination of vitamin D with hydrochlorothiazide. Switching from pharmaceutical drugs to nutrients for the management of hypertension requires diligent follow-up, informed consent, and documentation of beneficial clinical response and should be undertaken only by skilled and experienced clinicians.

Twilight of the Idiopathic Era and the Dawn of New Possibilities in Health and Healthcare

Alex Vasquez, D.C., N.D.

Originally published in *Naturopathy Digest* in 2006, this essay was slightly edited in 2010. http://www.naturopathydigest.com/archives/2006/mar/idiopathic.php

Among the perplexing paradoxes that exist in healthcare is coexistence of our adoration of allopathy for its "scientific method" along with the description of most chronic diseases as "idiopathic." If the allopathic use of the scientific method were so adroit, then why are so many conditions described as having "no known cause"? Is it that the scientific method is inadequate, or that the allopathic lens is incapable of bringing disease causation into focus? Perhaps a third option exists: that some groups—namely the allopaths and the pharmaceutical companies—benefit by convincing us that most diseases have "no known cause" and that therefore the best that doctors and patients can hope for is additive and endless pharmaceuticalization of all health problems. When the cause of our health problems is "unknown", we are disempowered, and we must depend on "experts" to help us. When the causes of our problems are known, we are empowered to take effective action. Certainly, some groups have financial and political interests in keeping us *as professionals* and *as patients* confused and disempowered.

The End of the Idiopathic Era
A stark contrast exists between primary research literature and the "facts" that are selectively reported in medical textbooks and which are used to buttress "conventional wisdom" and the resultant status quo. While I have been aware of this contrast for many years, the divergency was impressed upon me with renewed vigor during the preparation of a recent article[372] and the completion of my recent textbook *Integrative Rheumatology*.[373] Arthritis in general and autoimmune and rheumatic diseases in particular are frequently described as "idiopathic" and as having "no known cause" by most mainstream medical books like *The Merck Manual* and *Current Medical Diagnosis and Treatment*; these contentions are inconsistent with the abundant and diverse research showing that—rather than being *idiopathic*—most chronic musculoskeletal disorders are *multifactorial*. When a disease is codified as *idiopathic*, doctors lose their incentive to look for and treat the *causes* [plural] of the disease because the codified conventional wisdom has already stated that "The cause [singular] of the disease has not been identified." Similarly, patients are convinced to give up their hope of ever being *cured*; they chose what appears to be the second best option: lifelong medicalization. In these instances, acceptance of the codified conventional wisdom benefits doctors and patients by freeing them of the obligation to think, to

---

[372] **Vasquez A**. Reducing Pain and Inflammation Naturally. Part 6: Nutritional and Botanical Treatments Against "Silent Infections" and Gastrointestinal Dysbiosis, Commonly Overlooked Causes of Neuromusculoskeletal Inflammation and Chronic Health Problems. *Nutritional Perspectives* 2006; January http://www.optimalhealthresearch.com/part6
[373] **Vasquez A**. *Integrative Rheumatology. The Art of Creating Wellness While Effectively Managing Acute and Chronic Musculoskeletal Disorders*. 2006 http://www.optimalhealthresearch.com/rheumatology.html

mobilize their consciousness; the price paid for this exoneration from consciousness is perpetuated unconsciousness and drug dependence for doctors and patients. Being told by powerful institutions and ensconced authorities that "There's nothing else you can do, and nothing more to think about" lulls us all into apathy and conformity at the price of our individual and collective lives and consciousnesses.

Idiopathic, or Multifactorial?

Let's look at psoriasis and rheumatoid arthritis as two shining examples of *idiopathicity*. If one looks into a standard medical textbook, one sees that these conditions have no known cause and therefore the lifelong prescription of anti-inflammatory medications is presumptively justified. On the contrary, if one spends a few days in any medical library, one can find articles that point to the causes of these diseases and which then illuminate the path (and paths) by which doctors and patients can arrive at authentic improvement or permanent cure. Most patients can be cured of psoriasis, and a large percentage of rheumatoid arthritis patients can avoid the complications and medicalization associated with their disease, particularly if *the causes* of their condition are treated early. We now know that most autoimmune diseases are caused by and/or perpetuated by chronic infections, food allergies, a proinflammatory lifestyle, hormonal imbalances, and exposure to chemicals and metals that cause immune dysfunction. When the cause(s) of the disease is treated, the disease has the potential to be cured, provided that it is treated comprehensively and hopefully before the onset of irreversible damage. When the disease is cured, lifelong medicalization becomes unnecessary, the patient is free to fully resume his/her life, and doctors are liberated from their roles as drug representatives and can resume their proper positions as healers and creative free-thinking individuals.

Asserting an empowered stance toward disease prevention and treatment carries implications beyond those for the doctor and the patient. These implications also point to new ways of living and stewarding the world. When we look at a disease like Parkinson's disease and then determine that it is *idiopathic*, then nothing happens to change or shape our view of the world, our place in it, and the interconnected components of health and disease. Everyone agrees that that clinical manifestations of Parkinson's disease result from the death of dopaminergic neurons. From the allopathic perspective, the disease is *idiopathic*, while from an integrative naturopathic perspective, we see Parkinson's disease as a *multifaceted disorder* associated with defective mitochondrial function, impaired xenobiotic detoxification, and occupational and/or recreational exposure to toxicants, particularly pesticides. These associations align to create a new model for the illness based on exposure to neurotoxicants such as pesticides[374] which are ineffectively detoxified[375] and then accumulate in the brain[376] and induce mitochondrial dysfunction[377] and resultant oxidative stress[378] which leads to death of dopaminergic neurons. Therefore, from the perspective of both prevention and treatment, the clinical approach to Parkinson's disease would include pesticide avoidance and optimization of detoxification to prevent the neuronal accumulation of neurotoxic mitochondrial poisons. The plan must also include optimization of nutritional status, antioxidant capacity, and mitochondrial function.[379] Further, if our goal is to reduce the societal prevalence of Parkinson's disease, then we must begin living in better harmony with nature and thinking of ways to reduce our use of pesticides and herbicides, the chemicals that are consistently shown to cause premature neuronal death and which are increasingly pervasive in our home, work, and outdoor environments.

[374] Ritz B, Yu F. Parkinson's disease mortality and pesticide exposure in California 1984-1994. *Int J Epidemiol*. 2000 Apr;29(2):323-9.

[375] Menegon A, Board PG, Blackburn AC, Mellick GD, Le Couteur DG. Parkinson's disease, pesticides, and glutathione transferase polymorphisms. *Lancet*. 1998;352(9137):1344-6.

[376] Kamel F, Hoppin JA. Related Articles, Association of pesticide exposure with neurologic dysfunction and disease. *Environ Health Perspect*. 2004;112(9):950-8.

[377] Parker WD Jr, Swerdlow RH. Mitochondrial dysfunction in idiopathic Parkinson disease. *Am J Hum Genet*. 1998;62(4):758-62.

[378] Davey GP, Peuchen S, Clark JB. Energy thresholds in brain mitochondria. Potential involvement in neurodegeneration. *J Biol Chem*. 1998;273(21):12753-7.

[379] Kidd PM. Parkinson's disease as multifactorial oxidative neurodegeneration: implications for integrative management. *Altern Med Rev*. 2000 Dec;5(6):502-29.

The Dawn of New Possibilities in Health and Healthcare

The time is past when credible physicians can assert that most diseases are "of unknown origin." The truth is that we already have access to the information we need to help our patients. The truth is that we can often offer our patients the *probability of cure* rather than *lifelong and endless prescriptions for symptom-modifying drugs*. These truths imply that healthcare and our systems of healthcare delivery must change, because the pharmaceutical and medical icons that stand before us were built upon feet and legs of clay and interspersed lead. We stand at the dawn of a new era in healthcare—one in which patients with chronic diseases in general and autoimmune diseases in particular—have a tangible and authentic opportunity to regain their health.

Promoting Unhealthy Eating: Proatherosclerotic Recipes Endorsed by the US National Heart, Lung, and Blood Institute (NHLBI)

The following is a partial list of atherosclerosis-promoting recipes listed under the title "Stay Young at Heart: Cooking the Heart-Healthy Way"[380] advocated on the website of the NHLBI in December 2009. Notice the lack of nutrient density, the emphasis on simple carbohydrates, the frequent use of baking with oil to create the effect of frying, the lack of raw foods, and the scarcity of phytonutrients:

- "Stir-fried beef" with boiled potatoes and white rice
- "Beef stroganoff" with 6 cups of cooked macaroni pasta
- "Crispy oven-fried chicken" cooked in cornflakes and buttermilk
- "Classic macaroni and cheese"
- "Candied yams" with brown sugar, margarine, white flour, and orange juice
- "Oven French fries" (white potatoes oven-fried in vegetable oil)
- "White rice" cooked with vegetable oil and salt
- "Sunshine (white) rice" cooked with vegetable oil, orange juice, and lemon juice
- "Homestyle biscuits" made from white flour, salt, and sugar
- "Banana-nut bread" made from mashed ripe bananas, low-fat buttermilk, packed brown sugar, margarine, all-purpose white flour, egg and salt.
- "Apricot-orange bread" made from dried apricots, margarine, white sugar, egg, white flour, dry milk powder, salt and orange juice
- "Apple coffee cake" made with peeled apples (please note that >90% of the antioxidants contained in apples are in the peel—thus when the peel is removed, virtually all that remains is antioxidant-poor carbohydrate), one cup of sugar, one cup of dark raisins, one-quarter cup vegetable oil, 1 egg, and two-and-a-half cups of sifted all-purpose white flour
- "Frosted cake" with 2 1/4 cups cake flour, 4 tablespoons margarine, 1 1/4 cups sugar, 4 eggs, low fat cream cheese, and 2 cups sifted confectioners sugar!!
- "Topical fruit compote" with sugar
- "Peach cobbler" with sugar, white flour, margarine, canned peaches "packed in juice", peach nectar, and cornstarch
- "Rice pudding" with white rice, 3 cups of skim milk, and 2/3 cup sugar

The list goes on to include many other proatherosclerotic and prodiabetic meals. Any reasonable person—*the general public has the option but healthcare professionals have the obligation*—might ask why US National Heart, Lung, and Blood Institute would promote a diet plan that is ensured to contribute to the pandemics of hypertension, obesity, and diabetes mellitus.

---

[380] US National Heart, Lung, and Blood Institute (NHLBI). Stay Young at Heart: Cooking the Heart-Healthy Way. http://www.nhlbi.nih.gov/health/public/heart/other/syah/index.htm Accessed December 23, 2009

Thinking Outside the (Pill) Box: Is the "Battle Against Hypertension and Diabetes" Truly Meant to be "Won" for Patients…or for the Drug Companies?

The Most Profitable "Wars" are the ones that are Fought Indefinitely and which Require Reliance on Private Industry: As with most modern sociopolitical fights, wars, and missions, a keen observer (or any high-school student who read George Orwell's classic novel *1984*) might question whether the current "**Mission**: To **Combat** High Blood Pressure in America"[381] is actually meant to ever be won. The US National Heart, Lung, and Blood Institute (NHLBI) invokes the language of battle, e.g., "to **mobilize** all Americans in the **fight against high blood pressure** and reduce the more than 1 million heart attacks, strokes, and kidney failure cases that it causes each year. The CDC and the NHLBI have **joined forces** to **disseminate** these materials…"[382] Ironically, the NHLBI's document entitled "Physician Fact Sheet: What Every Physician Should Know" (http://hp2010.nhlbihin.net/mission/partner/physcian_factsheet.pdf) contains zero practical information on diet, exercise, or nutritional supplementation. Likewise, the document under the heading "Real Possibilities for America's Health Care Providers"[383] provides nothing that a clinician or patient could use to authentically correct the common causes of HTN; it provides near-meaningless mention of "diet and exercise" accompanied by a photo of people sitting at a table with food and encourages that doctors "Support Adherence to Treatment" accompanied by a photo of a woman taking pills.

"Common Objectives" …with Drug Companies: For more than a decade, the American Heart Association has been "advised" by their "Pharmaceutical Roundtable" (PRT) comprised of **monolithic drug companies which must each pay a least $1 million per year for each 3-year term of membership.**[384] According to the American Heart Association's website in a document updated August 2009[385], "The American Heart Association Pharmaceutical Roundtable (PRT) is a strategic coalition of 10 leading pharmaceutical companies and association volunteers and staff. It allows our association and members of the **pharmaceutical industry** to identify and pursue **common objectives** to improve cardiovascular health in the United States through research, patient education, and public and professional programs." Current (or recent) members of the American Heart Association Pharmaceutical Roundtable include:

1. AstraZeneca L.P.
2. Eli Lilly and Company
3. Bristol-Myers Squibb Company
4. GlaxoSmithKline
5. Merck/Schering-Plough Pharmaceuticals
6. Merck Pharmaceuticals
7. Novartis Pharmaceuticals Corporation
8. Pfizer, Inc.
9. Sanofi-Aventis
10. Takeda Pharmaceuticals

[381] National Heart, Lung, and Blood Institute (NHLBI). The Mission: To Combat High Blood Pressure in America http://hp2010.nhlbihin.net/mission/ Accessed December 22, 2009
[382] Centers for Disease Control and Prevention. State Heart Disease and Stroke Prevention Program Addresses High Blood Pressure. http://www.cdc.gov/dhdsp/library/fs_state_hbp.htm Accessed December 22, 2009
[383] National Heart, Lung, and Blood Institute (NHLBI). http://www.nhlbi.nih.gov/health/prof/heart/hbp/mp/mp_health.htm Accessed December 22, 2009
[384] "Each industry participant of the PRT will sign a separate agreement with AHA that will be binding only between the AHA and that individual industry member. The agreements will commit each industry member to contribute $1,000,000 per year for three years." Letter dated March 20, 1998 from Joel I. Klein (Assistant Attorney General), US Department of Justice Antitrust Division. http://www.justice.gov/atr/public/busreview/1608.htm Accessed December 23, 2009
[385] http://www.americanheart.org/presenter.jhtml?identifier=2366 Accessed December 23, 2009

Section 3:
Wellness Promotion
&
Re-Establishing the Foundation for Health

Introduction to Lifestyle Optimization, Wellness Promotion, and Disease Prevention

This section details the lifestyle modifications that support a wellness-promoting antihypertensive cardioprotective whole-health program.

Among the four major primary healthcare professions in the United States—chiropractic, osteopathy, naturopathy, and allopathy—the naturopathic profession stands preeminent in its emphasis upon wellness promotion and lifestyle optimization. This chapter reviews wellness promotion from the current author's perspective and experience—both personal and professional—which is consistent with but not officially representative of the naturopathic profession's concepts "re-establish the foundation of health" and "hierarchy of therapeutics."

This chapter originated many years ago as a handout for patients wherein it explained and described basic concepts that are foundational to health restoration, preservation, and optimization. Over the years that this handout has evolved into a chapter for my books, it has become more detailed and more relevant for clinicians treating patients. In essence, this chapter is a blueprint for the construction of a healthy lifestyle. While it may not cover every consideration, it covers the basics in sufficient detail so as to allow patients to change tracks from the downward descent of the disease-promoting lifestyle to the upward ascent of the health-promoting lifestyle.

Replacing the passive and disempowering drug-surgery paradigm with an active and empowering integrative/functional model of healthcare is one goal of this section.

This section can be thought of as a collection of essays. The review and consideration of a wide range of topics—which might otherwise appear random and nontopical to a reader accustomed to a more limited scope of discussion—is necessary due to the multifaceted nature of human experience and the widely ranging influences on health and disease outcomes.

<u>Topics</u>:

- **Re-establishing the Foundation for Health**
  - ○ **Healthcare, Health, and Wellness**
  - ○ **Daily living**
    - ▪ Lifestyle habits
    - ▪ Motivation: background and clinical applications
    - ▪ Exceptional living: the key to exceptional results
    - ▪ Recognize and affirm individual uniqueness
    - ▪ Individuation & conscious living: alternatives to common paradigms
    - ▪ Quality and quantity of sleep: concepts and clinical applications
    - ▪ Exercise, obesity, BMI, and proinflammatory activity of adipose tissue
  - ○ **Diet is a powerful tool for the prevention and treatment of disease**
    - ▪ Make "whole foods" the foundation of the diet
    - ▪ Increase consumption of fruits and vegetables
    - ▪ Phytochemicals: food-derived anti-inflammatory nutrients
    - ▪ Eat the right amount of protein
    - ▪ Reducing consumption of sugars: exceptions for supercompensation
    - ▪ Avoiding artificial sweeteners, colors, and other additives, reducing caffeine
    - ▪ To the extent possible, eat "organic" foods
    - ▪ Recognize the importance of avoiding food allergens
    - ▪ Supplement your healthy diet with vitamins, minerals, and fatty acids
    - ▪ General guidelines for the safe use of nutritional supplements
  - ○ **Advanced concepts in nutrition**
    - ▪ "Biochemical Individuality" and "Orthomolecular Medicine"
    - ▪ Nutrigenomics: Nutritional genomics
    - ▪ Putting it all together: *the supplemented Paleo-Mediterranean diet*
  - ○ **Emotional, mental, and social health**
    - ▪ Stress management and authentic living
    - ▪ Stress always has a biochemical/physiologic component
    - ▪ The body functions as a whole
    - ▪ Healing past experiences
    - ▪ Autonomization, intradependence, emotional literacy, corrective experience
  - ○ **Environmental health**
    - ▪ Environmental exposures and the importance of detoxification
    - ▪ Avoid unnecessary chemical medications and medical procedures
    - ▪ Intestinal health, bowel function, and introduction to dysbiosis
- **Natural holistic healthcare contrasted to standard medical treatment**
- **Opposite influences of health promotion vs. disease promotion**
- **Brief Overview of Integrative Primary Healthcare Disciplines**: Chiropractic, Naturopathic Medicine, Osteopathic Medicine, Functional Medicine
- **Previously published essays**
  - ○ Five-Part Nutritional Wellness Protocol That Produces Consistently Positive Results
  - ○ Implementing the Five-Part Nutritional Wellness Protocol for the Treatment of Various Health Problems
  - ○ Common Oversights and Shortcomings in the Study and Implementation of Nutritional Supplementation
  - ○ Revisiting the Five-Part Nutritional Wellness Protocol: The Supplemented Paleo-Mediterranean Diet

Introduction to Wellness Promotion:
Re-Establishing the Foundation for Health

> "The work of the naturopathic physician is to elicit healing by helping patients to create or recreate conditions for health to exist within them.
> **Health will occur where the conditions for health exist.**
> **Disease is the product of conditions which allow for it.**" *Jared Zeff, N.D.*[1]

One of the most important concepts within the philosophy and practice of naturopathic medicine is that of "re-establishing the foundation for health." This means that instead of first looking to a specific treatment or "magic bullet" to solve a health problem, we first look at the environment in which the problem arose to determine if the patient's environment has initiated or perpetuated the problem. The term *environment* as used here means much more than the patient's immediate surroundings at home and work; it includes all modifiable factors that may have an effect on the patient's health, such as lifestyle, diet, exercise, supplementation, chronic and situational stress, medications with positive and negative effects, exposure to toxicants and microbes, nutritionally-modifiable genetic factors[2], emotions, feelings, and unconscious assumptions[3], and many other considerations. Although the genes that we and our patients have inherited cannot be changed, we can very often modulate the expression of those genes (e.g., via nutrigenomics, described later) by modifying the biochemical, microbial, toxicologic, and neurohormonal milieu that bathes our cells and thus our genes; this concept was expressed in a statement by the US Centers for Disease Control and Prevention in its "Gene-Environment Interaction Fact Sheet" available on-line.[4]

`"Optimal health" does not and never will come in a pill or tonic—the human body and the interactions that we each have between our genes, outlooks, environments, and lifestyles are far too complex to ever be addressed wholly and completely by a simplistic paradigm or single treatment. Even a superficial observation of the complexity of human physiology and the complexity of our environments (including noise, toxins such as benzene and mercury, chemicals such as formaldehyde from building materials, work stress and multitasking, radiation

---

Environment—lifestyle, diet, stresses, microbes, toxins—influences genetic expression and the manifestation of health or disease

"Virtually all human diseases result from the interaction of genetic susceptibility factors and modifiable environmental factors, broadly defined to include infectious, chemical, physical, nutritional, and behavioral factors. …

"Even so-called single-gene disorders actually develop from the interaction of both genetic and environmental factors. …

"We do not inherit a disease state per se. Instead, we inherit a set of a susceptibility factors to certain effects of environmental factors and therefore inherit a higher risk for certain diseases."

Gene-Environment Interaction Fact Sheet by the Centers for Disease Control and Prevention, August 2000

---

[1] Zeff JL. The process of healing: a unifying theory of naturopathic medicine. *Journal of Naturopathic Medicine* 1997; 7: 122-5
[2] Kaput J, Rodriguez LR. Nutritional genomics: the next frontier in the postgenomic era. *Physiol Genomics* 16: 166–177 http://physiolgenomics.physiology.org/cgi/content/full/16/2/166
[3] Miller A. The truth will set you free: overcoming emotional blindness and finding your true adult self. New York: Basic Books; 2001
[4] Gene-Environment Interaction Fact Sheet by the Centers for Disease Control and Prevention, August 2000 http://www.ashg.org/pdf/CDC%20Gene-Environment%20Interaction%20Fact%20Sheet.pdf

exposure, microwaves, etc) shows that **our modern lifestyles subject the human body to many more "stressors" than ever before in the history of human existence.** Each of these stressors depletes our psychic and physiologic reserves, such that daily replenishment and protection are necessary.

Research in nutrition and physiology is revealing the mechanisms by which "simple" lifestyle practices and dietary interventions exert their powerful benefits. For example, whole foods such as fruits and vegetables contain over 8,000 phytochemicals with different physiologic effects[5], and simple practices such as meditation and massage can significantly alter hormone and neurotransmitter levels.[6,7] On the surface, a simple practice such as consumption of fruits and vegetables and a multivitamin/multimineral supplement may seem to be a way to provide merely "good nutrition"; however the clinical effects can include antidepressant[8] and anti-inflammatory benefits[9] by enhancing the efficiency of biochemical reactions[10] and by reducing excess activity of NF-kappaB[11], respectively. The power of interventional nutrition utilizing high-doses and/or synergistic formulations of nutraceuticals and phytonutraceuticals becomes much more clinically apparent when patients first (re)establish a healthy foundation of diet and lifestyle practices upon which these treatments can be added; **I estimate that the effectiveness of treatments for complex illness such as inflammatory diseases and cancer is *at least* doubled when patients implement these lifestyle changes in addition to specific treatments rather than relying on specific treatments alone without a healthy supportive lifestyle.** In other words, *"foundation for health* + specific treatments" is much more effective than *"**un**healthy lifestyle* + specific treatments." This explains, in part, the discrepancy between the relatively lackluster response seen in *single-intervention* clinical trials* compared to the better results that we attain clinically when using a holistic approach characterized by *multicomponent* treatment plans. The biochemical and "scientific" reasons for this positive/negative synergism will become more clear during the course of this chapter and textbook.

Single-intervention clinical trials (i.e., clinical trials that utilize only one treatment) are the "gold standard" in allopathic drug-based research because in that setting the goal is to quantify and qualify the nature of positive and negative responses to a single intervention, generally a drug. However, this approach loses much of its luster and relevance in clinical settings where neither patients nor their environments and treatment plans can be standardized due to the unique constitution, lifestyle, history, and other nuances of each patient. Single intervention clinical trials have a place in the researching of all treatments, including natural interventions. However, clinicians—especially recent graduates—must pry themselves away from this research

---

[5] "We propose that the additive and synergistic effects of phytochemicals in fruit and vegetables are responsible for their potent antioxidant and anticancer activities, and that the benefit of a diet rich in fruit and vegetables is attributed to the complex mixture of phytochemicals present in whole foods." Liu RH. Health benefits of fruit and vegetables are from additive and synergistic combinations of phytochemicals. *Am J Clin Nutr.* 2003 Sep;78(3 Suppl):517S-520S

[6] "The significant decrease of the catecholamine metabolite VMA (vanillic-mandelic acid) in meditators, that is associated with a reciprocal increase of 5-HIAA supports as a feedback necessity the "rest and fulfillment response" versus "fight and flight". Bujatti M, Riederer P. Serotonin, noradrenaline, dopamine metabolites in transcendental meditation-technique. *J Neural Transm.* 1976;39(3):257-67

[7] "By the end of the study, the massage therapy group, as compared to the relaxation group, reported experiencing less pain, depression, anxiety and improved sleep. They also showed improved trunk and pain flexion performance, and their serotonin and dopamine levels were higher." Hernandez-Reif M, Field T, Krasnegor J, Theakston H. Lower back pain is reduced and range of motion increased after massage therapy. *Int J Neurosci* 2001;106(3-4):131-45

[8] Benton D, Haller J, Fordy J. Vitamin supplementation for 1 year improves mood. *Neuropsychobiology.* 1995;32(2):98-105

[9] Church TS, Earnest CP, Wood KA, Kampert JB. Reduction of C-reactive protein levels through use of a multivitamin. *Am J Med.* 2003;115(9):702-7

[10] Ames BN, Elson-Schwab I, Silver EA. High-dose vitamin therapy stimulates variant enzymes with decreased coenzyme binding affinity (increased K(m)): relevance to genetic disease and polymorphisms. *Am J Clin Nutr.* 2002 Apr;75(4):616-58 http://www.ajcn.org/cgi/content/full/75/4/616

[11] **Vasquez A**. Reducing pain and inflammation naturally - part 4: nutritional and botanical inhibition of NF-kappaB, the major intracellular amplifier of the inflammatory cascade. A practical clinical strategy exemplifying anti-inflammatory nutrigenomics. *Nutritional Perspectives*, July 2005:5-12. www.OptimalHealthResearch.com/part4

tool when it comes to treating individual patients in clinical practice, where **single interventions are the antithesis of holistic treatment**.

<u>**Daily Living**</u>: Life occurs on a moment-to-moment and daily basis. Choices that we make in relationships, occupations, exercise, and diet have profound and powerful influence over the course of our lives—particularly our health and happiness. Despite the previous and current obfuscation of health information by allopathic groups[12,13,14,15,16] and the pharmaceutical industry[17,18], enough valid information and common sense is available to doctors and the public such that **ignorance is no longer a viable excuse for deferring responsibility for lifestyle-induced disease and misery**.[19] Eating too much sugar and fat while not eating enough fruits and vegetables is making a choice to have an increased probability of developing diabetes, cancer, heart disease, arthritis, and obesity. Exercising regularly, eating a healthy diet, and supplementing the diet with high-quality nutrients and botanicals is making the choice to greatly reduce one's risk of health problems[20,21] and to nurture one's life and one's body so that one can make the most of one's life experience and enjoy life, hobbies, life purpose(s), travel, creativity, community involvement, and time with friends and family.

When we were children, we looked to other people to provide for us and to "take care of us." **As adults, we have to assume responsibility for the course of our own lives, to make decisions based on long-term considerations rather than instant gratification and selective ignorance.** Of course, this does not mean that we have to abandon enjoyment; but it does mean that we can make decisions based on priorities, and if health is a priority then we should take steps to attain and maintain it. For people who have chosen to make their health a priority, sugar- and fat-laden food begins to lose its appeal, and exploring new health-building experiences such as healthy cooking, outdoor activities, and community involvement can become an empowering lifestyle that can be transformed into an art—one that is particularly amenable to building relationships and connections with other people. **The improved sense of well-being and improved physical and intellectual performance obtained from consumption of a health-promoting Paleo-Mediterranean diet (described later) supercedes any short-term gratification from the disease-promoting diet commonly referred to as the Standard American Diet (SAD).** When people want to be healthy, exercising and spending enjoyable time outdoors becomes more fun than the inactivity and passivity of watching television. When we consider that the average American watches at least 3-4 hours of television per day then we should not be surprised that, with physical inactivity as such a major component of the day, Americans show progressively

---

[12] Wolinsky H, Brune T. <u>The Serpent on the Staff: The Unhealthy Politics of the American Medical Association</u>. GP Putnam and Sons, New York, 1994
[13] Wilk CA. <u>Medicine, Monopolies, and Malice: How the Medical Establishment Tried to Destroy Chiropractic</u>. Garden City Park: Avery, 1996
[14] Carter JP. <u>Racketeering in Medicine: The Suppression of Alternatives</u>. Norfolk: Hampton Roads Pub; 1993
[15] National Alliance of Professional Psychology Providers. AMA Seeks To Control and Restrict Psychologist's Scope of Practice. http://www.nappp.org/scope.pdf Accessed November 25, 2006
[16] "In an effort to marshal the medical community's resources against the growing threat of expanding scope of practice for allied health professionals, the AMA has formed a national partnership to confront such initiatives nationwide… The committee will use $25,000..." Daly R, American Psychiatric Association. AMA Forms Coalition to Thwart Non-M.D. Practice Expansion. *Psychiatric News* 2006 March; 41: 17 http://pn.psychiatryonline.org/cgi/content/full/41/5/17-a?eaf Accessed November 25, 2006
[17] Angell M. <u>The Truth About the Drug Companies: How They Deceive Us and What to Do About it</u>. Random House; August 2004
[18] "It begins on the first day of medical school… It starts slowly and insidiously, like an addiction, and can end up influencing the very nature of medical decision-making and practice… Attempts to influence the judgment of doctors by commercial interests serving the medical industrial complex are nothing if not thorough." Editorial. Drug-company influence on medical education in USA. *Lancet*. 2000 Sep 2;356(9232):781
[19] "Error is not blindness, error is cowardice. Every acquisition, every step forward in knowledge is the result of courage, of severity towards oneself, of cleanliness with respect to oneself." Nietzsche FW. <u>Ecce Homo: How One Becomes What One Is</u>. [Translator: Hollingdale RJ] Penguin Books:1979,34
[20] Orme-Johnson DW, Herron RE. An innovative approach to reducing medical care utilization and expenditures. *Am J Manag Care*. 1997;3(1):135-44
[21] **Vasquez A**. Five-Part Nutritional Protocol that Produces Consistently Positive Results.*Nutr Wellness* 2005Sept. http://optimalhealthresearch.com/spmd

higher rates of obesity, cancer, heart disease, and diabetes. Such an inactive lifestyle also affects our children: on average, each American child watches more than 23 hours of television per week[22]—a national habit that unquestionably contributes to the high levels of obesity and (social) illiteracy demonstrated by America's youth. Adults who watch average amounts of television are exposed to—some might say "…indoctrinated by…") more than 30 hours of drug advertisements per year—far exceeding their exposure to

---

Health living: lifestyle as living art

"What one should learn from artists: How can we make things beautiful, attractive, and desirable for us when they are not?—and I rather think that in themselves they never are! ... This we should learn from artists, while being wiser than they are in other matters. For with them this subtle power usually comes to an end where art ends and life begins; but we want to be the poets of our lives—first of all in the smallest, most everyday matters."

Nietzsche FW. The Happy Science. 1882. Essay #299.

---

other, potentially more authentic, health-promoting health information.[23] Not only does television siphon time and energy that could be used more productively, more socially, or more enjoyably, but at a cost of $50-100 per month ($600 to $1,200 per year) **cable television subtracts from the available resources (i.e., time, money, and attention) that could be directed toward health-promoting choices**. Cable television—because of its financial cost and time commitment—is only one of many examples of how everyday lifestyle choices can have an impact on long-term health/disease outcomes. **Clinicians should encourage patients to become mindful of their choices and the impact these choices have on long-term health and vitality.**

Lifestyle habits: Without the conscious decision that **health is a priority** and the realization that **optimal health has to be earned rather than taken for granted**, patients and doctors alike can fall into the belief that healthcare and health maintenance are *burdens* and *inconveniences* rather than opportunities for fulfillment and self-care. Taking an **empowered** and **pro-active** role in one's healthcare may include a coordinated program of diet changes (i.e., eating certain foods, avoiding other foods, modulating total intake), regular exercise, nutritional supplementation, stress reduction, and relationship improvement. Unhealthy habits such as eating junk foods, using tobacco, and watching too much television rob people of the time, energy, motivation, and financial resources that could otherwise be used to improve health and prevent unnecessary illness. As described later in this chapter, the choices that are made on a daily basis from this point forward are the most powerful predictors of future health and are generally more powerful than past habits or genetic inheritance. We can all greatly increase our probability of enjoying a future of high-energy health rather than painful illness by consistently choosing health-promoting options instead of foods, behaviors, and emotional states that promote illness.

---

[22] "American children view over 23 hours of television per week. * Teenagers view an average of 21 to 22 hours of television per week. * By the time today's children reach age 70, they will have spent 7 to 10 years of their lives watching television." American Academy of Pediatrics http://www.aapca1.org/aapca1/tv.html accessed September 30, 2003

[23] "…many ads may be targeted specifically at women and older viewers. Our findings suggest that Americans who watch average amounts of television may be exposed to more than 30 hours of direct-to-consumer drug advertisements each year, far surpassing their exposure to other forms of health communication." Brownfield ED, Bernhardt JM, Phan JL, Williams MV, Parker RM. Direct-to-consumer drug advertisements on network television: an exploration of quantity, frequency, and placement. *J Health Commun.* 2004 Nov-Dec;9(6):491-7

One hour of time per day and/or about $2 - $8 per day:

Active self-care lifestyle	*Distraction & inactive lifestyle*
1. Meditation 2. Yoga, stretching 3. Walking, jogging, biking, no-cost calisthenics 4. Martial arts, Tai Chi 5. Hot bath 6. Cooking new healthy meals 7. Herbal teas (especially green tea) provide anti-inflammatory, anticancer, and antioxidant benefits 8. Basic nutritional supplementation (less than $2 per day): 1) High-potency multivitamin and multimineral supplement, 2) Complete balanced, fatty acid supplementation, 3) 2,000 – 4,000 IU vitamin D per day for adults, 4) probiotics and/or symbiotic.	1. Cable television 2. 1 pack of cigarettes per day 3. Designer coffee such as Grande Café Latte
Benefits 1. Increased flexibility and joint mobility 2. Reduction in blood pressure 3. Reduced risk of cancer 4. Increased strength 5. Improved cognitive function 6. New and enjoyable meals 7. Relaxation 8. New life skills 9. Improved heart health 10. The opportunity to develop social skills and more friends and a better social support network 11. Reduced risk for Alzheimer's and Parkinson's diseases	**Results** 1. Cable television: Cost $2 - $4 per day = average $1,095 per year) 2. 1 pack of cigarettes per day ($3 per day = $1,095 per year) 3. Grande Café Latte ($4 per day = average $1,460 per year)
Cost: At $2 per day for meditation, stretching, calisthenics, (etc.) and basic supplementation, the total comes to $730 per year.	**Cost:** For cable television, cafe coffee, and cigarettes, the total comes to approximately $3,600 per year.

Motivation: We all have a combination of reasons, feelings, inclinations, and unconscious influences that support and perpetuate our health behaviors.[24,25,26] Getting in touch with those motivations can help us to better understand the healthy/functional (health-promoting) and unhealthy/dysfunctional (illness-promoting) aspects of our psyches. Uncovering and "upgrading" these motivations can help us and our patients to develop more authentic lives and improved health. Self-defeating behaviors, such as 1) a willingness to remain ignorant of factors which influence health, 2) a willingness to frequently consume disease-promoting processed convenience foods, and 3) submission to confinement within the boundaries of one's insurance coverage (which often confines one to drugs and surgery as the only treatment options), reflect — *at best* — the willingness to settle for mediocrity and — *at worst* — an unconscious movement in the direction of illness and early death — masochism and suicide by lifestyle. Conversely, an unencumbered drive toward health will create the greatest opportunity for wellness. Since **actions originate from beliefs and goals**, we can surmise much about undisclosed beliefs and goals in others and ourselves simply by observing outward behavior. Effectively changing actions (such as diet and lifestyle choices) therefore must include not only behavior modification but also careful examination and reconsideration of largely unconscious goals and beliefs that motivate and underlie those behaviors. **When a fully empowered motivation toward health is matched with accurate informational insight, we have the *potential* for health-promoting change — *potential* which only becomes *manifest* after the habitual application of appropriate action.** Patients and doctors alike can benefit from considering the factors that incline them *toward* or *away* from behaviors that promote health or disease.

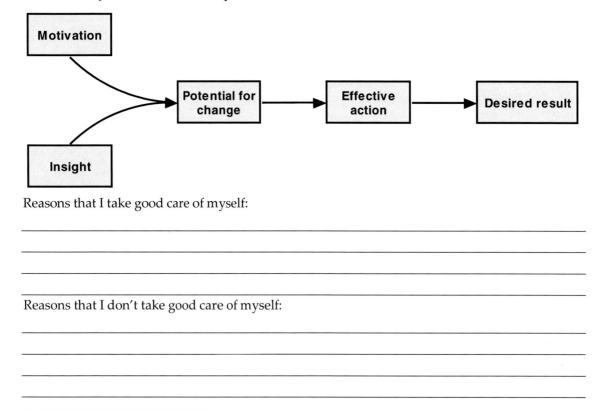

Reasons that I take good care of myself:

_____

_____

_____

_____

Reasons that I don't take good care of myself:

_____

_____

_____

_____

[24] Bradshaw J. Healing the Shame that Binds You [Audio Cassette (April 1990) Health Communications Audio; ISBN: 1558740430]
[25] Miller A. The Drama of the Gifted Child: The Search for the True Self. Basic Books: 1981
[26] Prochaska, JO, Norcross, JC, and DiClemente, CC (1994). Changing for Good: A Revolutionary Six-Stage Program for Overcoming Bad Habits and Moving Your Life Positively Forward. NY, William Morrow and Company; 1994

Motivation: moving from theory to practice: Many recently-graduated doctors start with the erroneous assumption that all patients actually want to become healthier, and furthermore, that all that the doctor has to do is "enlighten" them to the error of their ways and the patient will be dutifully compliant unto the attainment of his or her health-related goals. In reality, many people are surprisingly indifferent about their health. Many people do not care if they are 30 lbs overweight or have hypertension or will die early as a result of their

> **Action determines outcome**
> "Knowing is not enough;
> we must apply.
>
> Willing is not enough;
> we must do."
>
> Johann Wolfgang von Goethe,
> German novelist, poet, and scientist
> (1749 - 1832)

lifestyle; they often have to be encouraged to begin to *consider* making positive changes.

At our 2004 Functional Medicine Symposium, Dr. James Prochaska[27] elucidated the different stages of patient preparedness, and we note that each of these five levels of thought and action produces specific results and requires different types of support from the doctor. I have summarized and modified Dr. Prochaska's lecture in the following table; for additional information and insights, obtain his lecture from the Institute for Functional Medicine (functionalmedicine.org) or obtain his book *Changing for Good*.[28]

Level of preparedness and readiness for change

Stage: representative statement	*Doctor's interventions and social support*
1. **Pre-contemplation**: "I am not seriously thinking about making a change to be healthier."	▪ Outreach ▪ Retainment
2. **Contemplation**: "I am thinking about making a change, but I am not ready for action."	▪ Resolve resistance ▪ Emphasize benefits ▪ Address ambivalence
3. **Preparation**: "I am getting ready to make a change, but I am not taking effective action yet."	▪ Ensure adequate preparation ▪ Prevent relapse following initial action
4. **Action**: "I am beginning to make changes to become healthier."	▪ Support (group support is best) ▪ Encouragement ▪ Reward system
5. **Maintenance**: "I take action every day and on a consistent basis to reach my goals."	▪ Continued provision for continuation of health changes: facilities, supplements, social support, affirmation

Recognizing the different levels of patient preparedness and addressing individual patients with a customized approach not only for their *disease* but also for their *level of preparedness* for action can help doctors deliver more effective healthcare. Also, patients may have different levels of preparedness for different aspects of their treatment plans. He/she may be ready for **action** with regard to exercise, in **preparation** for dietary change, but in **precontemplation** for the use of supplements and botanicals.

---

[27] Prochaska JO. Changing for good: motivating diabetic patients. The Coming Storm: Reversing the Rising Pandemic of Diabetes and Metabolic Syndrome. The Eleventh International Symposium on Functional Medicine. May 13-15, 2004 in Vancouver, British Columbia, Canada. Pages 173-180. Presented by the Institute for Functional Medicine in Gig Harbor, Washington. www.FunctionalMedicine.org
[28] Prochaska, JO, Norcross, JC, and DiClemente, CC (1994). Changing for Good: A Revolutionary Six-Stage Program for Overcoming Bad Habits and Moving Your Life Positively Forward. NY, William Morrow and Company; 1994

The secret to being exceptionally healthy: *One has to live in an exceptional (unique, personalized) way.* We cannot expect to achieve the goal of being vibrantly healthy or exceptionally happy if we live in the same way as everyone else, particularly when our fellow citizens are likely to be overweight, depressed, socially isolated[29], requiring multiple pharmaceutical medications[30], and experiencing a state of progressively declining health.[31] *Healthy lifestyle* not only includes the basics of adequate sleep, healthy whole-foods diet, supportive relationships, and regular exercise, but it also includes preventive medicine and pro-active healthcare. **Despite the fact that we in the United States (US) spend more on medical treatments than does any other country in the world, Americans have the worst health outcomes of all the major industrialized countries.**[32,33,34] This is largely because *American medicine is centered on a disease-oriented model of medicine* which means that instead of having a healthcare system and social structure that proactively promotes health and prevents disease before it happens, our systems are *reactive*—treating disease *after* it occurs rather than emphasizing the prevention of disease *before* it occurs. The dominant allopathic model in the US is also reductionistic: focusing on the small problem (micromanagement) rather than the big picture (macromanagement).

Clearly, the most effective method for avoiding expensive and potentially dangerous medical procedures and drug treatments is for us as a nation and as individuals to shift our thinking from a *disease treatment* model of healthcare to a more logical program of aggressive *disease prevention* and *wellness promotion* via the use of safe natural treatments

---

Americans have poor health outcomes compared to citizens of other industrialized nations

"Basically, you die earlier and spend more time disabled if you're an American rather than a member of most other advanced countries."

Christopher Murray MD PhD, Director of World Health Organization's Global Program on Evidence for Health Policy. Press release on June 4, 2000. http://www.who.int/inf-pr-2000/en/pr2000-life.html

---

Approximately 493 Americans are killed each day by hospital injuries and drug-prescribing errors

"Recent estimates suggest that each year more than 1 million patients are injured while in the hospital and approximately 180,000 die because of these injuries. Furthermore, drug-related morbidity and mortality are common and are estimated to cost more than $136 billion a year."

Holland EG, Degruy FV. Drug-induced disorders. *Am Fam Physician*. 1997;56:1781-8, 1791-2

Medical drug (in)efficacy

"The vast majority of drugs —more than 90 percent— only work in 30 or 50 percent of the people."

Allen Roses, M.D., worldwide vice-president of genetics at GlaxoSmithKline. Published Dec 8, 2003 http://commondreams.org/headlines03/1208-02.htm

---

[29] McPherson M, Smith-Lovin L, Brashears ME. Social Isolation in America: Changes in Core Discussion Networks over Two Decades. *American Sociological Review* 2006; 71: 353-75 http://www.asanet.org/galleries/default-file/June06ASRFeature.pdf

[30] "According to the latest available data, total health care costs reached $1.3 trillion in 2000. This represents a per capita health care expenditure of $4,637. The total prescription drug expenditure in 2000 was $121.8 billion, or approximately $430 per person." Presentation to the U.S. Senate Commerce Committee April 23, 2002 "Drug Pricing & Consumer Costs" Kathleen D. Jaeger, R.Ph., J.D. http://commerce.senate.gov/hearings/042302jaegar.pdf

[31] Zack MM, Moriarty DG, Stroup DF, Ford ES, Mokdad AH. Worsening trends in adult health-related quality of life and self-rated health-United States, 1993-2001. *Public Health Rep*. 2004 Sep-Oct;119(5):493-505 http://www.pubmedcentral.nih.gov/articlerender.fcgi?tool=pubmed&pubmedid=15313113

[32] "[America] also has the fewest hospital days per capita, the highest hospital expenditures per day, and substantially higher physician incomes than the other OECD countries. On the available outcome measures, the United States is generally in the bottom half, and its relative ranking has been declining since 1960." Anderson GF, Poullier JP. Health spending, access, and outcomes: trends in industrialized countries. *Health Aff* (Millwood) 1999 May-Jun;18(3):178-92 http://content.healthaffairs.org/cgi/reprint/18/3/178.pdf

[33] "However, on outcomes indicators such as life expectancy and infant mortality, the United States is frequently in the bottom quartile among the twenty-nine industrialized countries, and its relative ranking has been declining since 1960." Anderson GF. In search of value: an international comparison of cost, access, and outcomes. *Health Aff* 1997 Nov-Dec;16(6):163-71

[34] "Basically, you die earlier and spend more time disabled if you're an American rather than a member of most other advanced countries," says Christopher Murray, MD, PhD, Director of WHO's Global Program on Evidence for Health Policy. http://www.who.int/inf-pr-2000/en/pr2000-life.html

rather than heroic interventions.[35],[36] Of course, this means that our concept and view of health and healthcare will have to change. As noted by Shi[37], **"Redesigning the system of health care delivery in the United States may be the only viable option to improve the quality of health care."** In the meantime, while we work for change on a national level, we are wise to change our personal habits and healthcare choices in favor of natural and preventive healthcare.

<u>Healthy lifestyle and biochemical individuality credo: Recognize and affirm that you are a unique individual with unique needs</u>: For each of us, our "personality" extends far beyond and far deeper than our sense of humor and our choice of clothing; we are very unique on a physiologic and biochemical level as well. So-called *normal* and *apparently healthy* individuals vary greatly in their biochemical efficiency and nutritional needs. This is the concept of "biochemical individuality" which was first detailed in 1956 by the renowned scientist Roger J Williams from the University of Texas. In his historic work *Biochemical Individuality: The Basis for the Genetotrophic Concept*, Dr. Williams[38] reviews research that conclusively proves that among *apparently healthy* individuals, we can objectively determine great differences in physiology, organ efficiency, enzyme function, and nutritional needs. For example, variables that promote health include increased enzyme efficiency and efficient digestion and assimilation of nutrients, while internal factors that reduce health can include inadequate digestion, inefficient absorption, increased excretion of nutrients, impaired detoxification, poor enzyme function and "partial genetic blocks"—a term now understood to imply single nucleotide polymorphisms[39] and related enzyme defects, which result in **supradietary requirements for specific vitamins and minerals** for the prevention of disease and maintenance of health.[40] What this means for us as doctors and for our patients in practical terms is that in order for us to become as healthy as possible, we will almost certainly have to give attention to each person's unique biochemical abilities/disabilities in order to maximize the function of the various body systems, enzymes, and to optimize genetic expression.[41] This means that what works for one's neighbor, spouse, or best friend in terms of exercise, diet and nutrition may not work for one's unique physiology. We must all muster the courage to affirm that, in order to attain the goal of stable or progressively better health, we will each have to learn about how our unique bodies work—what conditions of health must be created. We will have to learn to make changes in lifestyle and daily routine which reflect and honor our bodies' ways of working. This may mean modifying work, sleep, and exercise schedules, avoiding some foods and eating others, and customizing nutrient intake to meet the body's needs as they are *in the present*—the health program that appears to have worked last year may not be appropriate at the present time. The process of learning how a person's body works requires time, patience, and the process of trial and error—from patient and doctor—but achieving the goal of improved health and increased energy are well worth the effort.

---

[35] "Systematic access to managed chiropractic care not only may prove to be clinically beneficial but also may reduce overall health care costs." Legorreta A, Metz D, Nelson C, Ray S, Chernicoff H, DiNubile N. Comparative Analysis of Individuals With and Without Chiropractic Coverage. *Archives of Internal Medicine* 2004; 164: 1985-1992

[36] Orme-Johnson DW, Herron RE. An innovative approach to reducing medical care utilization and expenditures. *Am J Manag Care*. 1997;3(1):135-44

[37] Shi L. Health care spending, delivery, and outcome in developed countries: a cross-national comparison. *Am J Med Qual* 1997;12(2):83-93

[38] Williams RJ. <u>Biochemical Individuality : The Basis for the Genetotrophic Concept</u>. Austin and London: University of Texas Press, 1956

[39] Ames BN. Cancer prevention and diet: help from single nucleotide polymorphisms. *Proc Natl Acad Sci U S A*. 1999 Oct 26;96(22):12216-8

[40] Ames BN, Elson-Schwab I, Silver EA. High-dose vitamin therapy stimulates variant enzymes with decreased coenzyme binding affinity (increased K(m)): relevance to genetic disease and polymorphisms. *Am J Clin Nutr*. 2002 Apr;75(4):616-58 http://www.ajcn.org/cgi/content/full/75/4/616

[41] "The combination of biochemical individuality and known functional utilities of allelic variants should converge to create a situation in which nutritional optima can be specified as part of comprehensive lifestyle prescriptions tailored to the needs of each person." Eckhardt RB. Genetic research and nutritional individuality. *J Nutr* 2001;131(2):336S-9S

Individuation and the practice of conscious living: Our visions of reality are influenced by religious institutions, large corporations, advertising networks[42], corporate-owned mass media[43], and what Professors Stevens and Glatstein called "the medical-industrial complex."[44] Some of the paradigms that are advocated are both *unhistorical* (having no historical precedent) and *antihistorical* (contrary to the available historical precedent, which includes sustainability). Some of these companies and organizations offer us a view of reality and vision of our individual potentials that is fashioned in such a way as to promote the financial and political interests of the company or organization. Conversely, the actualization of our true physical, emotional, intellectual, and spiritual potentials may require that we separate from or at least attain a conscious appreciation of the (pseudo)reality that we have been advised to follow.[45,46] Critiques of and reasonable alternatives to our current paradigms of school[47], work[48,49], and money[50] have been discussed elsewhere and are worthy of consideration. Becoming mindful of the paradigms and assumptions under which we live is the first step in true individuation, characterized by choosing (*creating* the best option: freedom) rather than deciding (*selecting* one of the offered options: the illusion of freedom). Various conscious thoughts and unconscious assumptions create our "working reality" which represents the way that we see things and the paradigm by which we *act in* and *interact with* the larger world. These layers come from our own families, schools, teachers, churches, companies, friends, parents, and ourselves—our previous interpretations and misinterpretations of ourselves and events; in sum, our responses to outer events combined with our internal experiences meld into our perception of ourselves (known as "the genesis of personal identity") and how we as individuals relate to our inner ourselves and [our perception of] the outer world. Becoming conscious of these realities and illusions allows us the opportunity to discard those

> **The importance of living consciously**
>
> "Consciousness is our basic tool for successful adaptation to reality. The more conscious we are in any situation, the more possibilities we tend to perceive, the more options we have, the more powerful we are — perhaps even the longer we will live.
>
> Living consciously means seeking to be aware of everything that bears on our actions, purposes, values, and goals — and behaving in accordance with that which we see and know."
>
> Branden N. The Art of Living Consciously. http://nathanielbranden.com Accessed Feb 2011

views that are inaccurate, dysfunctional, and harmful and to accept a truer reality based on what we experience, feel, and know to be real—in the present, as adults. Once we are freed from *unreality*, we can live true to ourselves in a way that is authentically responsible to our own needs *and* the needs of our communities so that we can simultaneously sustain our obligations to society[51,52] while being free to be unique individuals.[53,54]

---

[42] "Patients' requests for medicines are a powerful driver of prescribing decisions. In most cases physicians prescribed requested medicines but were often ambivalent about the choice of treatment. If physicians prescribe requested drugs despite personal reservations, sales may increase but appropriateness of prescribing may suffer." Mintzes B, Barer ML, Kravitz RL, Kazanjian A, Bassett K, Lexchin J, Evans RG, Pan R, Marion SA. Influence of direct to consumer pharmaceutical advertising and patients' requests on prescribing decisions: two site cross sectional survey. *BMJ.* 2002 Feb 2; 324(7332): 278-9
[43] Manufacturing Consent: Noam Chomsky and the Media. Movie directed by Achbar M and Wintonick P. 1992. See also http://zeitgeistmovie.com/
Stevens CW, Glatstein E. Beware the Medical-Industrial Complex. *Oncologist* 1996;1(4):IV-V
http://theoncologist.alphamedpress.org/cgi/reprint/1/4/190-iv.pdf on July 4, 2004
[45] Breton D, Largent C. The Paradigm Conspiracy. Center City; Hazelden: 1996
[46] Pearce JC. Exploring the Crack in the Cosmic Egg: Split Minds and Meta-Realities. New York: Washington Square Press; 1974
[47] Gatto JT. Dumbing us down: the hidden curriculum of compulsory education. Gabriola Island, Canada; New Society Publishers: 2005
[48] "No one should ever work. In order to stop suffering, we have to stop working. That doesn't mean we have to stop doing things. It does mean creating a new way of life based on play..." Black B. The abolition of work and other essays. Port Townsend: Loompanics Unlimited; 1985, pages 17-33
[49] Jarow R. Creating the Work You Love: Courage, Commitment and Career; Inner Traditions Intl Ltd; 1995 [ISBN: 0892815426]
[50] Dominguez JR. Transforming Your Relationship With Money. Sounds True; Book and Cassette edition: 2001 Audio tape.
[51] Bly R. The Sibling Society. Vintage Books USA; Reprint edition (June 1, 1997) ISBN: 0679781285 (Abridged audio edition (May 1, 1996)
[52] Bly R. Where have all the parents gone? A talk on the Sibling Society. New York: Sound Horizons; 1996 Highly recommended.
[53] Bradshaw J. Healing the Shame that Binds You [Audio Cassette (April 1990) Health Communications Audio; ISBN: 1558740430]
[54] Miller A. The truth will set you free: overcoming emotional blindness and finding your true adult self. New York: Basic Books; 2001

Examples of commonly accepted paradigms and their reasonable alternatives

Commonly advocated/accepted paradigms ↳ *Implication and effect*	*Alternate paradigm* ↳ *Implication and effect*
It is OK to be irresponsible in daily choices and then blame health problems on bad luck, bad genes, or both. ↳ Many people fail to take responsibility for their lives and thereby become victims of circumstances—negative circumstances that they themselves helped to create.	**Lifestyle, especially diet and nutrition, is the most powerful influence on health outcomes. Therefore, an educated patient is empowered to direct his/her health destiny.** ↳ Optimal health *per individual* is attained when people take responsibility for their lives, seek health information, and then incorporate this information into their daily routine in the form of healthy living: health-promoting lifestyle, eating, exercise, supplementation, relationships, and occupational and social activities, including socio-political involvement to protect the environment and resist the privatization of life and the spoliation of the environment in which we live and upon which our lives and health depend.[55,56]
In general, chemical medications are the answer to nearly all health problems. ↳ The belief in medications as the primary treatment of disease creates a patient population that is apathetic, disempowered, and dependent upon the medical-pharmaceutical industry, which grows richer and more powerful despite so-called 'earnest' attempts at cost containment.[57]	**Many acute and chronic problems can be more effectively managed in terms of prevention, safety, efficacy, and cost-effectiveness when phytonutritional interventions are either used as primary therapy or, when necessary, used in conjunction with medications.** ↳ A reduction in disease prevalence via health-promoting diet and lifestyle along with integrative treatments offers the best opportunity for benefit to patients, doctors, and third-party payers.[58]

---

[55] "Your lack of interest in the past, your lack of involvement, your unwillingness to develop coherent strategies, your unwillingness to challenge authority - these have created a vacuum in decision-making, that has been filled by professional groups with close relationships with the chemical industries..." Samuel Epstein MD, 1993. Professor of Occupational and Environmental Medicine at the School of Public Health, University of Illinois Medical Center Chicago. http://www.converge.org.nz/pirm/pestican.htm accessed September 11, 2004

[56] Kristin S. Schafer, Margaret Reeves, Skip Spitzer, Susan E. Kegley. Chemical Trespass: Pesticides in Our Bodies and Corporate Accountability. Pesticide Action Network North America. May 2004 Available at http://www.panna.org/campaigns/docsTrespass/chemicalTrespass2004.dv.html on August 1, 2004

[57] "In this paper I offer four hypotheses to help explain why use of pharmaceuticals has continued to grow even as managed care and other cost containment efforts have flourished." Berndt ER. The U.S. pharmaceutical industry: why major growth in times of cost containment? *Health Aff* (Millwood). 2001 Mar-Apr;20(2):100-14

[58] "Hospital admission rates in the control group were 11.4 times higher than those in the MVAH group for cardiovascular disease, 3.3 times higher for cancer, and 6.7 times higher for mental health and substance abuse. ...MVAH patients older than age 45...had 88% fewer total patients days compared with control patients." Orme-Johnson DW, Herron RE. An innovative approach to reducing medical care utilization and expenditures. *Am J Manag Care*. 1997 Jan;3(1):135-44

Examples of commonly accepted paradigms and their reasonable alternatives —*continued*

Commonly accepted paradigms ↳ *Implication and effect*	Alternate paradigm ↳ *Implication and effect*
Work ethic: a belief that "hard work" has moral value and makes a person "better." ↳ Belief in the principle of "work ethic" encourages people to mindlessly engage in work for the sake of engaging in work without considering the implications of their actions or other alternatives that might produce a more beneficial outcome.[59]	**Work is the means rather than an end unto itself (except when the "work" is enjoyable, in which case it is no longer "work").** ↳ Occupations and professions can be designed for the enhancement of life (health, pleasure, relationships, the environment, care of the poor) rather than as an end to themselves at the expense of the individual, society, and the environment.
It is "normal" for adults to give 10.5-12 hours per day 5 days per week to work. ↳ In most corporate environments, employee's work at least 8.5 hours per day, with 1 additional hour spent in commuting[60] and another hour spent in preparation, transportation, and maintenance of work-related clothing, preparing work-related meals, maintaining the auto that is used for work-related tasks. With 10.5 hours given directly to work, 0.5-1 additional hours are needed for recuperation from work-related stress ("daily decompression"); thus the average amount of time given to work-related activities is much larger than commonly believed.[61] Because of the time and energies devoted to "work" the vast majority of people feel that they do not have sufficient time for themselves, their families and friends, their creativity, learning about the world, political involvement, and other more important aspects of life. "Not enough time" is the most common reason given by patients for not exercising.	**A paradigm of a 4-day workweek is just as valid and perhaps more valid than one that advocates a 5-day workweek. A paradigm of a 6-hour workday is at least as valid as one of an 8-10 hour workday.** ↳ Many people in our culture are chronically overworked, undernourished, tired and suffer from an insufficiency of time to simply be in community, to rest, to be creative. Living with such limitations and pressures should be expected to produce a population that is reactively hedonistic, impulsive, and prone to addiction. Behaviors that are addictive (e.g., drugs, alcohol) and destructive (e.g., over-eating, alcohol, sugar, fat) are simply frustrated and maladaptive coping strategies to combat the stress caused by a damaging, unnatural paradigm from which most people cannot escape.[62] Redesigning our societal structures and expectations in ways that conform to our natural humanity and biologic, nutritional, and emotional needs is more rational than forcing *en masse* all of humanity to contort and conform to an artificial posture and cadence of performance, productivity, "professionalism", and other unnatural expectations. Less time dedicated to work and all that it entails leaves more time for 1) healthy cooking, 2) relaxed, conscious, and enjoyable eating, 3) exercise, 4) creativity and hobbies, 5) keeping informed of and involved with political change, and 6) participation in social relationships.[63]

[59] "Conventional wisdom is the habitual, the unexamined life, absorbed into the culture and the fashion of the time, lost in the mad rush of accumulation, lulled to sleep by the easy lies of political hacks and newspaper scribblers, or by priests who wouldn't know a god if they met one." Nisker W. Crazy Wisdom. Berkeley; Ten Speed Press: 1990, page 7

[60] Monday, September 8, 2003 -- The average daily one-way commute to work in the United States takes just over 26 minutes, according to the Bureau of Transportation Statistics' Omnibus Household Survey. Omnibus Household Survey Shows Americans' Average Commuting Time is Just Over 26 Minutes. http://www.bts.gov/press_releases/2003/bts020_03/html/bts020_03.html on August 3, 2004

[61] Dominguez JR. Transforming Your Relationship with Money. Sounds True; Book and Cassette edition: 2001

[62] Breton D, Largent C. The Paradigm Conspiracy: Why Our Social Systems Violate Human Potential-And How We Can Change Them. Hazelden: 1998

Quality and quantity of sleep: A sleep duration of less than 8 hours of deep solid sleep each night is physiologically insufficient for most of people; many people feel best with 9 hours of sleep, yet some people appear to function well on about 6 hours of sleep per night. Not only is it important to get a sufficient *quantity* of sleep, but we need to ensure that the *quality* of the sleep receives appropriate attention, as well. Sleep should be mostly continuous, not "broken" or

> ### The Importance of Sleep
> Regulation of sleep-wake cycles and the regular satisfaction of sleep needs are important for preservation of immune function, intellectual performance, emotional stability, and the internal regulation of the body's inflammatory tendency.

interrupted. Some experts believe that people should be able to recall their dreams at night, as this may be a sign of proper neurotransmitter status, especially with regard to serotonin, which is affected by pyridoxine[64] as well as other factors. Going to bed at a regular hour (not later than 10 or 11 at night) helps to synchronize the daily schedule with the body's inherent hormonal rhythms and "physiological clock" which expects one to be in deep sleep by midnight and to be waking at approximately 8 o'clock in the morning. Recent research has shown that **sleep deprivation causes a systemic inflammatory response manifested objectively by increases in high-sensitivity C-reactive protein (hsCRP)**.[65] Correspondingly, sleep apnea, a condition associated with repetitive sleep disturbances, is also associated with an elevation of CRP[66], and effective treatment of sleep apnea results in a normalization of CRP levels.[67] We could therefore conclude that **sleep deprivation creates a proinflammatory condition**. Furthermore, **sleep deprivation has been proven to impair intellectual functioning, emotional state, and immune function**, with abnormalities in immune status already evident the morning after sleep deprivation.[68] Wakefulness and exposure to light at night result in a suppression of melatonin production and may therefore contribute to cancer development since melatonin has anticancer actions that would be abrogated by its reduced endogenous production.[69,70] Limited evidence also suggests that melatonin production is altered in patients with the inflammatory conditions

---

[63] "Take back your time" is a major U.S./Canadian initiative to challenge the epidemic of overwork, over-scheduling and time famine that now threatens our health, our families and relationships, our communities and our environment. http://www.simpleliving.net/timeday/ on August 3, 2004

[64] " …a significant difference in dream-salience scores (this is a composite score containing measures on vividness, bizarreness, emotionality, and color) between the 250-mg condition and placebo over the first three days of each treatment… An hypothesis is presented involving the role of B-6 in the conversion of tryptophan to serotonin." Ebben M, Lequerica A, Spielman A. Effects of pyridoxine on dreaming: a preliminary study. *Percept Mot Skills* 2002 Feb;94(1):135-40

[65] "CONCLUSIONS: Both acute total and short-term partial sleep deprivation resulted in elevated high-sensitivity CRP concentrations… We propose that sleep loss may be one of the ways that inflammatory processes are activated and contribute to the association of sleep complaints, short sleep duration, and cardiovascular morbidity observed in epidemiologic surveys." Meier-Ewert HK, Ridker PM, et al. Effect of sleep loss on C-reactive protein, an inflammatory marker of cardiovascular risk. *J Am Coll Cardiol*. 2004 Feb 18;43(4):678-83

[66] "OSA is associated with elevated levels of CRP, a marker of inflammation and of cardiovascular risk. The severity of OSA is proportional to the CRP level." Shamsuzzaman AS, Winnicki M, Lanfranchi P, Wolk R, Kara T, Accurso V, Somers VK. Elevated C-reactive protein in patients with obstructive sleep apnea. *Circulation*. 2002 May 28;105(21):2462-4

[67] "CONCLUSIONS: Levels of CRP and IL-6 and spontaneous production of IL-6 by monocytes are elevated in patients with OSAS but are decreased by nCPAP." Yokoe T, Minoguchi K, Matsuo H, Oda N, Minoguchi H, Yoshino G, Hirano T, Adachi M. Elevated levels of C-reactive protein and interleukin-6 in patients with obstructive sleep apnea syndrome are decreased by nasal continuous positive airway pressure. *Circulation*. 2003 Mar 4;107(8):1129-34 Available on-line at http://circ.ahajournals.org/cgi/reprint/107/8/1129.pdf on August 2, 2004

[68] "Taken together, SD induced a deterioration of both mood and ability to work, which was most prominent in the evening after SD, while the maximal alterations of the host defence system could be found twelve hours earlier, i.e., already in the morning following SD." Heiser P, Dickhaus B, Opper C, Hemmeter U, Remschmidt H, Wesemann W, Krieg JC, Schreiber W. Alterations of host defense system after sleep deprivation are followed by impaired mood and psychosocial functioning. *World J Biol Psychiatry* 2001 Apr;2(2):89-94

[69] "Observational studies support an association between night work and cancer risk. We hypothesise that the potential primary culprit for this observed association is the lack of melatonin, a cancer-protective agent whose production is severely diminished in people exposed to light at night." Schernhammer ES, Schulmeister K. Melatonin and cancer risk: does light at night compromise physiologic cancer protection by lowering serum melatonin levels? *Br J Cancer*. 2004 Mar 8;90(5):941-3

[70] "This is the first biological evidence for a potential link between constant light exposure and increased human breast oncogenesis involving MLT suppression and stimulation of tumor LA metabolism." Blask DE, Dauchy RT, Sauer LA, Krause JA, Brainard GC. Growth and fatty acid metabolism of human breast cancer (MCF-7) xenografts in nude rats: impact of constant light-induced nocturnal melatonin suppression. *Breast Cancer Res Treat*. 2003 Jun;79(3):313-20

eczema[71] and psoriasis[72] and that this sleep-related hormone has anti-inflammatory/anti-autoimmune benefits that may be relevant for the suppression of diseases such as multiple sclerosis[73] and sarcoidosis.[74]

Helping patients improve quality and quantity of sleep

- Reduce intake of stimulants such as caffeine, tobacco, and aspartame. Some patients will need to reduce intake only in the evening, while others will need to reduce intake even in the morning in order to have improved quality and quantity of sleep later at night.

- Exercise early in the day (morning or early afternoon) to promote restful sleep at night.[75]

- Avoid aggressive or arousing physical activity in the evening to avoid increases in norepinephrine, epinephrine, and cortisol, which can discourage sleep.

- Dim lights at night to promote melatonin production. Beginning one to two hours before bedtime, turn off bright lights and use only dim lighting. Bright lights reduce melatonin secretion and stimulate neocortical activity and thereby inhibit sleep.

- Have an evening ritual/pattern that helps the psyche recognize that the time for sleep has arrived. Such practices can include relaxing warm tea, meditation, prayer, and daily reflection.

- For patients with a pattern of falling asleep and then waking approximately 4-6 hours later with feelings of hunger or anxiety (nocturnal hypoglycemia), they should eat a small meal or snack of complex carbohydrates, protein, and fat before going to bed. For example, the combination of nuts (or nut butter) with whole fruit such as apples provides protein, fat, and complex carbohydrate with a low glycemic index to provide sustenance throughout the night. Protein powders and other sources of "predigested" amino acids should generally be avoided late at night because an excess consumption of high protein foods can reduce tryptophan entry into the brain and thus reduce serotonin and melatonin synthesis. Most amino acid-derived neurotransmitters such as dopamine, glutamate, and norepinephrine are excitatory/stimulatory in nature.

- Vitamin and mineral supplementation is commonly beneficial, particularly with thiamine[76], methylcobalamin (weak evidence[77]), and magnesium (particularly sleep disturbance associated with restless leg syndrome[78]). Vitamins should be taken earlier in the day (with breakfast and lunch; not before bed); however calcium and magnesium can be taken before bed.

- Earplugs, window covers, and a quiet, snore-free environment are generally conducive to better sleep.

- For patients with difficulty falling asleep, consider 5-hydroxytryptophan consumed with simple carbohydrate (50-200 mg for adults, up to 2 mg/kg[79] for children), melatonin (0.5-10 mg), valerian-hops tea or capsules[80] 60-90 minutes before bedtime.

---

[71] "In 6 patients exhibiting low serum levels of melatonin, the circadian melatonin rhythm was found to be abolished. In 8 patients a diminished nocturnal melatonin increase was observed compared with the controls (n = 40)." Schwarz W, Birau N, Hornstein OP, Heubeck B, Schonberger A, Meyer C, Gottschalk J. Alterations of melatonin secretion in atopic eczema. *Acta Derm Venereol*. 1988;68(3):224-9

[72] "Our results show that psoriatic patients had lost the nocturnal peak and usual circadian rhythm of melatonin secretion." Mozzanica N, Tadini G, Radaelli A, Negri M, Pigatto P, Morelli M, Frigerio U, Finzi A, Esposti G, Rossi D, et al. Plasma melatonin levels in psoriasis. *Acta Derm Venereol*. 1988;68(4):312-6

[73] "This hypothesis is supported by the observation that administration of melatonin (3 mg, orally) at 2:00 p.m., when the patient experienced severe blurring of vision, resulted within 15 minutes in a dramatic improvement in visual acuity and in normalization of the visual evoked potential latency after stimulation of the left eye." Sandyk R. Diurnal variations in vision and relations to circadian melatonin secretion in multiple sclerosis. *Int J Neurosci*. 1995 Nov;83(1-2):1-6

[74] Cagnoni ML, Lombardi A, Cerinic MC, Dedola GL, Pignone A. Melatonin for treatment of chronic refractory sarcoidosis. *Lancet*. 1995;346:1229-30

[75] "This is the first report to demonstrate that low intensity activity in an elderly population can increase deep sleep and improve memory functioning." Naylor E, Penev PD, Orbeta L, Janssen I, Ortiz R, Colecchia EF, Keng M, Finkel S, Zee PC. Daily social and physical activity increases slow-wave sleep and daytime neuropsychological performance in the elderly. *Sleep*. 2000 Feb 1;23(1):87-95

[76] Wilkinson TJ, Hanger HC, Elmslie J, George PM, Sainsbury R. The response to treatment of subclinical thiamine deficiency in the elderly. *Am J Clin Nutr*. 1997;66(4):925-8

[77] "However, because the percentage of improvement was low and significant improvement was inconsistent, Met-12 might be considered to have a low therapeutic potency and possible use as a booster for other treatment methods of the disorders." Takahashi K, et al. Double-blind test on the efficacy of methylcobalamin on sleep-wake rhythm disorders. *Psychiatry Clin Neurosci*. 1999 Apr;53(2):211-3

[78] "Our study indicates that magnesium treatment may be a useful alternative therapy in patients with mild or moderate RLS-or PLMS-related insomnia." Hornyak M, Voderholzer U, et al. Magnesium therapy for periodic leg movements-related insomnia and restless legs syndrome: an open pilot study. *Sleep*. 1998 Aug 1;21(5):501-5

[79] Bruni O, Ferri R, Miano S, Verrillo E. l-5-Hydroxytryptophan treatment of sleep terrors in children. *Eur J Pediatr*. 2004 May 14

[80] "Sleep improvements with a valerian-hops combination are associated with improved quality of life. Both treatments appear safe and did not produce rebound insomnia upon discontinuation during this study. Overall, these findings indicate that a valerian-hops combination and diphenhydramine might be useful adjuncts in the treatment of mild insomnia." Morin CM, Koetter U, Bastien C, Ware JC, Wooten V. Valerian-hops combination and diphenhydramine for treating insomnia: a randomized placebo-controlled clinical trial. *Sleep*. 2005 Nov 1;28(11):1465-71

Exercise: Human existence has changed radically over the past few millennia, centuries, and decades, and one of the most profound changes has been in our relationship to physical activity. Paleologists and historical scientists agree that physical activity among humans is at its all-time historical low, and that levels of exertion that we now call "vigorous and frequent exercise" would have been *completely normal* in the daily lives of our ancestors, who engaged in at least four times more physical activity than their modern-day progeny.[81] At one time—a time in which vigorous physical activity was a normal part of daily life—probably no word existed for what modern people describe and often resist as "exercise."

Daily exercise is health-promoting and restorative
"The health rewards of exercise extend far beyond its benefits for specific diseases." Exercise reduces blood clotting, lowers blood pressure, lowers cholesterol, improves glucose tolerance and insulin sensitivity, enhances self-image, elevates mood, reduces stress, creates a feeling of well-being, reinforces other positive life-style changes, stimulates creative thinking, increases muscle mass, increases basal metabolic rate, promotes improved sleep, stimulates healthy intestinal function, promotes weight loss, and enhances appearance. "Furthermore, **the ability of exercise to restore function to organs, muscles, joints, and bones is not shared by drugs or surgery**."
Harold Elrick, MD. Exercise is Medicine. *Physician and Sportsmedicine.* 1996: 24; 2 (February)

Daily exercise is the body's physiological expectation
"Although modern technology has made physical exertion optional, it is still important to exercise as though our survival depended on it, and in a different way it still does. **We are genetically adapted to live an extremely physically active lifestyle.**"
O'Keefe JH Jr, Cordain L. Cardiovascular disease resulting from a diet and lifestyle at odds with our Paleolithic genome: how to become a 21st-century hunter-gatherer. *Mayo Clin Proc.* 2004 Jan;79(1):101-8

Our current mode of compulsory primary and secondary education prioritizes "being still" over physical exertion/expression for the vast majority of students' time. Thus having been separated from their inherent tendency to be physically active and emotionally expressive, many children grow into adults who have to be *retaught to inhabit their bodies* and to engage in physical activity on a daily basis. Basic science has proven that this is true: when animals are restrained, they show less activity when freed and no longer tied down. Conversely, when animals are rigorously exercised, they show higher levels of *spontaneous physical activity* when left to their own discretion. A probable sociological parallel is at work in human cultures where, under the guise of *work* and *entertainment*, people are corralled into lifestyles of physical inactivity in a wide range of apparently divergent activities. Watching television, driving a car, seeing a movie, doing computer/desk work at the office, attending a sports event or educational lecture, seeing the opera—all of these are simply different forms of *sitting*, of physical inactivity. Changing our social structure in a way that prioritizes *life* over *work*, such as moving toward a 4-day work week and/or a 6-hour work day, would allow people more time to live their lives, to pursue healthy diets and relationships, to be creative, and to engage in more physical activity; thus, "escape entertainment" such as fiction books and movies and processed "fast foods"—the latter of which are inherently unhealthy[82]—would become less necessary and less attractive.

---

[81] Eaton SB, Cordain L, Eaton SB. An evolutionary foundation for health promotion. *World Rev Nutr Diet* 2001; 90:5-12
[82] For an additional perspective see movie by Morgan Spurlock (director). Super Size Me. www.supersizeme.com released in 2004

Exploring the spectrum of physical activity from inactivity to athleticism

Inactivity	Minimally active	Active	Healthy	Athletic
• Bed-ridden • Chair-ridden • Minimal activity, such as walking to car or bathroom or to buy groceries • Activity in this category is equivalent to or barely above that which is necessary to sustain life	• Periodic performance of more activity than the minimal needed to sustain life, such as walking around the block after dinner, or taking a brief stroll at a park or at the beach	• Regular performance of low/moderate levels of activity at work or leisure, at least 30-60 minutes of physical activity per day	• 60-120 minutes of vigorous activity such as running, swimming, or cycling 4-7 days per week	• More than 2 hours devoted to conditioning, strengthening, and skill-building 4-7 days per week

At least 30-45 minutes of exercise four days per week is the *absolute minimum*. Ideally, patients who have been sedentary and are over age 45 years would have a pre-exercise physical exam that might also include electrocardiography before embarking on a program of vigorous exercise. Patients who have been sedentary for many years can start slowly with their new exercise program, gradually increasing the duration and intensity. With the simple addition of regular exercise to their routine, patients will have significantly reduced risk for problems such as depression, chronic pain, cancer, coronary artery disease, stroke, hypertension, diabetes, arthritis, osteoporosis, dyslipidemia, obesity, chronic obstructive pulmonary disease, constipation, and

> **Industrialized Westernized societies' disregard for connection with the body**
>
> "That I deemed it an imposition to have to make use of my perfectly adequate coordination, or resented—from unexamined principle—the use of time to fill a need, was an arbitrary assignment of values that [this other culture] did not share."
>
> Liedloff J. <u>The Continuum Concept</u>. Cambridge, MA: Da Capo Press; 1977, page 15

other problems.[83] Furthermore, successful prevention and treatment of health problems with exercise and lifestyle modifications reduces dependency on pharmaceutical drugs, thereby further saving lives. O'Keefe and Cordain[84] report that **during the hunter-gatherer period, humans averaged 5-10 miles of daily running and walking**. Additionally, **other physical activities such as heavy lifting, digging, and climbing would have been considered "normal" aspects of daily life rather than "exercise"—an achievement for which modern/industrialized people seek recognition.** Thus, when sedentary patients achieve the first-step goal of walking around the block after dinner, we can commend them for making a significant stride forward in ultimately attaining better health, but we cannot stop there nor delude them into believing that this is adequate.

---

[83] Harold Elrick, MD. Exercise is Medicine. *The Physician and Sportsmedicine* - Volume 24 - No. 2 - February 1996
[84] O'Keefe JH Jr, Cordain L. Cardiovascular disease resulting from a diet and lifestyle at odds with our Paleolithic genome: how to become a 21st-century hunter-gatherer. *Mayo Clin Proc*. 2004 Jan;79(1):101-8. Available on line at http://www.thepaleodiet.com/articles/Hunter-Gatherer%20Mayo.pdf on May 19, 2004

Common physical activities: a buffet of options from which to choose
☑ **Walking**: easy, accessible, virtually free; allows for conversation and exploration; allows for time outdoors
☑ **Jogging and running**: easy, accessible, virtually free; allows for conversation and exploration; increases endorphin production and promotes a sense of well-being; detoxification via sweating
☑ **Hiking**: virtually free of expense; allows for conversation, exploration, and time in nature; mountains required
☑ **Swimming**: requires access to a pool or suitable body of water; excellent for promoting fitness in a way that is generally easy on joints and muscles and is without impact; requires and thus promotes coordination and timing
☑ **Indoor aerobics**: excellent for cardiovascular fitness and weight loss, requires and thus promotes coordination and timing
☑ **Indoor cycling**: excellent for cardiovascular fitness and weight loss, easy on the joints; accessible during inclement weather
☑ **Outdoor cycling (road)**: same as above with added bonus of being outdoors; promotes independence from automobiles and petroleum products – thereby reducing pollution and sustaining the environment
☑ **Outdoor cycling (mountain and trail)**: same as above; requires more balance and coordination
☑ **Weight lifting, bodybuilding, and powerlifting**: excellent for increasing lean body mass – one of the primary determinants of basal metabolic rate; promotes bone strengthening
☑ **Tennis and racket sports**: requires more balance, coordination, timing, strategy, endurance; the rapid stops, starts, and turns can be hard on joints; upper body exertion is asymmetric and can promote muscle imbalance
☑ **Aerobic machines such as elliptical runners and stair-climbing machines**: easy on joints; accessible during inclement weather; easy to integrate with weight-lifting which is commonly available at the same facility
☑ **Rock-climbing (indoor and outdoor)**: requires upper body and grip strength; promotes agility, resourcefulness, courage, and trust; good for building stronger relationships assuming that your partner does not drop the rope or get distracted; carries some inherent risk
☑ **Volleyball**: good team activity; not highly exertional in terms of either aerobic fitness nor strength acquisition
☑ **Baseball**: requires some skill in throwing and batting, but otherwise this is a very inactive sport
☑ **Football**: much of the game is spent in inactivity; most of the fitness comes from preparation for the game, not the game itself; high impact activity wherein injuries are expected
☑ **Soccer**: excellent for lower-body conditioning, teamwork, and coordination, the rapid stops and turns can be hard on joints
☑ **Yoga, Pilates, Calisthenics**: inexpensive, can be done alone or in groups; does not require much/any equipment, therefore costs are low and access is near universal
☑ **Martial arts**: requires more balance, coordination, timing, strategy, endurance; injuries are to be expected
☑ **Surfing**: paddling requires upper body endurance and strength; some leg strength is required but is not strongly developed during the riding portion of surfing, which is mostly technique and "style"; excellent proprioceptive training
☑ **Kayaking and canoeing**: excellent combination of relaxation and exertion; develops upper body strength and balance
☑ **"Boot camp"-style aerobics classes**: excellent variety and fast-pace maintains oxygen debt for the entire session (generally 60 minutes) even among reasonably well trained "healthy" people
☑ **Skiing, snowboarding, cross-country skiing**: Require balance and coordination, costly equipment, and appropriate season and climate; risk of traumatic injury due to speed in skiing and snowboarding. Cross-country skiing is generally safe from trauma and provides excellent cardiovascular exertion, in addition to exposure to nature

Obesity: Obesity is a major risk factor for cardiovascular disease, cancer, diabetes mellitus, depression, joint degeneration and pain. Obese people also commonly report difficulties with performing daily activities, and they also report higher rates of depression and social isolation than do people of normal weight.

"Body Mass Index" is a clinically valuable measure of height-weight proportionality and therefore adiposity, since an excess of height-proportionate weight is more commonly due to excess

adipose than to excess muscle. To calculate BMI simply chart height and weight in the table below. Numbers greater than 25 correlate with being "overweight" while numbers greater than 30 meet the criteria for "obesity." BMI determinations may not be reflective of disease risk for people who are pregnant, highly muscular, or for young children or the frail elderly.

Body mass index (BMI) interpretation

- Severely underweight: < 16.5
- Underweight: 16.5 - 18.4
- **Normal: 18.5 - 24.9**
- Overweight: 25 - 29.9
- Obese Class 1: 30 - 34.9
- Obese Class 2 (severe obesity): 35 - 39.9
- Obese Class 3 (morbid obesity): 40 - 47.9
- Obese Class 4 (supermorbid obesity): ≥ 48

WEIGHT in pounds

HEIGHT	100	110	120	130	140	150	160	170	180	190	200	210	220	230	240	250
5'0"	20	21	23	25	27	29	31	33	35	37	39	41	43	45	47	49
5'1"	19	21	23	25	26	28	30	32	34	36	38	40	42	43	45	47
5'2"	18	20	22	24	26	27	29	31	33	35	37	38	40	42	44	46
5'3"	18	19	21	23	25	27	28	30	32	34	35	37	39	41	43	44
5'4"	17	19	21	22	24	26	27	29	31	33	34	36	38	39	41	43
5'5"	17	18	20	22	23	25	27	28	30	32	33	35	37	38	40	42
5'6"	16	18	19	21	23	24	26	27	29	31	32	34	36	37	39	40
5'7"	16	17	19	20	22	23	25	27	28	30	31	33	34	36	38	39
5'8"	15	17	18	20	21	23	24	26	27	29	30	32	33	35	36	38
5'9"	15	16	18	19	21	22	24	25	27	28	30	31	32	34	35	37
5'10"	14	16	17	19	20	22	23	24	26	27	29	30	32	33	34	36
5'11"	14	15	17	18	20	21	22	24	25	26	27	28	30	32	33	35
6'0"	14	15	16	18	19	20	22	23	24	26	27	28	30	31	33	34
6'1"	13	15	16	17	18	20	21	22	24	25	26	28	29	30	32	33
6'2"	13	14	15	17	18	19	21	22	23	24	26	27	28	30	31	32
6'3"	12	14	15	16	17	19	20	21	22	24	25	26	27	29	30	31
6'4"	12	13	15	16	17	18	19	21	22	23	24	26	27	28	29	30

Overview of the proinflammatory and endocrinologic activity of adipose tissue

Cardiovascular disease (predisposition)

Increased CRP and fibrinogen

Inflammation

Joint pain and swelling (predisposition)

Increased secretion of adipokines, including tumor necrosis factor, leptin, and interleukin-6 (thus CRP)

Inadequate physical exercise causes sarcopenia

Activation of NF-kappaB

Insulin resistance (mediated in part by TNF-a)

Inadequate antioxidant intake

Receptor insensitivity due to oxidative stress and inadequate omega-3 fatty acid intake

Exaggerated postprandial hyperglycemia, elevated serum insulin

Fat gain and the accumulation of pro-inflammatory visceral/intra-abdominal adipose

Excess dietary calories, especially fat and sugar

Micronutrient insufficiencies, such as chromium, selenium, magnesium, calcium, vitamin D

Increased production of androgens

Conversion of androgens to estrone by aromatase in adipose

Increased levels of estrogens

Genetic predisposition (in some people)

Increased risk for hormone-related cancers: breast, prostate, endometrium, colon, gallbladder

The old view that fat (adipose) tissue was merely serving as an inert and inactive depot for lipid/energy storage is now replaced with the view that adipose tissue is biologically-active, influencing overall health via complex mechanisms that are biochemical-inflammatory-endocrinologic and not merely mechanical (i.e., excess weight, excess mass).[85] **Excess fat tissue—especially visceral/abdominal adipose—creates a systemic proinflammatory state** evidenced most readily by the elevations in hsCRP commonly seen in patients with obesity and the metabolic syndrome.[86] Adipokines are cytokines secreted by adipose tissue and include tumor necrosis factor-alpha, interleukin-6, and leptin—a cytokine derived from fat cells that promotes inflammation and immune activation; levels are higher in obese patients and decrease after weight loss. Obese patients also appear to have "leptin resistance" with regard to the suppression of appetite by leptin. **Adipose creates excess estrogens;** concomitant hyperglycemia increases androgen production[87], and these androgens are subsequently converted to estrogens by aromatase in the adipose tissue. For example, the adrenal gland makes androstenedione, which can be converted by aromatase in adipose tissue into estrone.[88] These proinflammatory and hormonal perturbations manifest clinically as an increased risk for breast, prostate, endometrial, colon and gallbladder cancers, and cardiovascular disease. This pattern of inflammation, reduced testosterone, and elevated estrogen is also a predisposition toward the development of autoimmune/inflammatory diseases.

---

[85] "The fat cell is a true endocrine cell that secretes a variety of factors, including metabolites such as lactate, fatty acids, prostaglandin derivatives and a variety of peptides, including cytokines (leptin, tumor necrosis factor, interleukin-1 and -6, adiponectin), angiotensinogen, complement D (adipsin), plasminogen activator inhibitor-1 and undoubtedly many others." Bray GA. The underlying basis for obesity: relationship to cancer. *J Nutr.* 2002 Nov;132(11 Suppl):3451S-3455S

[86] "Our results indicate a strong relationship between adipocytokines and inflammatory markers, and suggest that cytokines secreted by adipose tissue could play a role in increased inflammatory proteins secretion by the liver." Maachi M, Pieroni L, Bruckert E, Jardel C, Fellahi S, Hainque B, Capeau J, Bastard JP. Systemic low-grade inflammation is related to both circulating and adipose tissue TNFalpha, leptin and IL-6 levels in obese women. *Int J Obes Relat Metab Disord.* 2004;28:993-7

[87] Christensen L, Hagen C, Henriksen JE, Haug E. Elevated levels of sex hormones and sex hormone binding globulin in male patients with insulin dependent diabetes mellitus. Effect of improved blood glucose regulation. *Dan Med Bull.* 1997 Nov;44(5):547-50

[88] "The conversion of androstenedione secreted by the adrenal gland into estrone by aromatase in adipose tissue stroma provides an important source of estrogen for the postmenopausal woman. This estrogen may play an important role in the development of endometrial and breast cancer." Bray GA. The underlying basis for obesity: relationship to cancer. *J Nutr.* 2002 Nov;132(11 Suppl):3451S-3455S

The Daily Diet—Powerful Intervention for the Prevention and Treatment of Disease: "Whole foods" should form the foundation and majority of the diet. As doctors and patients, we should emphasize whole fruits, vegetables, nuts, seeds, berries, and lean sources of protein. "Whole foods" are foods that are found in nature, and they should be eaten as closely as possible to their natural state—preferably *unprocessed* and *raw*. Creating a diet based on whole, natural foods by emphasizing the consumption of fruits, vegetables, and lean meats and excluding high-fat factory meats, high-sugar foods like white potatoes, and milled grains like wheat and corn is essential for our efforts of promoting health by matching the human *diet* with the human *genome*.[89] Our genetic make-up was co-created over a period of more than 2.6 million years by interaction with the environment as it exists in its natural state. This environment mandated daily physical activity and a diet that was exclusively composed of 1) fresh fruits, 2) fresh vegetables (mostly uncooked), 3) raw nuts, seeds, berries, roots, and 4) generous portions of lean game meat that was rich in omega-3 fatty acids from free-living animals who were lean because they also ran, fasted, and dealt with limited food supplies. Humans have deviated from this original diet for the sake of ease, conformity, and short-term satisfaction at the expense of health and longevity. Peoples who consume traditional, natural diets have dramatically lower incidences *major* health problems such as cancer, cardiovascular disease, diabetes, obesity and also suffer much less from *milder* problems such as acne, psoriasis, dental cavities, oral malocclusion, and chronic sinus congestion. Societies that are free of

---

The Supplemented Paleo-Mediterranean Diet

My conclusion after reading several hundred articles on epidemiology, nutritional biochemistry, and dietary intervention studies is that the Paleo-Mediterranean diet—particularly its pesco-vegetarian version—is the single most healthy dietary regimen for the broadest range of patients and for the prevention of the widest range of diseases including cancer, hypertension, diabetes, dermatitis, depression, obesity, arthritis and all inflammatory and autoimmune diseases. By definition, this is a diet that helps patients increase their intake of fruits and vegetables (fiber, antioxidants, phytonutrients), increases their intake of fish (for the anti-inflammatory omega-3 fats EPA and DHA) while reducing intake of the pro-cancer and pro-inflammatory omega-6 fats linoleic acid and arachidonic acid), and it is naturally low in sugars and cholesterol (for alleviating hyperglycemia and dyslipidemia). This dietary pattern helps patients avoid grains, particularly wheat (a common allergen), and it reduces the intake of the high-fermentation carbohydrates in breads, pasta, pastries, potatoes, and sucrose which promote overgrowth of bacteria and yeast in the intestines. Supplementing this pesco-vegetarian diet with vitamins, minerals, fatty acids such as fish oil and GLA (from borage oil), and protein from soy and whey makes this diet effective for both the treatment and prevention of many conditions; I have called this "the Supplemented Paleo-Mediterranean Diet."

1. Vasquez A. A Five-Part Nutritional Protocol that Produces Consistently Positive Results. *Nutritional Wellness* 2005 September
2. Vasquez A. Implementing the Five-Part Nutritional Wellness Protocol for the Treatment of Various Health Problems. *Nutritional Wellness* 2005 November
3. Vasquez A. Revisiting the Five-Part Nutritional Wellness Protocol: The Supplemented Paleo-Mediterranean Diet. *Nutritional Perspectives* 2011 January

The complete texts of these articles are included within this book and on-line at http://optimalhealthresearch.com/spmd

---

these disorders become overwhelmed with them *within only one or two generations* as soon as they adopt the American/Western style of eating. These facts were conclusively documented by Weston Price in his famous 1945 masterpiece *Nutrition and Physical Degeneration*[90] and have been reiterated recently in an excellent review by O'Keefe and Cordain in *Mayo Clinic Proceedings*.[91]

---

[89] O'Keefe JH Jr, Cordain L. Cardiovascular disease resulting from a diet and lifestyle at odds with our Paleolithic genome: how to become a 21st-century hunter-gatherer. *Mayo Clin Proc.* 2004 Jan;79(1):101-8

[90] Price WA. Nutrition and Physical Degeneration. Santa Monica; Price-Pottinger Nutrition Foundation: 1945

[91] O'Keefe JH Jr,Cordain L.Cardiovascular disease resulting from a diet and lifestyle at odds with our Paleolithic genome. *Mayo Clin Proc.*2004;79:101-8

Most patients (and doctors) need to increase consumption of fruits and vegetables: Encourage consumption of collard greens, broccoli, kale, spinach, chard, lettuce, onions, red peppers, green beans, carrots, apples, oranges, nuts, blueberries and other fruits and vegetables. Patients can find or make a good low-carbohydrate dressing (such as lemon-garlic tahini[92]) to make these vegetables taste great. Fresh fruits and vegetables are best; but frozen fruits and vegetables are acceptable. Patients can buy a package of (organic) frozen vegetables; then when they are ready for a healthy-and-fast meal, simply thaw the vegetables or warm/steam them on the stovetop. In just a few minutes and with only minimal effort, by regularly eating vegetables, they will have significantly reduced their risk for heart disease, diabetes, cancer, hemorrhoids, constipation, and many other chronic health problems. Using frozen vegetables and eating vegetables only twice per day is not *optimal*—it is *minimal*. For many patients, consuming two servings of vegetables per day is a major lifestyle change. ***Ultimately, the goal is for fresh fruits and vegetables to form a major portion of the diet, to be the main course rather than simply a side dish.*** A diet based on fruits and vegetables is a powerful nutritional strategy for reducing the risk for cancer, heart disease, and autoimmune and inflammatory disorders.[93]

Phytochemicals—important antioxidant and anti-inflammatory nutrients from fruits, vegetables, nuts, seeds, berries, and many herbs and spices: While we have all commonly thought of the benefits of fruits and vegetables as being derived from the

---

Proteins, fruits, vegetables—not grains

"Historical and archaeological evidence shows hunter-gatherers generally to be lean, fit, and largely free from signs and symptoms of chronic diseases. When hunter-gatherer societies transitioned to an agricultural grain-based diet, their general health deteriorated. ... When former hunter-gatherers adopt Western lifestyles, obesity, type-2 diabetes, atherosclerosis, and other diseases of civilization become commonplace."

O'Keefe JH Jr, Cordain L. Cardiovascular disease resulting from a diet and lifestyle at odds with our Paleolithic genome. *Mayo Clin Proc.* 2004;79:101-8

---

vitamins, minerals, and fiber, we are learning from new research that many if not most of the health-promoting benefits of fruit and vegetable consumption comes from the unique plant-based chemicals—phytochemicals—contained therein. For example, while in the past we might have thought of the benefits of eating apples as being derived from the vitamin C content, we now know that vitamin C only provides 0.4% of the antioxidant action contained within a whole apple—obviously the other components of the apple, namely the phenolic compounds are responsible for most of an apple's antioxidant activity.[94] Recent research has shown that cranberries, apples, red grapes, and strawberries have the most antioxidant power of the fruits[95], while red peppers, broccoli, carrots, and spinach are the best antioxidant vegetables[96]; see the tables that follow. This is a very important concept to appreciate and remember: **the benefits**

---

[92] Mollie Katzen. The New Moosewood Cookbook Ten Speed Press; page 103

[93] "…one of the most consistent research findings is that those who consume higher amounts of fruits and vegetables have lower rates of heart disease and stroke as well as cancer…" Seaman DR. The diet-induced proinflammatory state: a cause of chronic pain and other degenerative diseases? *J Manipulative Physiol Ther.* 2002;25(3):168-79

[94] "We propose that the additive and synergistic effects of phytochemicals in fruit and vegetables are responsible for their potent antioxidant and anticancer activities, and that the benefit of a diet rich in fruit and vegetables is attributed to the complex mixture of phytochemicals present in whole foods." Liu RH. Health benefits of fruit and vegetables are from additive and synergistic combinations of phytochemicals. *Am J Clin Nutr.* 2003 Sep;78(3 Suppl):517S-520S

[95] "Cranberry had the highest total antioxidant activity (177.0 +/- 4.3 micromol of vitamin C equiv/g of fruit), followed by apple, red grape, strawberry, peach, lemon, pear, banana, orange, grapefruit, and pineapple." Sun J, Chu YF, Wu X, Liu RH. Antioxidant and antiproliferative activities of common fruits. *J Agric Food Chem.* 2002 Dec 4;50(25):7449-54

[96] "Red pepper had the highest total antioxidant activity, followed by broccoli, carrot, spinach, cabbage, yellow onion, celery, potato, lettuce, and cucumber." Chu YF, Sun J, Wu X, Liu RH. Antioxidant and antiproliferative activities of common vegetables. *J Agric Food Chem.* 2002 Nov 6;50(23):6910-6

derived from fruits and vegetables are *not* derived principally from the vitamins and therefore can never be obtained from the use of multivitamin pills as a substitute for whole foods. Multivitamin and multimineral supplements are valuable and worthwhile *supplements* to a whole-foods diet but should not be used as *substitutes for* a whole-foods diet.

Fruits and vegetables contain more than 8,000 phytochemicals, most of which have anti-inflammatory, anti-proliferative, and anti-cancer benefits[97]—the best and only way to benefit from these chemicals is to change the diet in favor of relying principally on fruits and vegetables as the major component of the diet, and the easiest way to do this is to eliminate carbohydrate-rich antioxidant-poor foods such as bread, pasta, rice, sweets, crackers, chips and "junk foods."

Phenolic content and antioxidant capacity of common vegetables and fruits

Vegetables		Fruits	
Phenolic content	*Antioxidant capacity*	*Phenolic content*	*Antioxidant capacity*
1. Broccoli	1. Red pepper	1. Cranberry	1. Cranberry
2. Spinach	2. Broccoli	2. Apple	2. Apple
3. Yellow onion	3. Carrot	3. Red grape	3. Red grape
4. Red pepper	4. Spinach	4. Strawberry	4. Strawberry
5. Carrot	5. Cabbage	5. Pineapple	5. Peach
6. Cabbage	6. Yellow onion	6. Banana	6. Lemon
7. Potato	7. Celery	7. Peach	7. Pear
8. Lettuce	8. Potato	8. Lemon	8. Banana
9. Celery	9. Lettuce	9. Orange	9. Orange
10. Cucumber	10. Cucumber	10. Pear	10. Grapefruit
		11. Grapefruit	11. Pineapple

Data from: Chu YF, Sun J, Wu X, Liu RH. Antioxidant and antiproliferative activities of common vegetables. *J Agric Food Chem*. 2002 Nov 6;50(23):6910-6 and Sun J, Chu YF, Wu X, Liu RH. Antioxidant and antiproliferative activities of common fruits. *J Agric Food Chem*. 2002 Dec 4;50(25):7449-54

Different fruits and vegetables contain different types, quantities, and ratios of vitamins, minerals, and phytochemicals; therefore, *dietary diversity* will therefore help patients obtain a broad spectrum of and maximum benefit from these different nutrients. Taking appropriate action with the data that a fruit/vegetable-based diet has powerful health-promoting benefits means that we as doctors and patients have to change our lifestyles with regard to how we plan our meals, what we buy, what we prepare, and what we eat. Behavior modification is a tremendous challenge for people, especially those who lack sufficient motivation or insight. This text is providing the *insight*—the data, references, and concepts. But without *motivation*—from doctors to help their patients attain the highest levels of health, and from patients to change their lifestyles to become as healthy as possible—the research itself does little to promote health.

Consuming the right amount of protein: Dietary protein is eaten to provide the body with amino acids, which are the fundamental components that the body uses to create new tissues (such as skin, mucosal surfaces, hair, and nails), heal wounds (e.g., formation of collagen), fight off infections (e.g., formation of immunoglobulin proteins, antibodies), and to create specific

---

[97] Liu RH. Health benefits of fruit and vegetables are from additive and synergistic combinations of phytochemicals. *Am J Clin Nutr*. 2003 Sep;78(3 Suppl):517S-520S

hormones (such as insulin and thyroid hormones) and neurotransmitters, such as dopamine, serotonin, norepinephrine, and gamma-aminobutyric acid (GABA). Amino acid profiles in meats, eggs, and milk is similar to that of the human body and such dietary sources have been described as containing relatively more "complete protein" than most plant-based protein sources. For plant-based diets without concomitant use of animal proteins to provide sufficient quantity and quality of protein, foods must be combined with respect to one another's amino acid profiles.

For most people (without kidney or liver problems) the goal for daily protein intake should be 0.50-0.75 grams of protein per pound of lean body weight, depending on activity level and other health needs (see table).

Recommended <u>Grams of Protein</u> Per <u>Pound of Body Weight</u> Per Day[98]	
Infants and children ages 1-6 years[99]	0.68-0.45
RDA for sedentary adult and children ages 6-18 years[100]	0.4
Adult recreational exerciser	**0.5-0.75**
Adult competitive athlete	0.6-0.9
Adult building muscle mass	0.7-0.9
Dieting athlete	0.7-1.0
Growing teenage athlete	0.9-1.0
Pregnant women need additional protein	Add 15-30 grams/day[101]

Sufficient dietary protein is essential for patients with musculoskeletal injuries because tissue healing relies on the constant availability of amino acids and micronutrients[102], which should be supplied by a healthy, balanced, whole-foods diet that may be supplemented with specific vitamins, minerals, and phytonutrients. Low-protein diets suppress immune function, reduce muscle mass, and impair healing[103,104] whereas intakes of higher amounts of protein safely facilitate healing and the maintenance of muscle mass. Increased protein intake does not adversely affect bone health as long as dietary calcium intake is adequate.[105] According to the 1998 review by Lemon[106]:

> "Those involved in strength training might need to consume as much as …1.7 g protein x kg(-1) x day(-1)…while those undergoing endurance training might need about 1.2 to 1.6 g x kg(-1) x day(-1)… …**there is no evidence that protein intakes in the range suggested will have adverse effects in healthy individuals.**"

[98] Slightly modified from Nancy Clark, MS, RD. Protein Power. *The Physician and Sportsmedicine* 1996, volume 24, number 4
[99] 1.5-1 g/kg/d (0.68-0.45 grams per pound of body weight. Younger people need proportionately more protein.) Brown ML (ed). Present Knowledge in Nutrition. Sixth Edition. Washington DC: International Life Sciences Institute Nutrition Foundation; 1990 page 68
[100] 0.83 g.kg-1.d-1 (equivalent to 0.37 grams per pound of body weight) Pellet PL. Protein requirements in humans. *Am J Clin Nutr* 1990 May;51:723-37
[101] Weinsier RL, Morgan SL (eds). Fundamentals of Clinical Nutrition. St. Louis: Mosby, 1993 page 50
[102] "Supplementation with protein and vitamins, specifically arginine and vitamins A, B, and C, provides optimum nutrient support of the healing wound." Meyer NA, Muller MJ, Herndon DN. Nutrient support of the healing wound. *New Horiz* 1994 May;2(2):202-14
[103] Castaneda C, Charnley JM, Evans WJ, Crim MC. Elderly women accommodate to a low-protein diet with losses of body cell mass, muscle function, and immune response. *Am J Clin Nutr* 1995 Jul;62(1):30-9 http://www.ajcn.org/cgi/reprint/62/1/30
[104] [No author listed]. Vegetarians and healing. *JAMA* 1995; 273: 910
[105] Heaney RP. Excess dietary protein may not adversely affect bone. *J Nutr* 1998 Jun;128(6):1054-7
[106] Lemon PW. Effects of exercise on dietary protein requirements. *Int J Sport Nutr 1998* Dec;8(4):426-47

For patients who are completely sedentary, multiply body weight in pounds by 0.4 and this will give the number of grams of protein that should be eaten each day.[107] For patients who are very active (frequent weight lifting, or competitive athlete), multiply body weight in pounds by 0.7-0.9 and this will give the number of grams of protein that should be eaten each day.

Again, compared with sedentary people, **sick people, injured people,** and *athletes* **need more protein** to maintain weight, fight infections, repair injuries, and build and maintain muscle. Not only can insufficient protein intake cause muscle weakness and loss of weight, but recent articles have also suggested that low-protein diets can cause suppression of the immune system[108] and impairment of healing after injury or surgery.[109]

For example, in most instances and according to the data presented in and reviewed for this section, a person weighing 120 pounds should aim for at least 60 grams of protein per day, or 90 grams of protein per day if he/she is more physically active, ill, or injured. A can of tuna has 30 grams of protein; one egg has 6 grams of protein. If she is going to eat eggs as a source of protein for a meal, she might have to eat as many as five eggs to reach a target of 30 grams of protein per meal. When eating meat, visualize the amount of meat in a can of tuna to estimate the amount of protein being eaten—for example, if the portion of meat at a given meal is about the size of a half can of tuna, then we can estimate that the serving contains 15-20 grams of high-quality protein. By knowing the "target intake" for the day, and by estimating the amount of protein eaten with each meal, patients will be able to modify their protein intake to ensure that they reach their protein intake goal.

Protein supplements—most common of which are based on concentrates of or isolated components of egg, soy, or cow's milk— can be used *in conjunction with a healthy diet.* Patients using a protein supplement should eat a healthy diet and then add protein supplements between regular meals. If they substitute a protein supplement for a regular meal, then they may not actually increase protein intake. Whole *real* foods should form the foundation for the diet—patients should not rely too heavily on *protein supplements* when patients can get better results *and improved overall health* with *whole foods.* Whey, casein, and lactalbumin are proteins from milk and dairy products, and may therefore be allergenic in people allergic to cow's milk. Soy protein is safe and a source of high-quality protein for adults[110], and research shows that consumption of soy protein can help reduce the risk of cancer and heart disease[111]; however, I do not recommend the use of large quantities of supplemental soy protein for pregnant women, or for children due to the potential for disrupting endocrine function. Patients may have to experiment with different products until they find one that is suitable in regard to taste, texture, digestibility, hypoallergenicity, nutritional effects, ease of preparation, and affordability.

Recall again that the goal is *improved health*, not simply *adequate protein intake.* If we focus solely on "grams of protein" then we might overlook adverse effects that are associated with certain protein sources. Cow's milk is a high quality protein, but it is commonly allergenic and can exacerbate joint pain in sensitive individuals.[112] Beef, liver, pork and other land animal meats

---

[107] Pellet PL. Protein requirements in humans. *Am J Clin Nutr* 1990 May;51(5):723-37
[108] Castaneda C, Charnley JM, Evans WJ, Crim MC. Elderly women accommodate to a low-protein diet with losses of body cell mass, muscle function, and immune response. *Am J Clin Nutr* 1995 Jul;62(1):30-9
[109] Vegetarians and healing. *Journal of the American Medical Association* 1995; 273: 910
[110] "These results indicate that for healthy adults, the isolated soy protein is of high nutritional quality, comparable to that of animal protein sources, and that the methionine content is not limiting for adult protein maintenance." Young VR, Puig M, Queiroz E, Scrimshaw NS, Rand WM. Evaluation of the protein quality of an isolated soy protein in young men: relative nitrogen requirements and effect of methionine supplementation. *Am J Clin Nutr.* 1984 Jan;39(1):16-24
[111] Lissin LW, Cooke JP. Phytoestrogens and cardiovascular health. *J Am Coll Cardiol.* 2000 May;35(6):1403-10
[112] Golding DN. Is there an allergic synovitis? *J R Soc Med* 1990 May;83(5):312-4

are excellent sources of protein, but they are also generally rich sources of arachidonic acid[113] (if not grass-fed) and iron[114], both of which have been shown to exacerbate joint pain and inflammation. Fish is an excellent source of protein, but fish are often poisoned with mercury and other toxicants, which can be ingested by humans to produce negative health effects.[115,116]

Eat complex carbohydrates to stabilize blood sugar, mood, and energy: Choose items with a "low glycemic index"[117] to stabilize blood sugar and—for many people—to lower triglycerides and cholesterol levels. Foods with a low Glycemic Index (GI < 55)[118] include yogurt, apple (36), whole orange (43), peach (28), legumes, lentils (28), and soybeans (18), cherries, dried apricots, nuts, most meats, and most vegetables. Healthy foods that have both a low *glycemic index* as well as a low *glycemic load* include: apples, carrots, chick peas, grapes, green peas, kidney beans, oranges, peaches, peanuts, pears, pinto beans, red lentils, and strawberries.[119]

Reduce or eliminate simple sugars from the diet (as necessary): Nearly everyone should minimize intake of table sugar (sucrose), fructose and high-fructose corn syrup, and all artificial sweeteners. Of important and recent note, high-fructose corn syrup has been shown to be contaminated by mercury due to the manufacturing process[120], and fructose has been shown to induce hypertension and the metabolic syndrome in humans.[121] Chronic overconsumption of refined carbohydrates promotes disease by 1) increasing urinary excretion of magnesium and calcium, 2) inducing oxidative stress, 3) promoting fat deposition and obesity, which then generally leads to insulin resistance and hyperinsulinemia with an increase in production of cholesterol, triglycerides, and proinflammatory adipokines[122], and 4) reducing function of leukocytes.[123] Among sweeteners, honey is the best choice since it is the only natural sweetener available with a wide range of health-promoting benefits including anti-inflammatory, antibacterial, antioxidant and anti-allergy effects.[124] Also consider the herb stevia as a non-caloric and nutritive sweetener. Occasional intake of sweets is likely to be of little consequence for people who are generally healthy and who are willing to sustain relatively short-term endothelial

---

[113] Adam O, Beringer C, Kless T, Lemmen C, Adam A, Wiseman M, Adam P, Klimmek R, Forth W. Anti-inflammatory effects of a low arachidonic acid diet and fish oil in patients with rheumatoid arthritis. *Rheumatol Int* 2003 Jan;23(1):27-36

[114] Dabbagh AJ, Trenam CW, Morris CJ, Blake DR. Iron in joint inflammation. *Ann Rheum Dis* 1993; 52:67-73

[115] "These fish often harbor high levels of methylmercury, a potent human neurotoxin." Evans EC. The FDA recommendations on fish intake during pregnancy. *J Obstet Gynecol Neonatal Nurs* 2002 Nov-Dec;31(6):715-20

[116] "Geometric mean mercury levels were almost 4-fold higher among women who ate 3 or more servings of fish in the past 30 days compared with women who ate no fish in that period.." Schober SE, Sinks TH, Jones RL, Bolger PM, McDowell M, Osterloh J, Garrett ES, Canady RA, Dillon CF, Sun Y, Joseph CB, Mahaffey KR. Blood mercury levels in US children and women of childbearing age, 1999-2000. *JAMA* 2003 Apr 2;289(13):1667-74

[117] For more information on glycemic index, consult a nutrition book or website such as http://www.stanford.edu/~dep/gilists.htm last accessed August 16, 2003

[118] Janette Brand-Miller, Kaye Foster-Powell. Diets with a low glycemic index: from theory to practice. *Nutrition Today* 1999 March. Accessed on-line at: http://www.findarticles.com/cf_dls/m0841/2_34/54654508/p1/article.jhtml on August 16, 2003.

[119] Mendosa D. Glycemic Values of Common American Foods http://www.mendosa.com/common_foods.htm Accessed on August 4, 2004

[120] "Average daily consumption of high fructose corn syrup is about 50 grams per person in the United States. With respect to total mercury exposure, it may be necessary to account for this source of mercury in the diet of children and sensitive populations." Dufault R, LeBlanc B, Schnoll R, Cornett C, Schweitzer L, Wallinga D, Hightower J, Patrick L, Lukiw WJ. Mercury from chlor-alkali plants: measured concentrations in food product sugar. *Environ Health*. 2009 Jan 26;8:2. See also: "High fructose corn syrup has been shown to contain trace amounts of mercury as a result of some manufacturing processes, and its consumption can also lead to zinc loss." Dufault R, Schnoll R, Lukiw WJ, Leblanc B, Cornett C, Patrick L, Wallinga D, Gilbert SG, Crider R. Mercury exposure, nutritional deficiencies and metabolic disruptions may affect learning in children. *Behav Brain Funct*. 2009 Oct 27;5:44.

[121] News release from American Heart Association's 63rd High Blood Pressure Research Conference. High-sugar diet increases men's blood pressure; gout drug protective. Abstract P127. Sept. 23, 2009. http://americanheart.mediaroom.com/index.php?s=43&item=829 Accessed December 19, 2009

[122] "Because visceral and subcutaneous adipose tissues are the major sources of cytokines (adipokines), increased adipose tissue mass is associated with alteration in adipokine production (eg, overexpression of tumor necrosis factor-a, interleukin-6, plasminogen activator inhibitor-1, and underexpression of adiponectin in adipose tissue)." Aldhahi W, Hamdy O. Adipokines, inflammation, and the endothelium in diabetes. *Curr Diab Rep*. 2003 Aug;3(4):293-8

[123] Sanchez A, Reeser JL, Lau HS, Yahiku PY, Willard RE, McMillan PJ, Cho SY, Magie AR, Register UD. Role of sugars in human neutrophilic phagocytosis. *Am J Clin Nutr*. 1973 Nov;26(11):1180-4

[124] Al-Waili NS. Effects of daily consumption of honey solution on hematological indices and blood levels of minerals and enzymes in normal individuals. *J Med Food*. 2003 Summer;6(2):135-4

dysfunction[125], oxidative stress[126], increased LDL oxidation[127], and activation of NF-kappaB[128] as a result of their self-induced hyperglycemia. Postexertional hyperglycemia can be used to enhance athletic performance by sustaining and inducing glycogen storage following and during exercise (i.e., carbohydrate loading for glycogen "supercompensation"[129,130]). Similarly, consumption of "simple" carbohydrate without protein can be used to promote entry of tryptophan across the blood-brain barrier and into the brain to promote serotonin synthesis.[131] In summary, *habitual overconsumption* of simple carbohydrates promotes disease by oxidative and proinflammatory mechanisms, while conversely *periodic consumption* of simple carbohydrates can be used to promote athletic performance and to increase intracerebral serotonin synthesis for the promotion of enhanced mood and cognitive performance and for the regulation of food intake.

<u>**Avoid artificial sweeteners, colors and other additives**</u>: Absolutely never use **aspartame**—this is a synthetic chemical that is easily converted to the toxin formaldehyde.[132] Aspartame causes cancer in animals and is strongly linked to brain tumors in humans.[133,134] **Sodium benzoate** is a food preservative that can cause asthma[135] and skin rashes[136] in sensitive individuals. **Tartrazine (yellow dye #5)** is a food/drug coloring agent that can cause asthma and skin rashes in sensitive individuals.[137] **Carrageenan** is a naturally-occurring carbohydrate extracted from red seaweed. Common sources of carrageenan are certain brands of "rice milk" and "soy milk." In addition to suppressing immune function[138], carrageenan causes intestinal ulcers and inflammatory bowel

---

[125] "Modest hyperinsulinemia, mimicking fasting hyperinsulinemia of insulin-resistant states, abrogates endothelium-dependent vasodilation in large conduit arteries, probably by increasing oxidant stress. These data may provide a novel pathophysiological basis to the epidemiological link between hyperinsulinemia/insulin-resistance and atherosclerosis in humans." Arcaro G, Cretti A, Balzano S, Lechi A, Muggeo M, Bonora E, Bonadonna RC. Insulin causes endothelial dysfunction in humans: sites and mechanisms. *Circulation*. 2002 Feb 5;105(5):576-82

[126] "Hyperglycemia increased plasma MDA concentrations, but the activities of GSH-Px and SOD were significantly higher after a larger dose of glucose only. Plasma catecholamines were unchanged. These results indicate that the transient increase of plasma catecholamine and insulin concentrations did not induce oxidative damage, while glucose already in the low dose was an important triggering factor for oxidative stress." Koska J, Blazicek P, Marko M, Grna JD, Kvetnansky R, Vigas M. Insulin, catecholamines, glucose and antioxidant enzymes in oxidative damage during different loads in healthy humans. *Physiol Res*. 2000;49 Suppl 1:S95-100

[127] "In conclusion, insulin at physiological doses is associated with increased LDL peroxidation independent of the presence of hyperglycemia." Quinones-Galvan A, Sironi AM, Baldi S, Galetta F, Garbin U, Fratta-Pasini A, Cominacini L, Ferrannini E. Evidence that acute insulin administration enhances LDL cholesterol susceptibility to oxidation in healthy humans. *Arterioscler Thromb Vasc Biol*. 1999 Dec;19(12):2928-32

[128] "These data show that the intake of a mixed meal results in significant inflammatory changes characterized by a decrease in IkappaBalpha and an increase in NF-kappaB binding, plasma CRP, and the expression of IKKalpha, IKKbeta, and p47(phox) subunit." Aljada A, Mohanty P, Ghanim H, Abdo T, Tripathy D, Chaudhuri A, Dandona P. Increase in intranuclear nuclear factor kappaB and decrease in inhibitor kappaB in mononuclear cells after a mixed meal: evidence for a proinflammatory effect. *Am J Clin Nutr*. 2004 Apr;79(4):682-90

[129] "A significant glycogen sparing, as well as supercompensation within 24 h of recovery, was observed after [carbohydrate] supplementation." Brouns F, Saris WH, Beckers E, Adlercreutz H, van der Vusse GJ, Keizer HA, Kuipers H, Menheere P, Wagenmakers AJ, ten Hoor F. Metabolic changes induced by sustained exhaustive cycling and diet manipulation. *Int J Sports Med*. 1989 May;10 Suppl 1:S49-62

[130] "The accepted method of increasing muscle glycogen stores is by "glycogen loading," which classically involves depletion of muscle glycogen, usually by exercise, followed by consumption of a high-CHO diet for several days (e.g., 3, 39). ...increase muscle glycogen concentrations ([glycogen]) to between 150 and 200% of normal resting levels." Robinson TM, Sewell DA, Hultman E, Greenhaff PL. Role of submaximal exercise in promoting creatine and glycogen accumulation in human skeletal muscle. *J Appl Physiol*. 1999 Aug;87(2):598-604

[131] "Our results suggest that high-carbohydrate meals have an influence on serotonin synthesis. We predict that carbohydrates with a high glycemic index would have a greater serotoninergic effect than carbohydrates with a low glycemic index." Lyons PM, Truswell AS. Serotonin precursor influenced by type of carbohydrate meal in healthy adults. *Am J Clin Nutr*. 1988 Mar;47(3):433-9

[132] Trocho C, Pardo R, Rafecas I, Virgili J, Remesar X, Fernandez-Lopez JA, Alemany M. Formaldehyde derived from dietary aspartame binds to tissue components in vivo. *Life Sci*. 1998;63(5):337-4949

[133] Compared to other environmental factors putatively linked to brain tumors, the artificial sweetener aspartame is a promising candidate to explain the recent increase in incidence and degree of malignancy of brain tumors. ...exceedingly high incidence of brain tumors in aspartame-fed rats compared to no brain tumors in concurrent controls..." Olney JW, Farber NB, Spitznagel E, Robins LN. Increasing brain tumor rates: is there a link to aspartame? *J Neuropathol Exp Neurol* 1996;55(11):1115-23

[134] Russell Blaylock MD. <u>Excitotoxins</u>. Health Press; December 1996 [ISBN: 0929173252] Pages 211-214

[135] "Adverse reactions to benzoate in this patient required avoidance of some drugs, some of those classically prescribed under the form of syrups in asthma." Petrus M, Bonaz S, Causse E, Rhabbour M, Moulie N, Netter JC, Bildstein G. [Asthma and intolerance to benzoates] [Article in French] *Arch Pediatr*. 1996;3(10):984-7

[136] Munoz FJ, Bellido J, Moyano JC, Alvarez M, Fonseca JL. Perioral contact urticaria from sodium benzoate in a toothpaste. *Contact Dermatitis*. 1996 Jul;35(1):51

[137] "Tartrazine sensitivity is most frequently manifested by urticaria and asthma... Vasculitis, purpura and contact dermatitis infrequently occur as manifestations of tartrazine sensitivity." Dipalma JR. Tartrazine sensitivity. *Am Fam Physician*. 1990 Nov;42(5):1347-50

[138] "Impairment of complement activity and humoral responses to T-dependent antigens, depression of cell-mediated immunity, prolongation of graft survival and potentiation of tumour growth by carrageenans have been reported." Thomson AW, Fowler EF. Carrageenan: a review of its effects on the immune system. *Agents Actions*. 1981;11(3):265-73

disease in animals[139] and some research indicates that carrageenan consumption is associated with an increased risk for cancer in humans.[140,141]

Consume sufficient daily water in the form of water and health-promoting teas and juices: Daily "water" intake should be approximately 30 ml/kg; thus, for a 150-lb (70-kg) person, fluid intake should be at least 2.1 liters, and for a person who weighs 220 lbs (100 kg) the daily intake should be approximately 3 liters. More fluids may be used during times of exercise, heat exposure, illness, or detoxification, while fluid restriction can be indicated in patients with heart failure, renal failure, anasarca, and hyponatremia.

Consider reducing or eliminating caffeine: This is especially important for people with reactive hypoglycemia, insomnia, anxiety, hypertension, low-back pain, and for women with fibrocystic breast disease. Caffeine ingestion also leads to the activation of brain noradrenergic receptors, which can cause inhibition of dopaminergic pathways.[142] For people who are in good health, 1-3 servings of caffeine per day are not harmful. Herbal teas and green tea appear to have significant health-promoting effects due to their phytonutrient components and antioxidant, anti-inflammatory, and anticancer properties.

To the extent possible, eat "organic" foods rather than industrially-produced foods: Organic foods (i.e., foods which are *naturally grown* rather than being treated with insect poisons, synthetic fertilizers, and chemicals to enhance shelf-life) tend to cost more than chemically-produced foods; but the increased phytonutrient content justifies the cost. Organic foods contain more nutrients than do chemically-produced foods.[143] More importantly, recent research has also indicated that organic foods are better able to prevent the genetic damage that can lead to cancer than are foods that have been grown in an environment of artificial fertilizers and pesticides.[144]

Recognize the importance of avoiding food allergens: Biomedical research has established that adverse food reactions, regardless of the underlying mechanisms or classification of allergy, intolerance, or sensitivity, can exacerbate a wide range of human illnesses, including thyroid disease[145], mental depression[146,147], asthma, rhinitis,[148] recurrent otitis media[149], migraine[150,151,152],

[139] Watt J, Marcus R. Experimental ulcerative disease of the colon. *Methods Achiev Exp Pathol*. 1975;7:56-71
[140] Tobacman JK. Review of harmful gastrointestinal effects of carrageenan in animal experiments. *Environ Health Perspect*. 2001 Oct;109(10):983-94
[141] "However, the gum carrageenan which is comprised of linked, sulfated galactose residues has potent biological activity and undergoes acid hydrolysis to poligeenan, an acknowledged carcinogen." Tobacman JK, Wallace RB, Zimmerman MB. Consumption of carrageenan and other water-soluble polymers used as food additives and incidence of mammary carcinoma. *Med Hypotheses*. 2001 May;56(5):589-98
[142] "The results suggest that noradrenergic innervation of dopamine cells can directly inhibit the activity of dopamine cells." Paladini CA, Williams JT. Noradrenergic inhibition of midbrain dopamine neurons. *J Neurosci*. 2004 May 12;24(19):4568-75
[143] Smith B. Organic Foods versus Supermarket Foods: element levels. *Journal of Applied Nutrition* 1993; 45(1), p35-9
[144] "Against BaP, three species of OC vegetables showed 30-57% antimutagenecity, while GC ones did only 5-30%." Ren H, Endo H, Hayashi T. The superiority of organically cultivated vegetables to general ones regarding antimutagenic activities. *Mutat Res*. 2001 Sep 20;496(1-2):83-8
[145] Sategna-Guidetti C, Volta U, Ciacci C, Usai P, Carlino A, De Franceschi L, Camera A, Pelli A, Brossa C. Prevalence of thyroid disorders in untreated adult celiac disease patients and effect of gluten withdrawal: an Italian multicenter study. *Am J Gastroenterol*. 2001 Mar;96(3):751-7
[146] "The detection and treatment of psychological dysfunction related to food intolerance with particular reference to the problem of objective evaluation is discussed... Long-term follow-up revealed maintenance of marked improvements in psychological and physical functioning." Mills N. Depression and food intolerance: a single case study. *Hum Nutr Appl Nutr*. 1986 Apr;40(2):141-5
[147] "OBJECTIVE: To describe a patient with food intolerance probably contributing to depressive symptoms, intolerance to psychotropic medication and treatment resistance... RESULTS: The patient's course improved considerably with an elimination diet." Parker G, Watkins T. Treatment-resistant depression: when antidepressant drug intolerance may indicate food intolerance. *Aust N Z J Psychiatry*. 2002 Apr;36(2):263-5
[148] Speer F. The allergic child. *Am Fam Physician*. 1975 Feb;11(2):88-94
[149] Juntti H, Tikkanen S, Kokkonen J, Alho OP, Niinimaki A. Cow's milk allergy is associated with recurrent otitis media during childhood. *Acta Otolaryngol*. 1999;119(8):867-73
[150] "Foods which provoked migraine in 9 patients with severe migraine refractory to drug therapy were identified... These observations confirm that a food-allergic reaction is the cause of migraine in this group of patients." Monro J, Carini C, Brostoff J. Migraine is a food-allergic disease. *Lancet*. 1984 Sep 29;2(8405):719-21

attention deficit and hyperactivity disorders[153], epilepsy[154,155,156], gastrointestinal inflammation[157], hypertension[158], joint pain and inflammation[159,160,161,162,163,164,165,166] and a wide range of other health problems. Any program of health promotion and health maintenance must include consideration of food allergies, food intolerances, and food sensitivities. The elimination-and-challenge technique is the most cost-effective and it also teaches patients how to identify their own food allergies and intolerances, which may change for the better or worse over time; when the patient is empowered with this technique, he/she can take an active and on-going role in his/her own healthcare. Patients may be allergic to foods that are generally considered healthy, including whole organic foods. The more common food allergens—exemplified here by a list of offending foods identified in a study of patients with migraine[167]—are wheat (78%), orange (65%), eggs (45%), tea and coffee (40% each), chocolate and milk (37%) each), beef (35%), and corn, cane sugar, and yeast (33% each).

Supplement the health-promoting whole-foods diet with specific vitamins, minerals, fatty acids, and probiotics: Despite the fact that America is one of the richest nations on earth, and that we produce more than enough food to feed ourselves and many other nations with a healthy diet, Americans tend to have poor dietary habits and inadequate levels of nutritional intake that do not meet the minimal standards, such as the Recommended Daily Allowance (RDA, now Daily Reference Intake (DRI)).[168] Many people are under the misperception that if they appear healthy or are even overweight then they could not possibly have nutritional deficiencies. The truths of this matter are that 1) gross/obvious nutritional deficiencies are common among "apparently healthy" individuals, 2) common situations like stress, poor diets, and use of medications predispose people to nutritional deficiencies, 3) hereditary/genetic disorders affect a large portion of the population and lead to an increased need for nutritional intake which can generally only be met with supplementation in addition to a healthy whole-foods diet. Taking a "one-a-day" multivitamin is insufficient for people who truly desire significant benefit from supplementation. These one-a-day preparations generally only provide the minimum daily

[151] Egger J, Carter CM, Wilson J, et al. Is migraine food allergy? A double-blind controlled trial of oligoantigenic diet treatment. *Lancet*. 1983 Oct 15;2(8355):865-9

[152] Monro J, Brostoff J, Carini C, Zilkha K. Food allergy in migraine. Study of dietary exclusion and RAST. *Lancet*. 1980 Jul 5;2(8184):1-4

[153] Boris M, Mandel FS. Foods and additives are common causes of the attention deficit hyperactive disorder in children. *Ann Allergy*. 1994 May;72(5):462-8

[154] Egger J, Carter CM, Soothill JF, Wilson J. Oligoantigenic diet treatment of children with epilepsy and migraine. *J Pediatr*. 1989;114(1):51-8

[155] Pelliccia A, Lucarelli S, Frediani T, D'Ambrini G, Cerminara C, Barbato M, Vagnucci B, Cardi E. Partial cryptogenetic epilepsy and food allergy/intolerance. A causal or a chance relationship? Reflections on three clinical cases. *Minerva Pediatr*. 1999 May;51(5):153-7

[156] Frediani T, Lucarelli S, Pelliccia A, Vagnucci B, et al. Allergy and childhood epilepsy: a close relationship? *Acta Neurol Scand*. 2001;104(6):349-52

[157] Marr HY, Chen WC, Lin LH. Food protein-induced enterocolitis syndrome: report of one case. *Acta Paediatr Taiwan*. 2001;42(1):49-52

[158] Grant EC. Food allergies and migraine. *Lancet*. 1979 May 5;1(8123):966-9

[159] "Food allergy appeared to be responsible for the joint symptoms in three patients and in one it was possible to precipitate swelling of a knee due to synovitis with effusion by drinking milk a few hours beforehand, the synovial fluid having mildly inflammatory features and a relatively high eosinophil count." Golding DN. Is there an allergic synovitis? *J R Soc Med*. 1990 May;83(5):312-4

[160] Panush RS. Food induced ("allergic") arthritis: clinical and serologic studies. *J Rheumatol*. 1990 Mar;17(3):291-4

[161] Pacor ML, Lunardi C, Di Lorenzo G, Biasi D, Corrocher R. Food allergy and seronegative arthritis: report of two cases. *Clin Rheumatol*. 2001;20(4):279-81

[162] Schrander JJ, Marcelis C, de Vries MP, van Santen-Hoeufft HM. Does food intolerance play a role in juvenile chronic arthritis? *Br J Rheumatol*. 1997 Aug;36(8):905-8

[163] van de Laar MA, van der Korst JK. Food intolerance in rheumatoid arthritis. I. A double blind, controlled trial of the clinical effects of elimination of milk allergens and azo dyes. *Ann Rheum Dis*. 1992 Mar;51(3):298-302

[164] Haugen MA, Kjeldsen-Kragh J, Forre O. A pilot study of the effect of an elemental diet in the management of rheumatoid arthritis. *Clin Exp Rheumatol*. 1994;12(3):275-9

[165] van de Laar MA, Aalbers M, Bruins FG, et al. Food intolerance in rheumatoid arthritis. II. Clinical and histological aspects. *Ann Rheum Dis*. 1992;51(3):303-6

[166] Panush RS, Stroud RM, Webster EM. Food-induced (allergic) arthritis. Inflammatory arthritis exacerbated by milk. *Arthritis Rheum* 1986; 29(2): 220-6

[167] Grant EC. Food allergies and migraine. *Lancet*. 1979 May 5;1(8123):966-9

[168] "Most people do not consume an optimal amount of all vitamins by diet alone. Pending strong evidence of effectiveness from randomized trials, it appears prudent for all adults to take vitamin supplements." Fletcher RH, Fairfield KM. Vitamins for chronic disease prevention in adults: clinical applications. *JAMA* 2002 Jun 19;287(23):3127-9

allowance—this dose is not large enough to provide truly preventive medicine results; also, such one-a-day products tend to contain low-quality nutrients, such as ergocalciferol rather than cholecalciferol[169], cyanocobalamin rather than the hydroxyl-, methyl-, or adenosyl- forms[170], and DL-tocopherol or exclusively L-alpha-tocopherol rather than a mix of tocopherols with a high concentration (generally approximately 40%) of gamma tocopherol.[171]

For people still not convinced of the importance of a multi-vitamin/mineral supplement as part of the basic foundation of the health plan, please consider the following data from the medical research:

- Many people think that eating a "healthy diet" will supply them with the nutrients that they need and that they do not need to take a vitamin supplement. This may have been true 2000 years ago, but today's industrially produced "foods" are generally stripped of much of their nutritional value long before they leave the factory. Industrially-produced fruits and vegetables contain lower quantities of nutrients than does naturally raised "organic" produce. [172]

- The reason that people can be of normal weight or can even be overweight and obese and still have nutrient deficiencies is that the body lowers the metabolic rate when the intake of vitamins and minerals is low. This is referred to as the "physiologic adaptation to marginal malnutrition." Even though people may eat enough calories and protein, they can still suffer from growth retardation and behavioral problems as a result of micronutrient malnutrition, even though they *appear* nourished.[173]

- Most nutrition-oriented doctors will agree that magnesium is one of the most important nutrients, especially for helping prevent heart attack and stroke. **Magnesium deficiency is an epidemic in so-called "developed" nations, with 20-40% of different populations showing objective laboratory evidence of magnesium deficiency.**[174,175,176,177]

- Add to the above that every day we are confronted with more chronic emotional stress and toxic chemicals than has ever before existed on the planet, and it becomes easy to see that basic nutritional support and an organic whole foods diet is just the start of attaining improved health.

---

[169] "Vitamin D(2) potency is less than one third that of vitamin D(3). Physicians resorting to use of vitamin D(2) should be aware of its markedly lower potency and shorter duration of action relative to vitamin D(3)." Armas LA, Hollis BW, Heaney RP. Vitamin D2 is much less effective than vitamin D 3 in humans. *J Clin Endocrinol Metab*. 2004 Nov;89(11):5387-91

[170] Freeman AG. Cyanocobalamin--a case for withdrawal: discussion paper. *J R Soc Med*. 1992 Nov;85(11):686–687 http://www.ncbi.nlm.nih.gov/pmc/articles/PMC1293728/pdf/jrsocmed00105-0046.pdf

[171] "gamma-tocopherol is the major form of vitamin E in many plant seeds and in the US diet, but has drawn little attention compared with alpha-tocopherol, the predominant form of vitamin E in tissues and the primary form in supplements. However, recent studies indicate that gamma-tocopherol may be important to human health and that it possesses unique features that distinguish it from alpha-tocopherol." Jiang Q, Christen S, Shigenaga MK, Ames BN. gamma-tocopherol, the major form of vitamin E in the US diet, deserves more attention. *Am J Clin Nutr*. 2001 Dec;74(6):714-22 http://www.ajcn.org/content/74/6/714.full.pdf

[172] Smith B. Organic Foods versus Supermarket Foods: element levels. *Journal of Applied Nutrition* 1993; 45(1), p35-9. I recently found that this article is also available on-line at http://journeytoforever.org/farm_library/bobsmith.html as of June 19, 2004

[173] Allen LH. The nutrition CRSP: what is marginal malnutrition, and does it affect human function? *Nutr Rev* 1993 Sep;51(9):255-67

[174] "The American diet is low in magnesium, and with modern water systems, very little is ingested in the drinking water." Innerarity S. Hypomagnesemia in acute and chronic illness. *Crit Care Nurs Q*. 2000 Aug;23(2):1-19

[175] "Altogether 43% of 113 trauma patients had low magnesium levels compared to 30% of noninjured cohorts." Frankel H, Haskell R, Lee SY, Miller D, Rotondo M, Schwab CW. Hypomagnesemia in trauma patients. *World J Surg*. 1999 Sep;23(9):966-9

[176] "There was a 20% overall prevalence of hypomagnesemia among this predominantly female, African American population." Fox CH, Ramsoomair D, Mahoney MC, Carter C, Young B, Graham R. An investigation of hypomagnesemia among ambulatory urban African Americans. *J Fam Pract*. 1999 Aug;48(8):636-9

[177] "Suboptimal levels were detected in 33.7 per cent of the population under study. These data clearly demonstrate that the Mg supply of the German population needs increased attention." Schimatschek HF, Rempis R. Prevalence of hypomagnesemia in an unselected German population of 16,000 individuals. *Magnes Res*. 2001 Dec;14(4):283-90

General Guidelines for the Safe Use of Nutritional Supplements: Supplementation with vitamins and minerals is generally safe, especially if the following guidelines are followed:

- <u>Vitamins and minerals should generally be taken with food in order to eliminate the possibility of nausea and to increase absorption</u>: Most vitamins and other supplements should be taken with food so that nausea is avoided.

- <u>Iron is potentially harmful</u>: Iron promotes the formation of reactive oxygen species ("free radicals") and is thus implicated in several diseases, such as infections, cancer, liver disease, diabetes, and cardiovascular disease. Iron supplements should not be consumed except by people who have been definitively diagnosed with iron deficiency by measurement of serum ferritin. Iron supplementation without documentation of iron deficiency by measurement of serum ferritin is inappropriate. [178]

- <u>Vitamin A is one of the only vitamins with the potential for serious toxicity even at low doses</u>: Attention should be given to vitamin A intake so that toxicity is avoided. Total intake of vitamin A must account for all sources—foods, fish oils, and vitamin supplements. Manifestations of vitamin A toxicity include: skin problems (dry skin, flaking skin, chapped or split lips, red skin rash, hair loss), joint pain, bone pain, headaches, anorexia (loss of appetite), edema (water retention, weight gain, swollen ankles, difficulty breathing), fatigue, and/or liver damage. Whenever vitamin A is used in high doses, it must be used for a defined period of time in order to avoid the toxicity that will result from high-dose long-term vitamin A supplementation.

  - <u>Adults</u>: Women who are pregnant or might become pregnant and who are planning to carry the baby to full term delivery should not ingest more than 10,000 IU of vitamin A per day. Vitamin A toxicity is seen with chronic ingestion of therapeutic doses (for example: 25,000 IU per day for 6 years, or 100,000 IU per day for 2.5 years[179]). Most patients should not consume more than 25,000 IU of vitamin A per day for more than 2 months without express supervision by a healthcare provider. Vitamin A is present in some multivitamins, in animal liver and products such as fish liver oil, and in other supplements—read labels to ensure that the total daily intake is not greater than 25,000 IU per day.

  - <u>Infants and Children</u>: Different studies have used either daily or monthly schedules of vitamin A supplementation. In a study with extremely low-birth weight infants, 5,000 IU of vitamin A per day for 28 days was safely used.[180] In another study conducted in sick children, those aged less than 12 months received 100,000 IU on two consecutive days, while children between ages 12-60 months received a larger dose of 200,000 IU on two consecutive days.[181]

---

[178] Hollán S, Johansen KS. Adequate iron stores and the 'Nil nocere' principle. *Haematologia* (Budap). 1993;25(2):69-84

[179] "The smallest continuous daily consumption leading to cirrhosis was 25,000 IU during 6 years, whereas higher daily doses (greater than or equal to 100,000 IU) taken during 2 1/2 years resulted in similar histological lesions. ... The data also indicate that prolonged and continuous consumption of doses in the low "therapeutic" range can result in life-threatening liver damage." Geubel AP, De Galocsy C, Alves N, Rahier J, Dive C. Liver damage caused by therapeutic vitamin A administration: estimate of dose-related toxicity in 41 cases. *Gastroenterology*. 1991 Jun;100(6):1701-9

[180] "Infants with birth weight < 1000 g were randomised at birth to receive oral vitamin A supplementation (5000 IU/day) or placebo for 28 days." Wardle SP, Hughes A, Chen S, Shaw NJ. Randomised controlled trial of oral vitamin A supplementation in preterm infants to prevent chronic lung disease. *Arch Dis Child Fetal Neonatal Ed*. 2001 Jan;84(1):F9-F13 Available on-line at http://adc.bmjjournals.com/cgi/content/full/fetalneonatal%3b84/1/F9

[181] "Children were assigned to oral doses of 200 000 IU vitamin A (half that dose if <12 months) or placebo on the day of admission, a second dose on the following day, and third and fourth doses at 4 and 8 months after discharge from the hospital, respectively." Villamor E, Mbise R, Spiegelman D, Hertzmark E, Fataki M, Peterson KE, Ndossi G, Fawzi WW. Vitamin A supplements ameliorate the adverse effect of HIV-1, malaria, and diarrheal infections on child growth. *Pediatrics*. 2002 Jan;109(1):E6

- <u>Preexisting kidney problems (such as renal insufficiency) increase the risks associated with nutritional supplementation</u>: Supplementation with vitamins and minerals does not cause kidney damage. However, if a patient already has kidney problems, then nutritional supplementation may become hazardous; this is particularly true with magnesium and potassium and perhaps also with vitamin C. Assessment of renal function with serum or urine tests is encouraged before beginning an aggressive plan of supplementation. Conditions which cause kidney damage include:
  - Use of specific medications—acetaminophen, aspirin, contrast and chemotherapy agents
  - Hypertension, high blood pressure
  - Diabetes mellitus
  - Use of recreational drugs, such as cocaine
  - Other diseases, such as lupus (SLE) and polycentric kidney disease
- <u>Pre-existing medical conditions may make supplementation unsafe</u>: A few rare medical conditions may cause nutritional supplementation to be unsafe, including severe liver disease, renal failure, electrolyte imbalances, hyperparathyroidism and other vitamin D hypersensitivity syndromes.
- <u>Several drugs/medications may adversely interact with vitamin/mineral supplements and with botanical medicines</u>: Vitamins/minerals may reduce the effectiveness of some prescription medications. For example, taking certain antibiotics such as ciprofloxacin or tetracycline with calcium reduces absorption of the drugs, therefore rendering the drugs much less effective. Taking botanical medicines with medications may make the drugs dangerously less effective (such as when St. John's Wort is combined with protease inhibitor drugs[182]) or may make the drug dangerously more effective (such when Kava is combined with the anti-anxiety drug alprazolam[183]). If vitamin D is used in doses greater than 1,000 IU/d in patients taking hydrochlorothiazide or other calcium-retaining drugs, serum calcium should be monitored at least monthly until safety (i.e., lack of hypercalcemia) has been established per patient.[184] Patients should not combine nutritional or botanical medicines with chemical/synthetic drugs without specific advice from a knowledgeable doctor. Do not increase vitamin K consumption from supplements or dietary improvements in patients taking coumadin/warfarin. A reasonable recommendation is that nutritional supplements be taken 2 hours away from pharmaceutical medications to avoid complications such as intraintestinal drug-nutrient binding.

---

[182] Piscitelli SC, Burstein AH, Chaitt D, Alfaro RM, Falloon J. Indinavir concentrations and St John's wort. *Lancet*. 2000 Feb 12;355(9203):547-8
[183] Almeida JC, Grimsley EW. Coma from the health food store: interaction between kava and alprazolam. *Ann Intern Med*. 1996 Dec 1;125(11):940-1
[184] **Vasquez A**, Manso G, Cannell J. The clinical importance of vitamin D (cholecalciferol): a paradigm shift with implications for all healthcare providers. *Altern Ther Health Med*. 2004 Sep-Oct;10(5):28-36 http://optimalhealthresearch.com/monograph04

Advanced concepts in nutrition—an introduction

Biochemical Individuality and Orthomolecular Medicine: "Biochemical individuality" was the term coined by biochemist Dr. Roger Williams of the University of Texas[185] to describe the genetic and physiologic variations in human beings that produced different nutritional needs among individuals. Because we all have different genes, each of our bodies therefore creates different protein enzymes, and many of these enzymes—which are essential for proper cellular function—are adversely affected by defects in their construction (i.e., amino acid sequence) that reduce their efficiency. Dr. Linus Pauling[186] noted that single amino acid substitutions could produce dramatic alterations in protein function. Pauling discovered that sickle cell disease was caused by a single amino acid substitution in the hemoglobin molecule, and for this discovery he won the Nobel Prize in Chemistry in 1954.[187] With recognition of the importance of individual molecules in determining health or disease, Pauling coined the phrase "orthomolecular medicine" based on his thesis that many diseases could be effectively prevented and treated if we used the "right molecules" to correct abnormal physiologic function. Pauling contrasted the clinical use of nutrients for the improvement of physiologic function (orthomolecular medicine) with the use of chemical drugs, which generally work by interfering with normal physiology (toximolecular medicine). Since nutrients are the fundamental elements of the human body from which all enzymes, chemicals, and cellular structures are formed, Pauling advocated that the use of customized nutrition and nutritional supplements could promote optimal health by optimizing cellular function and efficiency. More recently, Dr. Bruce Ames has thoroughly documented the science of the orthomolecular precepts[188] and has advocated optimal diets along with nutritional supplementation as a highly efficient and cost-effective method for

---

Orthomolecular precepts

- The functions of the body are dependent upon thousands of enzymes. Because of genetic defects that are common in the general population, some of these enzymes are commonly defective – even if only slightly – in large portions of the human population.
- Enzyme defects reduce the function and efficiency of important chemical reactions. Because enzymes are so important for normal function and the prevention of disease, defects in enzyme function can result in disruptions in physiology and the creation of what later manifests as "disease."
- Rather than treating these diseases with synthetic chemical drugs, it is commonly possible to prevent and treat disease with high-doses of vitamins, minerals, and other nutrients to compensate for or bypass metabolic dysfunctions, thus allowing for the promotion of optimal health by promoting optimal physiologic function.

Recent independent review: Ames BN, Elson-Schwab I, Silver EA. High-dose vitamin therapy stimulates variant enzymes with decreased coenzyme binding affinity (increased K(m)): relevance to genetic disease and polymorphisms. _Am J Clin Nutr_. 2002 Apr;75(4):616-58

---

[185] "Every individual organism that has a distinctive genetic background has distinctive nutritional needs which must be met for optimal well-being. …[N]utrition applied with due concern for individual genetic variations…offers the solution to many baffling health problems." Williams RJ. Biochemical Individuality : The Basis for the Genetotrophic Concept. Austin and London: University of Texas Press, 1956. Page x

[186] "…the concentration of coenzyme [vitamins and minerals] needed to produce the amount of active enzyme required for optimum health may well be somewhat different for different individuals. …many individuals may require a considerably higher concentration of one or more coenzymes than other people do for optimum health…" Pauling L. On the Orthomolecular Environment of the Mind: Orthomolecular Theory. In: Williams RJ, Kalita DK. A Physician's Handbook on Orthomolecular Medicine. New Cannan; Keats Publishing: 1977. Page 76

[187] http://www.nobel.se/chemistry/laureates/1954/pauling-bio.html on April 4, 2004

[188] "About 50 human genetic dis-eases due to defective enzymes can be remedied or ameliorated by the administration of high doses of the vitamin component of the corresponding coenzyme, which at least partially restores enzymatic activity." Ames BN, Elson-Schwab I, Silver EA. High-dose vitamin therapy stimulates variant enzymes with decreased coenzyme binding affinity (increased K(m)): relevance to genetic disease and polymorphisms. _Am J Clin Nutr_. 2002 Apr;75(4):616-58

preventing disease and optimizing health.[189,190] In sum, we see that 1) the foundational diet must be formed from whole foods such as fruits, nuts, seeds, vegetables, and lean meats, 2) processed and artificial foods should be avoided, and 3) the use of nutritional supplements is necessary to provide sufficiently high levels of nutrition to overcome defects in enzymatic activity.

Molecular rationale for high-dose nutrient supplementation
"As many as **one-third of mutations** in a gene result in the corresponding enzyme having an increased Michaelis constant, or Km, (decreased binding affinity) for a coenzyme, resulting in a lower rate of reaction. **About 50 human genetic dis-eases due to defective enzymes can be remedied or ameliorated by the administration of high doses of the vitamin component of the corresponding coenzyme**, which at least partially restores enzymatic activity." "**High doses of vitamins are used to treat many inheritable human diseases**. The molecular basis of disease arising from as many as one-third of the mutations in a gene is an increased Michaelis constant, or Km, (decreased binding affinity) of an enzyme for the vitamin-derived coenzyme or substrate, which in turn lowers the rate of the reaction." Ames BN, Elson-Schwab I, Silver EA. High-dose vitamin therapy stimulates variant enzymes with decreased coenzyme binding affinity (increased K(m)): relevance to genetic disease and polymorphisms. *Am J Clin Nutr*. 2002 Apr;75(4):616-58 http://www.ajcn.org/cgi/content/full/75/4/616

Nutrigenomics—Nutritional Genomics: "Genome" refers to all of the genetic material in an organism, and "genomics" is the field of study of this information. The field of nutritional genomics—nutrigenomics—refers to the clinical synthesis of 1) research on the human genome (e.g., the Human Genome Project[191]), and 2) the advancing science of clinical nutrition, including research on nutraceuticals (nutritional medicines) and phytomedicinals (botanical medicines). Nutrigenomics represents a major advance in our understanding of the underlying biochemical and physiologic mechanisms of the effects of nutrition.

Nutrition is far more than "fuel" for our biophysiologic machine; we know now that nutrition—the consumption of specific proteins, amino acids, vitamins, minerals, fatty acids, and phytochemicals—can alter genetic expression and can thus either promote health or disease at the very fundamental level of genetic expression. The commonly employed excuse that many patients use—"I just have bad genes"—now takes on a whole new meaning; it may be that these patients suffer from the expression of "bad genes" *because of the food that they eat.*

The concept and phenomenon of nutrigenomics can be described by saying that each of us has the genes for health, as well as the genes for disease; what largely determines our level of health is how we treat our genes with environmental inputs, especially nutrition. We appear able, to a large extent, to "turn on" disease-promoting genes with poor nutrition and a pro-inflammatory lifestyle[192,193], while, to a lesser extent, we are able to activate or "turn on" health-

---

[189] "An optimum intake of micronutrients and metabolites, which varies with age and genetic constitution, would tune up metabolism and give a marked increase in health, particularly for the poor and elderly, at little cost." Ames BN. The metabolic tune-up: metabolic harmony and disease prevention. *J Nutr*. 2003 May;133(5 Suppl 1):1544S-8S

[190] "Optimizing micronutrient intake [through better diets, fortification of foods, or multivitamin-mineral pills] can have a major impact on public health at low cost." Ames BN. Cancer prevention and diet: help from single nucleotide polymorphisms. *Proc Natl Acad Sci* U S A. 1999 Oct 26;96(22):12216-8

[191] "Begun formally in 1990, the U.S. Human Genome Project is a 13-year effort coordinated by the U.S. Department of Energy and the National Institutes of Health. The project originally was planned to last 15 years, but rapid technological advances have accelerated the expected completion date to 2003. Project goals are to identify all the approximate 30,000 genes in human DNA..." See the official Human Genome website at http://www.ornl.gov/sci/techresources/Human_Genome/home.shtml

[192] Rusyn I, Bradham CA, Cohn L, Schoonhoven R, Swenberg JA, Brenner DA, Thurman RG. Corn oil rapidly activates nuclear factor-kappaB in hepatic Kupffer cells by oxidant-dependent mechanisms. *Carcinogenesis*. 1999 Nov;20(11):2095-100 http://carcin.oxfordjournals.org/cgi/content/full/20/11/2095

promoting genes with a healthy diet[194] and with proper nutritional supplementation.[195] For additional details, see the literature cited in this section and the review article by Vasquez available on-line.[196]

Nutrigenomics—a conceptual diagram: Nutrients influence gene transcription as well as post-translational metabolism.

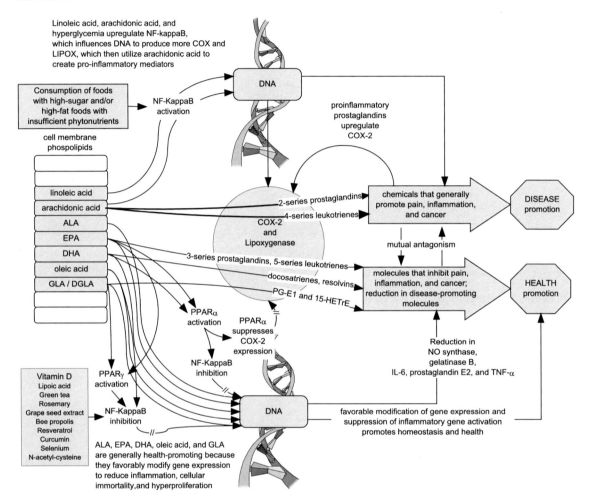

Putting it all together with "the supplemented Paleo-Mediterranean diet": The health-promoting diet of choice for the majority of people is a diet based on abundant consumption of fruits, vegetables, seeds, nuts, omega-3 and monounsaturated fatty acids, and lean sources of protein such as lean meats, fatty cold-water fish, soy and whey proteins. This diet prohibits and obviates overconsumption of chemical preservatives, artificial sweeteners, and carbohydrate-

[193] Aljada A, Mohanty P, Ghanim H, Abdo T, Tripathy D, Chaudhuri A, Dandona P. Increase in intranuclear nuclear factor kappaB and decrease in inhibitor kappaB in mononuclear cells after a mixed meal: evidence for a proinflammatory effect. *Am J Clin Nutr.* 2004 Apr;79(4):682-90
[194] OKeefe JH Jr,Cordain L.Cardiovascular disease resulting from a diet and lifestyle at odds with our Paleolithic genome.*Mayo Clin Proc.*2004;79:101-8
[195] Kaput J, Rodriguez LR. Nutritional genomics: the next frontier in the postgenomic era. *Physiol Genomics* 16: 166–177
http://physiolgenomics.physiology.org/cgi/content/full/16/2/166
[196] **Vasquez A**.Reducing pain and inflammation naturally - Part 4: Nutritional and Botanical Inhibition of NF-kappaB, the Major Intracellular Amplifier of the Inflammatory Cascade.A Clinical Strategy Exemplifying Anti-Inflammatory Nutrigenomics.*Nutr Perspec* 2005;Jul:5-12
http://optimalhealthresearch.com/part4

dominant foods such as candies, pastries, breads, potatoes, grains, and other foods with a high glycemic load and high glycemic index. This "Paleo-Mediterranean Diet" is a combination of the "Paleolithic" or "Paleo diet" and the well-known "Mediterranean diet", both of which are well described in peer-reviewed journals and the lay press. The Mediterranean diet is characterized by increased proportions of legumes, nuts, seeds, whole grain products, fruits, vegetables (including potatoes), fish and lean meats, and monounsaturated and n-3 fatty acids.[197] Consumption of the Mediterranean diet is associated with improvements in insulin sensitivity and reductions in cardiovascular disease, diabetes, cancer, and all-cause mortality when contrasted to the effects of *ad libitum* eating, particularly in the standard American diet (SAD) eating pattern.[198] The Paleolithic diet detailed by collaborators Eaton[199], O'Keefe[200], and Cordain[201] is similar to the Mediterranean diet except for stronger emphasis on fruits and vegetables (preferably raw or minimally cooked), omega-3-rich lean meats, and reduced consumption of starchy foods such as potatoes and grains, the latter of which were not staples in the human diet until the last few thousand years. Emphasizing the olive oil and red wine of the Mediterranean diet and the absence of grains and potatoes per the Paleo diet appears to be the way to get the best of both dietary worlds; the remaining diet is characterized by fresh whole fruits, vegetables, nuts (especially almonds), seeds, berries, olive oil, lean meats rich in n-3 fatty acids, and red wine in moderation. In sum, this dietary plan along with the inclusion of garlic and dark chocolate (a rich source of cardioprotective, antioxidative, antihypertensive, and anti-inflammatory polyphenolic flavonoids[202,203]) is expected to reduce adverse cardiovascular events by more than 76%.[204] Biochemical justification for this type of diet is ample and is well supported by numerous long-term studies in humans wherein both Mediterranean and Paleolithic diets result in statistically significant and clinically meaningful reductions in disease-specific and all-cause mortality.[205,206,207,208] Diets rich in fruits and vegetables are sources of more than 8,000 phytochemicals, many of which have antioxidant, anti-inflammatory, and anti-cancer properties.[209] Oleic acid, squalene, and phenolics in olive oil and phenolics and resveratrol in red wine have antioxidant, anti-inflammatory, and anti-cancer properties and also protect against cardiovascular disease.[210] N-3 fatty acids have numerous health benefits via multiple mechanisms as described in the sections that follow. Increased intake of dietary fiber from fruits and vegetable favorably modifies gut flora, promotes xenobiotic elimination (via flora modification, laxation,

[197] Curtis BM, O'Keefe JH Jr. Understanding the Mediterranean diet. Could this be the new "gold standard" for heart disease prevention? *Postgrad Med*. 2002 Aug;112(2):35-8, 41-5 http://www.postgradmed.com/issues/2002/08_02/curtis.htm

[198] Knoops KT, de Groot LC, Kromhout D, Perrin AE, Moreiras-Varela O, Menotti A, van Staveren WA. Mediterranean diet, lifestyle factors, and 10-year mortality in elderly European men and women: the HALE project. *JAMA*. 2004 Sep 22;292(12):1433-9

[199] Eaton SB, Shostak M, Konner M. The Paleolithic Prescription: A program of diet & exercise and a design for living, New York: Harper & Row, 1988

[200] O'Keefe JH Jr, Cordain L. Cardiovascular disease resulting from a diet and lifestyle at odds with our Paleolithic genome: how to become a 21st-century hunter-gatherer. *Mayo Clin Proc*. 2004 Jan;79(1):101-8

[201] Cordain L. The Paleo Diet: Lose Weight and Get Healthy by Eating the Food You Were Designed to Eat. Indianapolis; John Wiley and Sons, 2002

[202] Schramm DD, Wang JF, Holt RR, Ensunsa JL, Gonsalves JL, Lazarus SA, Schmitz HH, German JB, Keen CL. Chocolate procyanidins decrease the leukotriene-prostacyclin ratio in humans and human aortic endothelial cells. *Am J Clin Nutr*. 2001;73(1):36-40

[203] Engler MB, Engler MM, Chen CY, et al. Flavonoid-rich dark chocolate improves endothelial function and increases plasma epicatechin concentrations in healthy adults. *J Am Coll Nutr*. 2004;23(3):197-204

[204] Franco OH, Bonneux L, de Laet C, Peeters A, Steyerberg EW, Mackenbach JP. The Polymeal: a more natural, safer, and probably tastier (than the Polypill) strategy to reduce cardiovascular disease by more than 75%. *BMJ*. 2004;329(7480):1447-50

[205] de Lorgeril M, Salen P, Martin JL, Monjaud I, Boucher P, Mamelle N. Mediterranean dietary pattern in a randomized trial: prolonged survival and possible reduced cancer rate. *Arch Intern Med*. 1998 Jun 8;158(11):1181-7

[206] Knoops KT, de Groot LC, Kromhout D, Perrin AE, Moreiras-Varela O, Menotti A, van Staveren WA. Mediterranean diet, lifestyle factors, and 10-year mortality in elderly European men and women: the HALE project. *JAMA*. 2004 Sep 22;292(12):1433-9

[207] Lindeberg S, Cordain L, and Eaton SB. Biological and clinical potential of a Paleolithic diet. *J Nutri Environ Med* 2003; 13:149-160

[208] O'Keefe JH Jr, Cordain L, Harris WH, Moe RM, Vogel R. Optimal low-density lipoprotein is 50 to 70 mg/dl: lower is better and physiologically normal. *J Am Coll Cardiol*. 2004 Jun 2;43(11):2142-6

[209] Liu RH. Health benefits of fruit and vegetables are from additive and synergistic combinations of phytochemicals. *Am J Clin Nutr*. 2003;78(3 Sup):517S-520S

[210] Alarcon de la Lastra C, Barranco MD, Motilva V, Herrerias JM. Mediterranean diet and health: biological importance of olive oil. *Curr Pharm Des*. 2001;7:933-50

and overall reductions in enterohepatic recirculation), and is associated with reductions in morbidity and mortality. Such a "Paleolithic diet" can also lead to urinary alkalinization (average urine pH of ≥ 7.5 according to Sebastian et al[211]) which increases renal *retention of minerals* for improved musculoskeletal health[212,213,214] and which increases *urinary elimination of many toxicants and xenobiotics* for a tremendous reduction in serum levels and thus adverse effects from chemical exposure or drug overdose.[215] Furthermore, therapeutic alkalinization was recently shown in an open trial with 82 patients to reduce symptoms and disability associated with low-back pain and to increase intracellular magnesium concentrations by 11%.[216] **Ample intake of amino acids via dietary proteins supports phase-2 detoxification** (amino acid and sulfate conjugation) for proper xenobiotic elimination[217,218], **provides amino acid precursors for neurotransmitter synthesis** and maintenance of mood, memory, and cognitive performance[219,220,221,222], **and prevents the immunosuppression and decrements in musculoskeletal status caused by low-protein diets.**[223] Described originally by the current author[224], the "supplemented Paleo-Mediterranean diet" provides patients the best of current knowledge in nutrition by relying on a foundational diet plan of fresh fruits, vegetables, nuts, seeds, berries, fish, and lean meats which is adorned with olive oil for its squalene, phenolic antioxidant/anti-inflammatory and monounsaturated fatty acid content. Inclusive of medical foods such as red wine, garlic, and dark chocolate which may synergize to effect at least a 76% reduction in cardiovascular disease[225], this diet also reduces the risk for cancer[226] and can be an integral component of a health-promoting lifestyle.[227] Competitive athletes are allowed increased carbohydrate consumption before and after training and competition to promote glycogen storage supercompensation.[228,229,230]

---

[211] Sebastian A, Frassetto LA, Sellmeyer DE, Merriam RL, Morris RC Jr. Estimation of the net acid load of the diet of ancestral preagricultural Homo sapiens and their hominid ancestors. *Am J Clin Nutr* 2002;76:1308-16

[212] Sebastian A, Harris ST, Ottaway JH, Todd KM, Morris RC Jr. Improved mineral balance and skeletal metabolism in postmenopausal women treated with potassium bicarbonate. *N Engl J Med*. 1994;330(25):1776-81

[213] Tucker KL, Hannan MT, Chen H, Cupples LA, Wilson PW, Kiel DP. Potassium, magnesium, and fruit and vegetable intakes are associated with greater bone mineral density in elderly men and women. *Am J Clin Nutr*. 1999;69(4):727-36

[214] Whiting SJ, Boyle JL, Thompson A, Mirwald RL, Faulkner RA. Dietary protein, phosphorus and potassium are beneficial to bone mineral density in adult men consuming adequate dietary calcium. *J Am Coll Nutr*. 2002;21(5):402-9

[215] Proudfoot AT, Krenzelok EP, Vale JA. Position Paper on urine alkalinization. *J Toxicol Clin Toxicol*. 2004;42(1):1-26

[216] "The results show that a disturbed acid-base balance may contribute to the symptoms of low back pain. The simple and safe addition of an alkaline multimineral preparate was able to reduce the pain symptoms in these patients with chronic low back pain." Vormann J,Worlitschek M,Goedecke T,Silver B. Supplementation with alkaline minerals reduces symptoms in patients with chronic low back pain. J Trace Elem Med Biol. 2001;15:179-83

[217] Liska DJ. The detoxification enzyme systems. *Altern Med Rev*. 1998;3:187-9

[218] Anderson KE, Kappas A. Dietary regulation of cytochrome P450. *Annu Rev Nutr*. 1991;11:141-67

[219] Rogers RD, Tunbridge EM, Bhagwagar Z, Drevets WC, Sahakian BJ, Carter CS. Tryptophan depletion alters the decision-making of healthy volunteers through altered processing of reward cues. *Neuropsychopharmacology*. 2003;28:153-62 Accessed at http://www.acnp.org/sciweb/journal/Npp062402336/default.htm on November 10, 2004

[220] Arnulf I, Quintin P, Alvarez JC, Vigil L, Touitou Y, Lebre AS, Bellenger A, Varoquaux O, Derenne JP, Allilaire JF, Benkelfat C, Leboyer M. Mid-morning tryptophan depletion delays REM sleep onset in healthy subjects. *Neuropsychopharmacology*. 2002;27(5):843-51 http://www.nature.com/npp/journal/v27/n5/pdf/1395948a.pdf

[221] Thomas JR,Lockwood PA,Singh A, Deuster PA.Tyrosine improves working memory in a multitasking environment.*Pharmacol Biochem Behav*.1999;64:495-500

[222] Markus CR, Olivier B, Panhuysen GE, Van Der Gugten J, Alles MS, Tuiten A, Westenberg HG, Fekkes D, Koppeschaar HF, de Haan EE. The bovine protein alpha-lactalbumin increases the plasma ratio of tryptophan to the other large neutral amino acids, and in vulnerable subjects raises brain serotonin activity, reduces cortisol concentration, and improves mood under stress. *Am J Clin Nutr*. 2000;71:1536-44

[223] Castaneda C, Charnley JM, Evans WJ, Crim MC. Elderly women accommodate to a low-protein diet with losses of body cell mass, muscle function, and immune response. *Am J Clin Nutr*. 1995;62:30-9

[224] **Vasquez A**. Five-Part Nutritional Protocol that Produces Consistently Positive Results. *Nutritional Wellness* 2005 Sept. http://optimalhealthresearch.com/protocol

[225] Franco OH, Bonneux L, de Laet C, Peeters A, Steyerberg EW, Mackenbach JP. The Polymeal: a more natural, safer, and probably tastier (than the Polypill) strategy to reduce cardiovascular disease by more than 75%. *BMJ*. 2004;329(7480):1447-50

[226] "The combination of 4 low risk factors lowered the all-cause mortality rate to 0.35 (95% CI, 0.28-0.44). In total, lack of adherence to this low-risk pattern was associated with a population attributable risk of 60% of all deaths, 64% of deaths from coronary heart disease, 61% from cardiovascular diseases, and 60% from cancer." Knoops KT, de Groot LC, Kromhout D, et al. Mediterranean diet, lifestyle factors, and 10-year mortality in elderly European men and women: the HALE project. *JAMA*. 2004 Sep 22;292(12):1433-9

[227] Orme-Johnson DW, Herron RE. An innovative approach to reducing medical care utilization and expenditures. *Am J Manag Care*. 1997;3(1):135-44

[228] Cordain L, Friel J. The Paleo Diet for Athletes : A Nutritional Formula for Peak Athletic Performance: Rodale Books (September 23, 2005)

[229] "A significant glycogen sparing, as well as supercompensation within 24 h of recovery, was observed after [carbohydrate] supplementation." Brouns F, Saris WH, Beckers E, Adlercreutz H, van der Vusse GJ, Keizer HA, Kuipers H, Menheere P, Wagenmakers AJ, ten Hoor F. Metabolic changes induced by sustained exhaustive cycling and diet manipulation. *Int J Sports Med*. 1989 May;10 Suppl 1:S49-62

[230] "The accepted method of increasing muscle glycogen stores is by "glycogen loading," which classically involves depletion of muscle glycogen, usually by exercise, followed by consumption of a high-CHO diet for several days (e.g., 3, 39). …increase muscle glycogen concentrations ([glycogen]) to between 150 and 200% of normal resting levels." Robinson TM, Sewell DA, Hultman E, Greenhaff PL. Role of submaximal exercise in promoting creatine and glycogen accumulation in human skeletal muscle. *J Appl Physiol*. 1999 Aug;87(2):598-604

Profile of the Supplemented Paleo-Mediterranean Diet[231]

Foods to consume: whole, natural, minimally processed foods include:	Foods to avoid: factory products, high-sugar foods, and chemicals
☺ **Lean sources of protein** • Fish (avoiding tuna which is commonly loaded with mercury) • Chicken and turkey • Lean cuts of free-range grass-fed meats: beef, buffalo, lamb are occasionally acceptable • Soy protein[232] and whey protein[233,234] ☺ **Fruits and fruit juices** ☺ **Vegetables and vegetable juices** ☺ **Nuts, seeds, berries** ☺ **Generous use of olive oil**: On sautéed vegetables and fresh salads ☺ **Daily vitamin/mineral supplementation**: With a high-potency broad-spectrum multivitamin and multimineral supplement[235] ☺ **Sun exposure or vitamin D3 supplementation**: To ensure provision of 2,000-5,000 IU of vitamin D3 per day for adults[236] ☺ **Balanced broad-spectrum fatty acid supplementation**: With ALA, GLA, EPA, and DHA[237] ☺ **Water, tea, home-made fruit/vegetable juices**: Commercial vegetable juices are commonly loaded with sodium chloride; choose appropriately. Fruit juices can be loaded with natural and superfluous sugars. Herbal teas can be selected based on the medicinal properties of the plant that is used.	☒ **Avoid as much as possible fat-laden arachidonate-rich meats like beef, liver, pork, and lamb, as well as high-fat cream and other dairy products with emulsified, readily absorbed saturated fats and arachidonic acid** ☒ **High-sugar pseudofoods**: • Corn syrup • Cola and soda • Donuts, candy, etc…."junk food" ☒ **Grains such as wheat, rye, barley**: These have only existed in the human diet for less than 10,000 years and are consistently associated with increased prevalence of degenerative diseases due to the allergic response they invoke and because of their high glycemic load and high glycemic index. ☒ **Potatoes and rice**: High in sugar, low in phytonutrients ☒ **Avoid allergens**: Determined per individual ☒ **Chemicals to avoid**: • Pesticides, Herbicides, Fungicides • Carcinogenic sweeteners: aspartame[238] • Artificial flavors • Artificial colors: tartrazine • Preservatives: benzoate • Flavor enhancers: carrageenan and monosodium glutamate

[231] **Vasquez A**. Five-Part Nutritional Protocol that Produces Consistently Positive Results. *Nutritional Wellness* 2005 Sept. and Vasquez A. Revisiting the Five-Part Nutritional Wellness Protocol: The Supplemented Paleo-Mediterranean Diet. *Nutritional Perspectives* 2011 January. Both of these articles are included in this textbook and/or on-line at http://optimalhealthresearch.com/spmd

[232] "These results indicate that for healthy adults, the isolated soy protein is of high nutritional quality, comparable to that of animal protein sources, and that the methionine content is not limiting for adult protein maintenance." Young VR, Puig M, Queiroz E, Scrimshaw NS, Rand WM. Evaluation of the protein quality of an isolated soy protein in young men: relative nitrogen requirements and effect of methionine supplementation. *Am J Clin Nutr*. 1984 Jan;39(1):16-24

[233] Bounous G. Whey protein concentrate (WPC) and glutathione modulation in cancer treatment. *Anticancer Res*. 2000 Nov-Dec;20(6C):4785-92

[234] Markus CR, Olivier B, Panhuysen GE, Van Der Gugten J, Alles MS, Tuiten A, Westenberg HG, Fekkes D, Koppeschaar HF, de Haan EE. The bovine protein alpha-lactalbumin increases the plasma ratio of tryptophan to the other large neutral amino acids, and in vulnerable subjects raises brain serotonin activity, reduces cortisol concentration, and improves mood under stress. *Am J Clin Nutr*. 2000 Jun;71(6):1536-44 http://www.ajcn.org/cgi/content/full/71/6/1536

[235] "Most people do not consume an optimal amount of all vitamins by diet alone. …it appears prudent for all adults to take vitamin supplements." Fletcher RH, Fairfield KM. Vitamins for chronic disease prevention in adults: clinical applications. *JAMA*. 2002;287:3127-9

[236] Vasquez A, MansoG,CannellJ.The clinical importance of vitamin D (cholecalciferol).*Altern Ther Health Med*.2004Sep10:28-36 www.optimalhealthresearch.com

[237] **Vasquez A**. New Insights into Fatty Acid Supplementation and Its Effect on Eicosanoid Production and Genetic Expression. *Nutr Perspectives* 2005; Jan: 5-16

[238] "In the past two decades brain tumor rates have risen in several industrialized countries, including the United States... Compared to other environmental factors putatively linked to brain tumors, the artificial sweetener aspartame is a promising candidate to explain the recent increase in incidence and degree of malignancy of brain tumors." Olney JW, Farber NB, Spitznagel E, Robins LN. Increasing brain tumor rates: is there a link to aspartame? *J Neuropathol Exp Neurol* 1996 Nov;55(11):1115-23

Emotional, Mental, and Social Health

__Stress management and authentic living__: Mental, emotional, and physical "stress" describes any unpleasant living condition which can lead to negative effects on health, such as increased blood pressure, depression, apathy, increased muscle tension, and, according to some research, increased risk of serious health problems such as early death from cardiovascular disease and cancer. Many people find that their modern lives are characterized by excess amounts of multitasking, job responsibilities, family responsibilities, commuter traffic, financial pressures in combination with an insufficient amount of relaxation, sleep, community support, exercise, time in nature, healthy nutrition, and time to simply _be_ rather than _do_. Stress comes in many different forms and includes malnutrition, trauma, insufficient exercise (epidemic), excess exercise (rare), sleep deprivation, emotional turmoil, and exposure to chemicals and radiation. When most people talk about "stress" they are referring to either chronic anxiety (such as with high-pressure work situations or dysfunctional interpersonal relationships) or the acute stress reaction that is typical of unpredictable rapid-onset events such as an injury, accident, or other physically threatening situation. **These "different types of stress" are not separate from each other; rather, they are interconnected:**

- Emotional stress causes nutritional depletion[239],
- Sleep deprivation alters immune response[240],
- Chemical exposure can disrupt endocrine function.[241]

Therefore, **any type of stress can cause other types of stress**. Avoiding stressful situations is, of course, an effective way to avoid being bothered or harmed by them. If work-related stress is the problem, then finding a new position or occupation is certainly an option worth considering and implementing. High-stress jobs are often high-paying jobs; but if in the process of making money, a person ruins her health and loses years from her life, then no one would ever say, "It was worth it." **Money, success, and freedom only have value for the person alive and healthy to enjoy them.**

Toxic relationships, whether at home or work, are relationships that cause more harm than good by re-injuring old emotional wounds and by creating new emotional injuries. We can all benefit from affirming our right to a happy and healthy life by minimizing/eliminating contact with people who cause emotional harm to us—this requires conscious effort.[242] Engel[243] provides a clear articulation and description of abusive relationships, along with checklists for their recognition and exercises for their remediation. Healthy relationships are difficult to create and maintain these days, and probably a few basic components contribute to this phenomenon. ❶ With the society-wide disintegration of the extended family, most people in our society have never even seen a healthy family unit and therefore have no model and no available mentors to help them recreate a lasting family structure. ❷ Due specifically to the structure of our educational systems and (pseudo)culture of entertainment, most people have very short attention spans and are accustomed to inattention, distraction, and externally derived entertainment and gratification. ❸ Modern schools and fragmented families both fail to teach conflict resolution and relationship skills. ❹ Poor nutritional status—very common in the general population—promotes impulsivity, irritability, depression, and mood instability.

> "Good relationships make you feel loved, wanted, and cared for."
>
> Malcolm LL. Health Style. London; Thorsons: 2001, p 133

---

[239] Ingenbleek Y, Bernstein L. The stressful condition as a nutritionally dependent adaptive dichotomy. _Nutrition_ 1999 Apr;15(4):305-20

[240] Heiser P, Dickhaus B, Opper C, Hemmeter U, Remschmidt H, Wesemann W, Krieg JC, Schreiber W. Alterations of host defense system after sleep deprivation are followed by impaired mood and psychosocial functioning. _World J Biol Psychiatry_ 2001 Apr;2(2):89-94

[241] "Evidence suggests that environmental exposure to some anthropogenic chemicals may result in disruption of endocrine systems in human and wildlife populations." http://www.epa.gov/endocrine on March 7, 2004

[242] Bryn C. Collins. _How to Recognize Emotional Unavailability and Make Healthier Relationship Choices_. [Mjf Books; ISBN: 1567313442] Recently reprinted as: Emotional Unavailability: Recognizing It, Understanding It, and Avoiding Its Trap [McGraw Hill - NTC (April 1998); ISBN: 0809229145]

[243] Engel B. _The Emotionally Abusive Relationship: How to Stop Being Abused and How to Stop Abusing_. Wiley Publishers: 2003

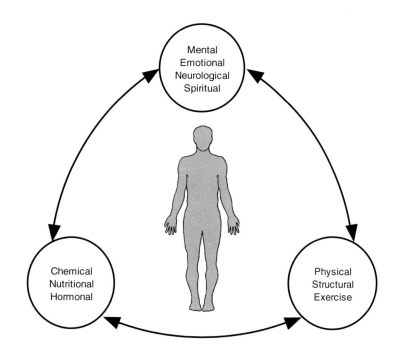

Stress affects the whole body.

Therefore, a complete stress management program must address the whole body:

Physical Structural

Biochemical Hormonal Nutritional

Mental Emotional Spiritual

An important concept is that **stress is a "whole body" phenomenon**: affecting the mind, the brain, emotional state, the physical body (including musculoskeletal, immune, and cardiovascular systems), as well as the nutritional status of the individual. The adverse effects of stress can be reduced with an integrated combination of therapeutics that addresses each of the major body systems affected by stress, which are 1) mental/emotional, 2) physical, and 3) nutritional/biochemical.

Approaching stress management from a tripartite perspective

	Mental/emotional	**Physical**	**Nutritional/biochemical**
Therapeutic considerations	• Social support • Re-parenting • Conversational style[244] • Meditation, prayer • Healthy boundaries • Books, tapes, groups • Expressive writing[245] • Time to simply rest and relax	• Yoga • Massage • Exercise • Stretching • Swimming • Resting • Biking • Hiking • Affection	• Vitamins, including vitamin C[246] • Fish oil[247] • Hormones, cytokines, neurotransmitters, and eicosanoids • Tryptophan, pyridoxine • Botanical medicines such as *kava*[248], *Ashwaganda,* and *Eleurherococcus*

[244] Rick Brinkman ND and Rick Kirschner ND. *How to Deal With Difficult People* [Audio Cassette. Career Track, 1995]

[245] Smyth JM, Stone AA, Hurewitz A, Kaell A. Effects of writing about stressful experiences on symptom reduction in patients with asthma or rheumatoid arthritis: a randomized trial. *JAMA*. 1999 Apr 14;281(14):1304-9

[246] Brody S, Preut R, Schommer K, Schurmeyer TH. A randomized controlled trial of high dose ascorbic acid for reduction of blood pressure, cortisol, and subjective responses to psychological stress. *Psychopharmacology* (Berl). 2002 Jan;159(3):319-24

[247] Hamazaki T, Itomura M, Sawazaki S, Nagao Y. Anti-stress effects of DHA. *Biofactors*. 2000;13(1-4):41-5

[248] Cagnacci A, et al. Kava-Kava administration reduces anxiety in perimenopausal women. *Maturitas*. 2003 Feb 25;44(2):103-9

Sometimes a stressful situation can be modified into one that is less stressful or dysfunctional, so that the benefits are retained, yet the negative aspects are reduced. Of course, the best example of this is interpersonal relationships, which easily lend themselves to improvement with the application of conscious effort. Many audiotapes, books, and seminars are available for people interested in having improved interpersonal relationships. Selected resources are listed here:

- Men and Women: Talking Together by Deborah Tannen and Robert Bly [Sound Horizons, 1992. ISBN: 1879323095] A lively discussion of the different communication and relationship styles of men and women by two respected experts in their fields.
- How to Deal with Difficult People by Drs. Rick Brinkman and Rick Kirschner. [Audio Cassette. Career Track, 1995] An entertaining format with solutions to common workplace and situational difficulties. Authored and performed by two naturopathic physicians.
- Men are From Mars, Women are From Venus by John Gray. [Audio Cassette and Books]. Phenomenally popular concepts in understanding, accepting, and effectively integrating the differences between men and women.
- The ManKind Project (www.mkp.org). An international organization hosting events for men and women. The men's events, formats, and groups are authentic, clear, and healthy. The ManKind Project has an organization for women called The WomanWithin (www.womanwithin.org). No book or tape can substitute for the dynamics and personal attention that can be experienced by a conscious, empowered, and well-intended group.

When "the problem" cannot be avoided, and the interaction/relationship with the problem cannot be improved, a remaining option is to supplement the internal environment so that it is somewhat "strengthened" to deal with the stress of the bothersome event or situation. For example, when dealing with emotional stress, we can use counseling, support groups, or various relaxation techniques.[249] If we determine that the emotional stress has a biochemical component, then we can use specific botanical and nutritional supplementation to safely and naturally support and restore normal function. Moving deeper into the issue of "stress management" requires that we ask why a person is in a stressful situation to begin with. Of course, with *random acts of chaos* like car accidents, we cannot always ascribe the problem to the person, unless the accident resulted from their own negligence. But **when people are chronically stressed and unhappy about their jobs and/or relationships, then we need to employ more than stress reduction techniques**, and as clinicians we need to offer more than the latest adaptogen. **We have to ask why a person would subject himself/herself to such a situation, and what fears or limitations (self-imposed and/or externally applied) keep him/her from breaking free into a life that works.**[250,251,252,253,254,255]

[249] Martha Davis PhD, Matthew McKay MSW, Elizabeth Robbins Eshelman PhD. The Relaxation & Stress Reduction Workbook 5th edition. New Harbinger Publishers; 2000. [ISBN: 1572242140]
[250] Rick Jarow. Creating the Work You Love: Courage, Commitment and Career; Inner Traditions Intl Ltd; 1995 [ISBN: 0892815426]
[251] Breton D, Largent C. The Paradigm Conspiracy: Why Our Social Systems Violate Human Potential-And How We Can Change Them. Hazelden: 1998
[252] Dominguez JR. Transforming Your Relationship With Money. Sounds True; Book and Cassette edition: 2001 Audio tape.
[253] Miller A. The truth will set you free: overcoming emotional blindness and finding your true adult self. New York: Basic Books; 2001
[254] Bradshaw J. Healing the Shame that Binds You [Audio Cassette (April 1990) Health Communications Audio; ISBN: 1558740430]
[255] Miller A. The Drama of the Gifted Child: The Search for the True Self. Basic Books: 1981

Stress always has a biochemical/physiologic component: Regardless of its origins, stress always takes a toll on the body—*the whole body*. Well-documented effects of stress include:

1. Increased levels of cortisol—higher levels are associated with osteoporosis, memory loss, slow healing, and insulin resistance.
2. Reduced function of thyroid hormones[256] (i.e., induction of peripheral/metabolic hypothyroidism)
3. Reduced levels of testosterone (in men)
4. Increased intestinal permeability and "leaky gut"[257]
5. Increased excretion of minerals in the urine
6. Increased need for vitamins, minerals, and amino acids
7. Suppression of immune function and of natural killer cells that fight viral infections and tumors
8. Decreased production of sIgA—the main defense of the lungs, gastrointestinal tract, and genitourinary tract
9. Increased populations of harmful bacteria in the intestines and an associated increased rate of lung and upper respiratory tract infections
10. Increased incidence of food allergies[258]
11. Sleep disturbance

The body functions as a whole—not as independent, autonomous organ systems: Problems with one aspect of health create problems in other aspects of health. Treatment of disease and promotion of wellness must therefore improve overall health and functioning while simultaneously addressing the disease or presenting complaint.

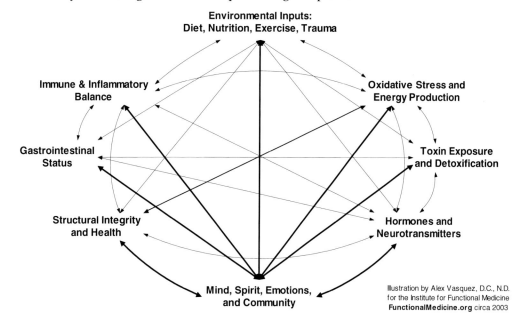

Illustration by Alex Vasquez, D.C., N.D. for the Institute for Functional Medicine **FunctionalMedicine.org** circa 2003

---

[256] Ingenbleek Y, Bernstein L. The stressful condition as a nutritionally dependent adaptive dichotomy. *Nutrition* 1999 Apr;15(4):305-20
[257] Hart A, Kamm MA. Review article: mechanisms of initiation and perpetuation of gut inflammation by stress. *Aliment Pharmacol Ther* 2002;16(12):2017-28
[258] Anderzen I, Arnetz BB, Soderstrom T, Soderman E. Stress and sensitization in children: a controlled prospective psychophysiological study of children exposed to international relocation. *Journal of Psychosomatic Research* 1997; 43: 259-69

Autonomization, intradependence, emotional literacy, corrective experience:

> "None of us are completely developed people when we reach adulthood.
> We are each incomplete in our own way." *Merle Fossum*[259]

Consciousness-raising is a keystone gift that holistic physicians can impart to their patients and one which may be necessary for true healing to be manifested and maintained. Healthcare providers are quick to enlighten their patients to the details of diet, exercise, nutrition, medications, surgeries, and other *biomechanical* and *biochemical* aspects of health, but are routinely negligent when it comes to sharing with patients the emotional tools that may be necessary to repair or construct the "self" which is supposed to implement the treatment plan that the doctor has designed. Passivity and ignorance are not hindrances to the success of the *medical paradigm*, which requires that patients are "compliant" rather than self-directed; however, for *authentic, holistic healthcare* to be successful, it must empower the patient sufficiently such that he/she attains/regains appropriate *autonomy*—an "internal locus of control"—sufficient for lifelong internally-driven health maintenance. Health implications of autonomy (or its absence) are obvious and intuitive. Patients with an underdeveloped internal locus of control appear to

experience greater degrees of social stress which can lead to hypercortisolemia and hippocampal atrophy.[260] A developed internal locus of control correlates strongly with the success of weight-loss programs, and for nonautonomous patients it is necessary to encourage the development of autonomous self-care behavior in addition to the provision of information about diet and exercise.[261]

Six fundamental components of self-esteem
1. Living consciously
2. Self-acceptance
3. Self-responsibility
4. Self-assertiveness
5. Living purposefully
6. Personal integrity
Branden N. The Six Pillars of Self-Esteem. Bantam: 1995

Completely formed internal identities are the natural result of the *continuum* of positive childhood experiences (inclusive of stability, "unconditional love", healthy parenting, and active, conscious intergenerational social contact) which are ideally merged into adolescent and adulthood experiences of success, acceptance, inclusion, independence, interdependence, and intradependence with the end result being a socially-conscious adult with an internal locus of control. Where the patient has experienced a relative absence of these natural and expected prerequisites, a truncated—wounded, reactive, shame-based, dissatisfied—self is likely to result. The failure to develop self-esteem and an internal locus of control largely explains why so many adult patients feign that they are incapable of action, "can't exercise", and "can't leave" their abusive jobs and relationships, and "can't resist" the dietary habits which daily contribute to their physical and psychoemotional decline. Thus, for more than a few patients, a therapeutic path must be explored which helps to re-create the foundation from which an autonomous adult and authentic self can grow—it is a *process* (not an event) of **emotional recovery**.[262] To this extent, interventional or therapeutic *autonomization* resembles a *recovery program* that can include various forms of conscious action, including goal-setting, positive reinforcement, developing emotional

---

[259] Fossum M. Catching Fire: Men Coming Alive in Recovery. New York; Harper/Hazelden: 1989, 4-7

[260] "Cumulative exposure to high levels of cortisol over the lifetime is known to be related to hippocampal atrophy... Self-esteem and internal locus of control were significantly correlated with hippocampal volume in both young and elderly subjects." Pruessner JC, Baldwin MW, Dedovic K, Renwick R, Mahani NK, Lord C, Meaney M, Lupien S. Self-esteem, locus of control, hippocampal volume, and cortisol regulation in young and old adulthood. *Neuroimage*. 2005 Dec;28(4):815-26

[261] "Their weight loss was significant and associated with an internal locus of control orientation (P < 0.05)... Participants with an internal orientation could be offered a standard weight reduction programme. Others, with a more external locus of control orientation, could be offered an adapted programme, which also focused on and encouraged the participants' internal orientation." Adolfsson B, Andersson I, Elofsson S, Rossner S, Unden AL. Locus of control and weight reduction. *Patient Educ Couns*. 2005 Jan;56(1):55-61

[262] Bradshaw J. Healing the Shame that Binds You [Audio Cassette (April 1990) Health Communications Audio; ISBN: 1558740430]

literacy[263] and emotional intelligence[264], and consciousness-raising experiences such as therapy and group work—all of which serve to intentionally (re)create and maintain the necessary climate for authentic selfhood. Therewith, the patient can accept challenges to further develop an *empowered self* by participating in exercises in which the ability to decide, choose, and act responsibly and appropriately are reinforced to eventually become second nature, replacing passivity, inaction, and ineffectiveness.[265]

"Empowerment" can only be authentic if it is built on the foundation of a developed self. While *emotional recovery* and *personal empowerment* are separate spheres of activity and attention, they are not mutually exclusive and indeed are synergistic. However, emotional recovery—that process of recounting one's own history, delving into the depths of one's own psyche, and integrating what is found into a cohesive, functional and healthy whole—must occur before the program of personal development emphasizes empowerment. *Empowerment* cannot succeed without *recovery* because otherwise the so-called "empowerment" is likely to add to the defense mechanisms that protect against pain and thereby block the development of an authentic self. Stated concisely by Janov[266], **"Anything that builds a stronger defense system deepens the neurosis."**

> **Primary, secondary, and tertiary means for developing an autonomous, authentic self**: Ideally, positive childhood experiences (A) merge into adolescent and adult experiences of confidence and maturity (B) for the development of a true adult (C). If A or B is lacking or insufficient, the result is an incomplete self often incapable of *effective* and *appropriate* action. Corrective experiences must then be pursued to re-establish the foundation from which an authentic self can arise.

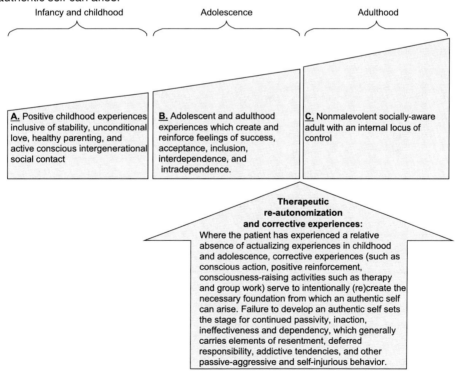

[263] Dayton T. <u>Trauma and Addiction: Ending the Cycle of Pain through Emotional Literacy</u>. Deerfield Beach; Health Communications, 2000
[264] Goleman D. <u>Emotional Intelligence</u>. New York; Bantam Books: 1995. Although the book as a whole was considered pioneering for its time, and the book continues to make a valuable contribution, a few of the concepts and author's personal stories are embarrassingly simplistic.
[265] Gatto JT. <u>A Schooling Is Not An Education: interview by Barbara Dunlop</u>. http://www.johntaylorgatto.com/bookstore/index.htm
[266] Janov A. <u>The Primal Scream</u>. New York; GP Putnam's Sons: 1970, page 20

Patients lacking an internal locus of control are much more likely to succumb to the tantalizing barrage of direct-to-consumer drug advertising[267] which infantilizes patients by 1) oversimplifying diseases, their causes, and treatments, 2) exonerating patients from responsibility and reinforcing the

Integration promotes health

"The object of healing is…to move closer to wholeness."

Kreinheder A. Body and soul: the other side of illness. Toronto, Canada; Inner City Books: 1991, page 38

illusion of victimization and helplessness, and 3) encouraging a dependent, passively receptive role by telling patients that they have no proactive role other than to "ask your doctor if a prescription is right for you." Americans consume more prescription and OTC medications per capita than people in any other country.[268,269] With the combined and synergistic effects of 1) the dissolution of first the extended family and now the nuclear family[270], 2) a society-wide famine of mentors, elders, and community[271,272,273], 3) a dearth of autonomous, genuine exploration from childhood to adulthood, and 4) primary and secondary "educational" institutions designed to squelch independence and autonomy in favor of the more efficient, predictable, and controllable conformity and "standardization"[274,275], **industrialized societies have raised generations of people who lack completely formed internal identities**. Lacking an internal locus of control and identity from which to think independently and critically, these "adults" are easy prey for slick and flashy drug advertisements that promise the illusion of perfect health in exchange for passivity, abdication, and lifelong medicalization. That the typical American watches four hours of television per day[276] is bad enough, what makes this worse is that "Americans who watch average amounts of television may be exposed to more than 30 hours of direct-to-consumer drug advertisements each year, far surpassing their exposure to other forms of health communication."[277] If we are to wean our suckling culture from undue dependence on the pharmaceutical industry, we have to address our patient population directly and transform them from *passive, nonautonomous, and ignorant about health and disease* to pro-active, autonomous, and well-informed about health and the means required to obtain and sustain it.

Insight into a patient's internal dynamic can provide the clinician with an understanding that explains the phenomena of *non-compliance* and *disease identification*. Rather than seeing non-compliance as "weakness of will", non-compliance as a form of "disobedience" may be a reflection of the patient's unconscious need to wrestle with and resolve parental introjects. For example, if a patient had a rejecting, nonaffirming parent, he/she may need to find another rejecting authority figure in order to continue playing the role of the child; by assuming this role and "setting the stage", the patient is unconsciously attempting to create a situation wherein the primary relationship can be healed.[278] Complicating this is *disease identification*—in which patients use their disease as a source of identity and secondary gain for martyrdom, social support, group participation, acceptance, admiration, purpose, excitement, and drama.

[267] Aronson E. The Social Animal. San Fransisco; WH Freeman and company: 1972: 21-22, 53

[268] America the medicated. http://www.cbsnews.com/stories/2005/04/21/health/printable689997.shtml and http://www.msnbc.msn.com/id/7503122/ . See also http://usgovinfo.about.com/od/healthcare/a/usmedicated.htm Accessed September 17, 2005.

[269] Kivel P. You Call This a Democracy? Apex Press (August, 2004). ISBN: 1891843265 http://www.paulkivel.com/

[270] Bly R. Iron John. Reading, Mass.: Addison Wesley, 1990

[271] Bly R. The Sibling Society. Vintage Books USA; Reprint edition (June 1, 1997) ISBN: 0679781285 (Abridged audio edition (May 1, 1996), ASIN: 0679451609)

[272] Bly R. Where have all the parents gone? A talk on the Sibling Society. New York: Sound Horizons, 1996 Highly recommended.

[273] Bly R, Hillman J, Meade M. Men and the Life of Desire. Oral Tradition Archives. ISBN: 1880155001. Audio Cassette

[274] Gatto JT. Dumbing Us Down: the Hidden Curriculum of Compulsory Education. Gabriola Island, Canada; New Society Publishers: 2005

[275] Gatto JT. The Paradox of Extended Childhood. [From a presentation in Cambridge, Mass. October 2000] http://www.johntaylorgatto.com/bookstore/index.htm

[276] "American children view over 23 hours of television per week. Teenagers view an average of 21 to 22 hours of television per week. By the time today's children reach age 70, they will have spent 7 to 10 years of their lives watching television." American Academy of Pediatrics http://www.aapca1.org/aapca1/tv.html See also TV-Turnoff Network. Facts and Figures About our TV Habit http://www.tvturnoff.org/factsheets.htm Accessed September 17, 2005

[277] Brownfield ED, Bernhardt JM, Phan JL, Williams MV, Parker RM. Direct-to-consumer drug advertisements on network television: an exploration of quantity, frequency, and placement. J Health Commun. 2004 Nov-Dec;9(6):491-7

[278] Miller A. The Drama of the Gifted Child: The Search for the True Self. Basic Books: 1981, page 88

Helping patients create and maintain authentic selves

An absent or underdeveloped locus of control is the key problem that underlies many anxiety disorders, addictive behavioral traits such as overeating, overworking, codependency, as well as chronic ineffectiveness in the pursuit of one's goals. The solutions to this problem are logical, practical, and accessible to everyone; the major costs associated with each are open-mindedness, attentiveness, discipline and persistence. There is scant mention of this concept and its intervention in the biomedical literature; however, it is well described in the psychological literature, particularly that which focuses on various types of "recovery" such as that from addiction, co-dependence, and low self-esteem, the latter two of which are virtually synonymous with an insufficient internal locus of control.

There is no single path here. There are many paths. The goal is not to choose the right path; rather the goal is to travel several paths to the degree necessary, implement what has been learned, travel other paths, and return to the same path again to retrace one's steps in new ways. The process is similar to that of *ceremonial initiation*, the purpose of which is to formally mark the *beginning* of a process that is *ongoing* and *infinite*.[279] Each path and each process has its gifts, significance, and limitations. However, the ultimate goal of each must be a tangible and positive change in the ways which the patient feels and/or behaves in and interacts with the world on a day-to-day basis.

In no particular order (since the proper sequence will have to be customized to the situation and willingness of the patient), the following are some of the more commonly cited exercises, processes, and sources of additional information:

Apprenticeship and Mentoring: books, tapes, and lectures: Children and non-autonomous adults are pulled into authentic adulthood by mentors, elders, and true adults. The therapeutic encounters thus provided—whether interpersonal or vicarious in the form of lectures, books, or audiotapes— serve as sources of information from which new possibilities can be gleaned, and these therefore serve as infinitely valuable resources for expanding the narrow horizons that characterize an underdeveloped internal locus of control. In essence, books, tapes, and lectures allow the patient to become a student and to choose a vicarious mentor. *Advantages*: Books and tapes allow access to many of the best minds in psychology; books and tapes are inexpensive; allow patients to explore and benefit from many different perspectives; books and tapes are always available and are therefore amenable to various schedules of work and responsibility. *Disadvantages*: Books and tapes do not re-create the interpersonal bridge which is essential for authentic recovery; do not provide a direct and objective means of accountably, thus potentially allowing patients to delude themselves about the effectiveness (or lack thereof) of their recovery process. Examples of better-known books, tapes and recorded lectures on the *process* of emotional recovery:

- ***The Six Pillars of Self-Esteem*** by Nathaniel Branden PhD. This is a very accessible yet very structured work in which Dr Branden brilliantly elucidates key concepts in psychology relevant to self-efficacy and self-esteem; also available as an audiobook excellently narrated by Dr Branden.
- ***Healing the Shame that Binds You*** by John Bradshaw [Audio Cassette (April 1990) Health Communications Audio; ISBN: 1558740430] Available as book and cassette with identical titles and different content.
- ***A Little Book on the Human Shadow*** by Robert Bly. Certainly among the most concise, accessible, and complete books ever written on the processes involved in losing and recovering the self; also available as an audio presentation.
- ***The Drama of the Gifted Child*** by Alice Miller. This internationally acclaimed book is considered a true classic among therapists and patients alike. Available as book and a brilliantly performed audio cassette.
- ***You Can Heal Your Life*** by Louise Hay. Another standard for recovery; very "new age."
- ***Codependent No More: How to Stop Controlling Others and Start Caring for Yourself*** by Melody Beattie. Pioneering for its time.
- ***The Artist's Date Book*** by Julia Cameron. Each page has a new creative idea for creative expression and "creative recovery."
- ***The Psychology of Self-Esteem*** by Nathaniel Branden PhD. More advanced and perhaps less widely relevant than his "six pillars" work, this is also an excellent encapsulation of important concepts in personal psychology.

---

[279] Hillman J, Meade M, Some M. Images of initiation. Oral Tradition Archives; 1992

Therapy: *"Therapy is a conversation that matters."* Therapy in this context specifically means face-to-face, active interaction, either one-on-one or in a group setting, with the specific intention to give and/or provide support for personal growth. Whether 12-step groups such as Codependents Anonymous qualify as a form of therapy depends entirely upon the level of engagement of the participant; sitting in a room while *other people* do *their* work provides slow or no benefit for the passive observer. **Recovery is an *active* process, which is why it is antithetical to depression, which is a *passive* state of being.** Patients should go in knowing that this is a *process* and to not expect to be "fixed" after the first hour or even the first month. ***Advantages***: Therapists can provide crucial support and insight while the client wrestles with undecipherable and convoluted emotional and psychic data. Therapists can help the client set goals ("stretches" and "homework") by which the client reaches beyond his/her comfort zone to attain the next expansion in being and experience. Therapists must create a safe space or "container" in which ideas and feelings can be brought forth to intermingle and be consciously appreciated. ***Disadvantages***: Requires a flexible and disciplined schedule; costs money; bad therapists can do more harm than good if they misdirect their clients away from volatile and core issues and authentic expression.[280,281,282,283] Therapy can be disempowering if the patient continues to project his/her locus of control onto the therapist.

Some of the more commonly used tools of the psychotherapeutic trade include:
- **Active listening**
- **Insight, explanation of events**: their origins, reasons, and significance
- **Reminders** of previous conclusions and stories
- **Challenge old ideas and habits**: Therapy that generally or completely lacks confrontation and accountability is ineffective.
- **Encourage exploration and new modes of being and interacting**
- **Creating a safe container wherein the client can review the details, significance, and feelings associated with past events**
- **Modeling the expression of feeling**
- **Defining goals and helping the client focus on what is significant**
- **Correcting distortions of reality**
- **Asking patients to get in touch with and then express their feelings**
- **Support and encourage clients to take calculated risks for the sake of self-expansion**
- **Pointing out errors in logic**
- **Coaching patients in the proper and responsible use of emotional language**
- **Discouraging evasiveness; requiring accountability**[284]

Creativity: All types of self-expression reinforce and validate the patient's sense of self. Creative self-expression, such as writing about thoughts and feelings about significant experiences, can reduce symptomatology in patients with rheumatoid arthritis and asthma.[285]

Experiential: Corrective experiences can be obtained in therapy, with friends and family, in integration groups, and during "experiential" retreats. ***Advantages***: Experiential events orchestrated by therapists and various groups such as ManKind Project (mkp.org) and WomanWithin.org can rapidly facilitate personal growth while also providing an ongoing container and support system that encourages self-development rather than the ego-inflation that accompanies short-term events. ***Disadvantages***: "Adventures" like driving across the nation or climbing a mountain are unconscious and largely impotent attempts at self-initiation; authentic initiation has always been supervised by community elders. However, once a well-founded initiation has taken place, preferably with an on-going community that facilitates continued refinement and self-exploration, then "adventures" can be undertaken consciously to maintain and reinforce the experience of autonomy and competent selfhood. Eventually, transformative and sustentative experiences can be integrated and created in the daily life experience so that dramatic adventures become unnecessary for the continued renewal and "recharging" of the self.

[280] Lee J. Expressing Your Anger Appropriately (Audio Cassette). Sounds True (June 1, 1990); ISBN: 1564550338
[281] Bradshaw J. Healing the Shame that Binds You [Audio Cassette (April 1990) Health Communications Audio; ISBN: 1558740430]
[282] Miller A. The Drama of the Gifted Child: The Search for the True Self. Basic Books: 1981
[283] Miller A. The truth will set you free: overcoming emotional blindness and finding your true adult self. New York: Basic Books; 2001
[284] Kottler JA. The Compleat Therapist. San Francisco; Jossey-Bass publishers; 1991, pages 134-174
[285] Smyth JM, Stone AA, Hurewitz A, Kaell A. Effects of writing about stressful experiences on symptom reduction in patients with asthma or rheumatoid arthritis: a randomized trial. JAMA. 1999 Apr 14;281(14):1304-9

Creating and Re-creating the Self: An on-going process that involves various types of "therapy" such as healthy formal/informal interpersonal and group relationships, creative expression and exploration, the periodic infusion of new ideas from teachers and mentors, attendance in workshops and seminars (or other forms of on-going consciousness-raising), reflection, and the integration of transformative and sustentative significance into everyday life, in such a way that daily life itself becomes *therapeutic* and *affirmative*.

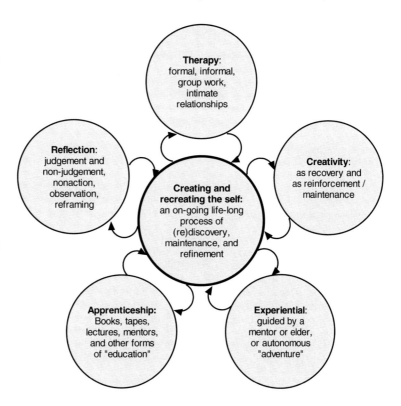

One possible sequence of events for effective, lasting, and authentic autonomization: The caterpillar does not blossom into a butterfly without spending time in its cocoon. The airborne seed descends into the earth for its nourishment before it sprouts and searches for the sun. Similarly, gratification of our ascentionist and impatient ego must be deferred for the sake of allowing the time and descent that provide "grounding" and developing of a solid foundation from which authentic growth can arise. The Western view of "personal development" idealizes a life course of constant ascension that is generally inconsistent with living in a real world fraught with imperfections; two of the major complications arising from such a perfectionistic paradigm are 1) that it causes people to feel anxious and ashamed when confronted with otherwise normal delays and failures, and 2) that it biases people into believing that improvement comes only from advancement rather than also from the return and short-term regression that are characteristic of most historically-proven societal traditions. With modification of the stepwise model proposed by Bradshaw[286], here I propose the following sequence:

1. *Short-term behavior modification*: For people whose behavior is acutely dysfunctional or harmful to themselves or others, they must stop the "acting out" that is the symptom of the underlying emotional injury or schism. Accepting abuse—at work or home—is a form of **acting out** that perpetuates old wounds and saps the strength required for recovery. Enacting addictive behavior is injurious to the psyche because self-injurious behavior reinforces the image of oneself as an object of contempt while also reinforcing the image of psychological dependency and emotional helplessness.

---

[286] Bradshaw J. Healing the Shame that Binds You [Audio Cassette (April 1990) Health Communications Audio; ISBN: 1558740430]

2. *Emotional recovery*: Complete healing is only possible when consciously pursued, and conscious healing can only be pursued after one has become conscious of the wounds, injuries, absences, dynamics, and events that lead to the current state. This process of recovery is referred to mythologically as the "descent" or the time of "eating ashes" that is a recurrent theme in various fairy tales ("Cinderella" literally means "ash girl") and cultural-religious histories (such as Jesus' *descent* into the tomb).[287] The biggest blockades to this process are 1) the ego, which prefers to ascend and to deny intrapersonal "negativity"[288], and 2) the challenge in finding elders and mentors in a society that constantly perpetuates and encourages immaturity, materialism, and superficiality.[289] In the words of famed psychologist Carl Jung, "One does not become enlightened by imagining figures of light, but by making the darkness *conscious*. The latter procedure, however, is disagreeable, and therefore unpopular." People often have tremendous resistances to the process of self-exploration and internal learning; as Jeffrey Kottler[290] wrote of his own experience in The Compleat Therapist, "…like most prospective consumers of therapy, I made up a bunch of excuses for why I could handle this on my own… I was smiling like an idiot…"

3. *Long-term behavior modification and integration*: Insight allows for an illumination of the internal mental-emotional landscape, and effective insight must then be manifested externally by changes/modifications in behavior, habits, and interaction in the world. **Externalized behaviors simultaneously reflect and reinforce thoughts and feelings.** According to Grieneeks[291], patients (and their healthcare providers) can "*think* their way into new ways of *acting*" and "*act* their way into new ways of *thinking*." Eventually, a consciously designed life can be created so that actions, interactions, thoughts, and feelings are melded together in such ways that everyday life itself becomes simultaneously *therapeutic*, *affirmative*, *sustentative*, and *empowering*. In this way, the person and his/her life are unified in such ways as to become self-perpetuating and self-sustaining cycles of ascents and descents, thought-feeling and action, reflection and courage, independence and interdependence—in sum: "a wheel rolling from its own center."[292] At this point the self is established, though it must be maintained and developed with the continuous application of consciousness, reflection, and action.

4. *Metapersonal involvement in community, religion, spirituality, and the world*: Many people are tempted to move from a state of woundedness, relative incompleteness and the feelings of shame and disempowerment to a state of illusory *perfection*, *enlightenment* and *omnipotence* without doing the requisite hard work that makes authentic personal growth possible. People with unhealed emotional wounds often seek to camouflage those deficiencies by becoming pious and projecting an image of completeness and of "having it all figured out" and "having it all together"; religion and the acquisition of power are often misused for this purpose. Many people are successful in wearing this mask for many years; but its crumbling—often manifested as the "midlife crisis"—heralds an opportunity for personal growth if not medicated with anti-depressants, vacations, affairs, gambling, or other distractions.[293] The temptation to bypass Stages 2 [emotional recovery] and 3 [integration] and leapfrog from

---

[287] Bly R, Hillman J, Meade M. Men and the Life of Desire. Oral Tradition Archives. ISBN: 1880155001
[288] Robert Bly. The Human Shadow. Sound Horizons, New York 1991 [ISBN: 1879323001] and Bly R. A Little Book on the Human Shadow.[ISBN: 0062548476]
[289] Bly R. Where have all the parents gone? A talk on the Sibling Society. New York: Sound Horizons, 1996
[290] Kottler JA. The Compleat Therapist. San Francisco; Jossey-Bass publishers; 1991, pages 2-3
[291] Keith Grieneeks PhD. "Psychological Assessment" taught in 1998 at Bastyr University.
[292] Friedrich Wilhelm Nietzsche, Walter Kaufmann (Translator). Thus Spoke Zarathustra. Penguin USA; 1978, page 27
[293] Robinson JC. Death of a Hero, Birth of a Soul: Answering the Call of Midlife. Council Oak Books, March 1997 ISBN: 1571780432

Stage 1 [woundedness] to Stage 4 [spirituality] should be resisted because the religion or spirituality is then used as a shield *against authenticity* and as a tool for illusory control. Religion can be misused in this way by providing an "identity" and sense of redemption for people with incompletely formed identities and for those with incompletely reconciled shadows and unresolved childhood-parental introjects.[294,295,296] Nietzsche's[297] response to this problem was to encourage self-knowledge and self-reconciliation as prerequisites to religious devotion, hence his admonition, "By all means love your neighbor as yourself – but *first* be such that you love yourself." Historical and recent events remind us of how religion can be misused for misanthropic ends.[298] What is commonly referred to as "spiritual development"—a level of resolution, reconciliation, and autonomy that allows for compassionate interdependence with people, the planet and the larger "world"—is synergistic with and can be supported by religion; but the latter is not a substitute for the former.[299,300] Religion and other forms of metapersonal involvement (e.g., community participation and social generosity) are *important* and *necessary* extensions of self-development. In order for personal development to blossom from the germ of necessary narcissism into its flower of functional completeness, it must eventually manifest in the larger community and the world.

5. *Acceptance of mortality and death*: No individual person or any system of thought, whether scientific or religious, can feign completeness without accounting for the end of life and incorporating this account into its overarching paradigm. The event is too significant, and the fear and concerns it provokes are too weighty to not be addressed directly and held in consciousness on a periodic—if not frequent—basis. This topic is of practical importance, too, not only in our own lives and those of our friends and family, but also to the national healthcare system, which currently spends the bulk of its money and resources vainly attempting to preserve life in the last few years and months after which disease or age call unrelentingly for the end of life. Perhaps if we as individuals and as participants in the healthcare system could accept and deal with our own deaths, then we would not

> "**The event of death is not a tragedy**—to rabbit, fox or man. But **the *concept* of death *is* a tragedy**, for man, and *indirectly* for poor fox, rabbit, bush, bird, just anything and everything in man's path."
>
> Pearce JC, <u>Exploring the Crack in the Cosmic Egg</u>. Washington Square Press; 1974, page 59

have to panic and participate in such superfluous expenditures of time, energy, emotion, and money when death seeks to arrive, either for our patients, our friends and family, or ourselves. Proximal to the panic and aversion that characterizes the West's relationship to death is the "subclinical" panic and aversion that infiltrate the lives, practices, and policies that we experience every day. Surely, many unconscious events and subconscious influences contribute to the "lives of quiet desperation"[301] and "universal anxiety"[302] that subtly yet

[294] Bradshaw J. <u>Healing the Shame that Binds You</u> [Audio Cassette (April 1990) Health Communications Audio; ISBN: 1558740430]
[295] Miller A. <u>The Drama of the Gifted Child: The Search for the True Self</u>. Basic Books: 1981
[296] Miller A. <u>The truth will set you free: overcoming emotional blindness and finding your true adult self</u>. New York: Basic Books; 2001
[297] Nietzsche N. <u>Thus spoke Zarathustra</u>. Read by Jon Cartwright and Alex Jennings and published by Naxos AudioBooks. I think this is among the more brilliant achievements in human history. http://naxosaudiobooks.com/nabusa/pages/432512.htm
[298] Bonhoeffer. (movie documentary by director/writer Martin Doblmeier) <u>http://www.bonhoeffer.com/</u>
[299] Lozoff B. <u>It's a Meaningful Life : It Just Takes Practice</u>. March 1, 2001. ISBN: 0140196242
[300] Bradshaw J. <u>Healing the Shame that Binds You</u> [Audio Cassette (April 1990) Health Communications Audio; ISBN: 1558740430]
[301] Threoau HD, (Thomas O, ed). <u>Walden and Civil Disobedience</u>. New York: WW Norton and Company; 1966, page 5
[302] Becker E. <u>The Denial of Death</u>. New York: Free Press; 1973, pages 11 and 21

powerfully afflict most people; surely, lack of reconciliation with death is a major contributor. Especially in western cultures, death is commonly seen as some type of failure or shortcoming, either on behalf of the patient or his/her doctors, and the most common questions asked on the topic of death are "*how can this be avoided*?" before the event and "*who is to blame*?" after the event. Other cultures accept death as a natural part of life, and indeed, people are seen to have an obligation to die so that the next generations can have their turn in the cycle of life. Alternatives to western hysteria are founded on acceptance of death, and the prerequisites for the acceptance of death are 1) the dedication of sufficient time for its consideration (most people would rather watch a bad movie or attend spectator sports), 2) reframing the event in terms of its being a natural part of our lives, certainly nothing to be ashamed of (discussed below), 3) making necessary logistical preparations (e.g., writing of wills, providing for dependents, and other obvious technicalities), and 4) living as completely, consciously, compassionately, effectively, and authentically as possible so that remorse can be minimized, perhaps completely mitigated. Reframing the event of death begins with its description in general terms so that its enigma, from which its power over the hearts and minds of humanity is derived, can be deciphered and thus deflated. The main characteristics of death which precipitate its fear are 1) the unpredictability of its arrival, 2) the duration of the dying process, and 3) the quality of that process, for example whether it is painful or associated with or precipitated by severe illness or injury. The first characteristic of *timeliness*—the unpredictability of its arrival—stresses people because of their inadequate preparation and the feeling that they have only recently begun to live or have not quite yet begun to live their authentic lives. These concerns are allayed by preparation, both logistical and intrapersonal. Each of us has the responsibility to "become authentically whole" so that we do not inflict our incompleteness onto others, either directly through various forms of transference or deprivation or indirectly though the more subtle means of politics and cultural mores.[303,304] If a person can live with vitality, authenticity, compassion and effectiveness then little is left to want, and fears of death and its untimely arrival are diminished. The remaining variables are both controllable and uncontrollable; they are uncontrollable to the extent that we are all subject to chaos and accidents, whether in cars, planes, or bathtubs. *Duration* and *quality* are both controllable on an inpatient setting to the extent that palliative care and autonomous decision-making is made available.[305,306]

Life can only be authentically and completely experienced after one has created an authentic self and has thereafter accepted life *as it is*. Since death is part of life, the full engagement of life requires *acceptance of* and *reconciliation with* death. Acceptance of death does not necessarily entail that life becomes permeated with nihilistic resignation; on the contrary, it infuses daily events with significance and makes all experiences unique and worthy of appreciation.

> "Once accepted, death is an integral component of every event, as the left hand to the right. The cultural death concept could only be instilled in a mind split from its own life flow."
>
> Pearce JC. Exploring the Crack in the Cosmic Egg: Split Minds and Meta-Realities. New York: Washington Square Press; 1974, page 59

---

[303] Miller A. The Drama of the Gifted Child: The Search for the True Self. Basic Books: 1981

[304] Robert Bly. The Human Shadow. Sound Horizons, New York 1991 [ISBN: 1879323001] and Bly R. A Little Book on the Human Shadow.[ISBN: 0062548476

[305] Steinbrook R. Medical marijuana, physician-assisted suicide, and the Controlled Substances Act. *N Engl J Med*. 2004 Sep 30;351(14):1380-3

[306] "Failure to give an effective therapy to seriously ill patients, either adults or children, violates the core principles of both medicine and ethics... Therefore, in the patient's best interest, patients and parents/surrogates, have the right to request medical marijuana under certain circumstances and physicians have the duty to disclose medical marijuana as an option and prescribe it when appropriate." Clark PA. Medical marijuana: should minors have the same rights as adults? *Med Sci Monit*.2003;9:ET1-9 www.medscimonit.com/pub/vol_9/no_6/3640.pdf

Growth, integration, and acceptance: Starting at the top, the progression of personal growth, emotional recovery, integration and daily practice is followed by the more advanced integration of one's chosen purpose, mission, and life work with one's chosen spiritual/religious practice, family and community involvement, and acceptance of and preparation for the end of life and the continuity of society and the environment.

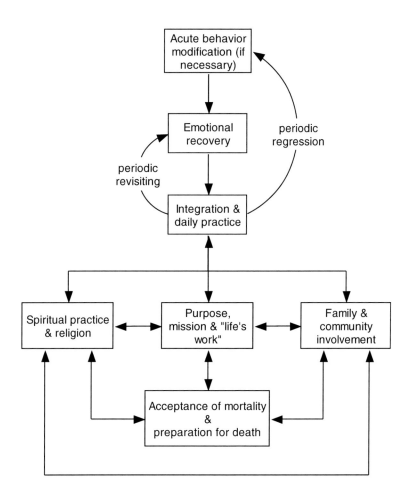

"They say there's no future for us.
They're right,
which is fine with us." Rumi[307]

---

[307] Rumi in Barks C (translator). <u>The Essential Rumi</u>. HarperSanFransisco: 1995, page 2

Environmental Health, Toxicity, and Detoxification

> "Man's attitude toward nature is today critically important simply because we have now acquired a fateful power to alter and destroy nature. But man is a part of nature, and his war against nature is inevitably a war against himself."   *Rachel Carson*[308]

Environmental exposures to chemicals and toxic substances: Studies using blood tests and tissue samples from Americans across the nation have consistently shown that all Americans have toxic chemical accumulation whether or not they work in chemical factories or are obviously exposed at home or work.[309,310] **The recent report from the CDC found toxic chemicals such as pesticides in all Americans, especially minorities, women, and children.**[311] Nearly all of these chemicals are known to contribute to health problems in humans—problems such as cancer, fatigue, poor memory, endocrinopathy, subfertility/infertility, Parkinson's disease, autoimmune diseases like lupus, and many other serious conditions. Therefore, *detoxification programs are a necessity—not a luxury*.

Examples of toxicants commonly found in Americans

Environmental pollutant (population frequency)	Biologic effects as quoted from HSDB: Hazardous Substances Data Bank. National Library of Medicine, NIH[312] or other reference as noted
DDE (found in 99% of Americans): DDE is the main metabolite of DDT, a pesticide that was presumably banned in the US in 1972	<ul><li>DDT is known to be immunosuppressive in animals.</li><li>A study published in 2004 showed that increasing levels of DDE in African-American male farmers in North Carolina correlated with a higher prevalence of antinuclear antibodies and up to 50% reductions in serum IgG.[313]</li><li>Other studies in humans have suggested an estrogenic or anti-androgenic effect.[314]</li><li>Virtually all US women have evidence of DDT/DDE accumulation. Women with higher levels of DDT and/or its metabolites show pregnancy and childbirth complications and have higher rates of infant mortality.[315]</li></ul>

---

[308] Rachel Carson. *Silent Spring*. Boston, Houghton Mifflin Company (2002). ISBN: 0395683297. See also Rachel Carson Dies of Cancer; 'Silent Spring' Author Was 56. New York Times 1956. http://www.rachelcarson.org/ on August 1, 2004

[309] "The average concentration of 2,3,7,8-tetrachlorodibenzo-p-dioxin in the adipose tissue of the US population was 5.38 pg/g, increasing from 1.98 pg/g in children under 14 years of age to 9.40 pg/g in adults over 45." Orban JE, Stanley JS, Schwemberger JG, Remmers JC. Dioxins and dibenzofurans in adipose tissue of the general US population and selected subpopulations. *Am J Public Health* 1994 Mar;84(3):439-45

[310] "Although the use of HCB as a fungicide has virtually been eliminated, detectable levels of HCB are still found in nearly all people in the USA." Robinson PE, Leczynski BA, Kutz FW, Remmers JC. An evaluation of hexachlorobenzene body-burden levels in the general population of the USA. *IARC Sci Publ* 1986;77:183-92

[311] "Many of the pesticides found in the test subjects have been linked to serious short- and long-term health effects including infertility, birth defects and childhood and adult cancers." http://www.panna.org/campaigns/docsTrespass/chemicalTrespass2004.dv.html July 25, 2004

[312] Primary source for this data is the Hazardous Substances Data Bank. National Library of Medicine, National Institutes of Health: http://toxnet.nlm.nih.gov/cgi-bin/sis/htmlgen?HSDB accessed on August 1, 2004

[313] Cooper GS, Martin SA, Longnecker MP, Sandler DP, Germolec DR. Associations between plasma DDE levels and immunologic measures in African-American farmers in North Carolina. *Environ Health Perspect.* 2004 Jul;112(10):1080-4

[314] Dalvie MA, Myers JE, Lou Thompson M, Dyer S, Robins TG, Omar S, Riebow J, Molekwa J, Kruger P, Millar R. The hormonal effects of long-term DDT exposure on malaria vector-control workers in Limpopo Province, South Africa. *Environ Res.* 2004 Sep;96(1):9-19

[315] "The findings strongly suggest that DDT use increases preterm births, which is a major contributor to infant mortality. If this association is causal, it should be included in any assessment of the costs and benefits of vector control with DDT." Longnecker MP, Klebanoff MA, Zhou H, Brock JW. Association between maternal serum concentration of the DDT metabolite DDE and preterm and small-for-gestational-age babies at birth. *Lancet.* 2001 Jul 14;358(9276):110-4

Examples of toxicants commonly found in Americans—*continued*

Environmental pollutant (population frequency)	Biologic effects as quoted from HSDB: Hazardous Substances Data Bank. National Library of Medicine, NIH[316] or other reference
2,5-dichlorophenol (88% nationally and up to 96% in select children populations): Dichlorophenols can occur in tap water as a result of standard chlorination treatment. General population may be exposed to 2,5-dichlorophenol through oral consumption or dermal contact with chlorinated tap water. 2,5-Dichlorophenol was identified in 96% of the urine samples of children residing in Arkansas near an herbicide plant at concentrations of 4-1,200 ppb. The sole manufacturer for herbicide use is Sandoz (Clariant Corporation).	• Human Toxicity Excerpts: 1. Burning pain in mouth and throat. White necrotic lesions in mouth, esophagus, and stomach. Abdominal pain, vomiting ... and bloody diarrhea. 2. Pallor, sweating, weakness, headache, dizziness, tinnitus. 3. Shock: Weak irregular pulse, hypotension, shallow respirations, cyanosis, pallor, and a profound fall in body temperature. 4. Possibly fleeting excitement and confusion, followed by unconsciousness. ... 5. Stentorous breathing, mucous rales, rhonchi, frothing at nose and mouth and other signs of pulmonary edema are sometimes seen. Characteristic odor of phenol on the breath. 6. Scanty, dark-colored ... urine ... moderately severe renal insufficiency may appear. 7. Methemoglobinemia, Heinz body hemolytic anemia and hyperbilirubinemia have been reported. ... 8. Death from respiratory, circulatory or cardiac failure. 9. If spilled on skin, pain is followed promptly by numbness. The skin becomes blanched, and a dry opaque eschar forms over the burn. When the eschar sloughs off, a brown stain remains.
Chlorpyrifos (found in 93% of Americans): Insecticide used on corn and cotton and for termite control. Conservative estimates hold that 80% of the chlorpyrifos in the US was produced directly or indirectly by Dow Chemical Corporation.[317] **This pesticide is routinely used in schools and is thus found in blood and tissue samples of nearly all American children.**	• Toxic if inhaled, in contact with skin, and if swallowed. • All the organophosphorus insecticides have a cumulative effect by progressive inhibition of cholinesterase. • The symptoms of chronic poisoning due to organophosphorus pesticides include headache, weakness, feeling of heaviness in head, decline of memory, quick onset of **fatigue**, **disturbed sleep**, loss of appetite, and loss of orientation. Other manifestations of accumulation include **tension, anxiety, restlessness, insomnia, headache, emotional instability, fatigue**… • Chlorpyrifos is a suspected endocrine disruptor.[318] • **Higher chlorpyrifos levels in children correlate with higher incidences attention problems, attention-deficit/hyperactivity disorder, and pervasive developmental disorder.**[319]

[316] Primary source for this data is the Hazardous Substances Data Bank, National Institutes of Health: http://toxnet.nlm.nih.gov/cgi-bin/sis/htmlgen?HSDB accessed on August 1, 2004
[317] Kristin S. Schafer, Margaret Reeves, Skip Spitzer, Susan E. Kegley. Chemical Trespass: Pesticides in Our Bodies and Corporate Accountability. Pesticide Action Network North America. May 2004 Available at http://www.panna.org/campaigns/docsTrespass/chemicalTrespass2004.dv.html on August 1, 2004
[318] http://www.panna.org/resources/documents/factsChlorpyrifos.dv.html accessed August 1, 2004
[319] "Highly exposed children (chlorpyrifos levels of >6.17 pg/g plasma) scored, on average, 6.5 points lower on the Bayley Psychomotor Development Index and 3.3 points lower on the Bayley Mental Development Index at 3 years of age compared with those with lower levels of exposure. Children exposed to higher, compared with lower, chlorpyrifos levels were also significantly more likely to experience Psychomotor Development Index and Mental Development Index delays, attention problems, attention-deficit/hyperactivity disorder problems, and pervasive developmental disorder problems at 3 years of age." Rauh VA, Garfinkel R, Perera FP, Andrews HF, Hoepner L, Barr DB, Whitehead R, Tang D, Whyatt RW. Impact of prenatal chlorpyrifos exposure on neurodevelopment in the first 3 years of life among inner-city children. *Pediatrics.* 2006 Dec;118(6):e1845-59

Examples of toxicants commonly found in Americans—*continued*

Environmental pollutant (population frequency)	Biologic effects as quoted from HSDB: Hazardous Substances Data Bank. National Library of Medicine, NIH[320] or other reference as noted
Mercury (8% of American women of reproductive age have mercury levels high enough to cause adverse health effects)	▪ Mercury is a well-known neurotoxin, immunotoxin, and nephrotoxin. Mercury toxicity is also a known cause of hypertension in humans. ▪ A recent study published in *JAMA—Journal of the American Medical Association*[321] noted that "Humans are exposed to methylmercury, a well-established neurotoxin, through fish consumption. The fetus is most sensitive to the adverse effects of exposure. … **approximately 8% of women had concentrations higher than the US EPA's recommended reference dose (5.8 microg/L),** below which exposures are considered to be without adverse effects." **The most obvious interpretation of this data published in *JAMA* is that 8% of American women have chronic mercury poisoning—poisoning in this case refers specifically to elevated blood levels of a known toxicant that consistently demonstrates adverse effects on human health.** Logical deduction holds that such a high prevalence of human poisoning should be unacceptable and should lead directly to legislative restrictions on corporate emissions to protect and salvage the health of the public.
2,4-dichlorophenol (found in 87% of Americans): Pesticide	▪ Human Toxicity Excerpts: same as for 2,5-dichlorophenol ▪ In males, significant increases in relative risk ratios for lung cancer, rectal cancer, and soft tissue sarcomas were reported; in females, there were increases in the relative risk of cervical cancer.

"The only thing necessary for the triumph of evil is for good men to do nothing."
Edmond Burke (1729 – 1797)

"Your lack of interest in the past, your lack of involvement, your unwillingness to develop coherent strategies, your unwillingness to challenge authority - these have created a vacuum in decision-making, that has been filled by professional groups with close relationships with the chemical industries…"

Samuel Epstein, M.D.[322]

---

[320] Primary source for this data is the Hazardous Substances Data Bank, National Institutes of Health: http://toxnet.nlm.nih.gov/cgi-bin/sis/htmlgen?HSDB accessed on August 1, 2004

[321] Schober SE, Sinks TH, Jones RL, Bolger PM, McDowell M, Osterloh J, Garrett ES, Canady RA, Dillon CF, Sun Y, Joseph CB, Mahaffey KR. Blood mercury levels in US children and women of childbearing age, 1999-2000. *JAMA*. 2003 Apr 2;289(13):1667-74

[322] Samuel Epstein MD, 1993. Professor of Occupational and Environmental Medicine at the School of Public Health, University of Illinois Medical Center Chicago. http://www.converge.org.nz/pirm/pestican.htm accessed September 11, 2004

<u>**Toxicity and detoxification—basics**</u>: The physiologic processes by which toxins—whether chemicals or metals—are referred to generally as "detoxification." Clinically, doctors can implement treatment interventions to promote and facilitate the removal of chemical and metal toxins; this, too, is generally referred to as detoxification or clinical/therapeutic detoxification programs. Detoxification programs are popular with patients and some doctors and are most often misused and misapplied.

The recent findings that mercury poisoning can result from once-weekly consumption of tuna[323] and that **the average American has 13 pesticides in his/her body**[324] should be seen as an indication of how dangerously toxic our environment has become, largely due to irresponsible corporate and government policies that value profitability over sustainability.

<u>**Detoxification procedures**</u>: Though a detailed clinical explanation of detoxification procedures will not be included here (see Chapter 4 of *Integrative Rheumatology*[325]), the general concepts for detoxification are as follows:
1. *Avoidance*: reduced exposure = reduced problem
   a. If there were less chemical pollution, then our environment would be less toxic and therefore we would not have such problems with environmental poisoning.
   b. Limit or eliminate exposure to paint fumes, car exhaust, new carpet, solvents, adhesives, artificial foods, synthetic chemical drugs, copier fumes, pesticides, herbicides, chemical fertilizers, etc.
2. *Depuration*: "The act or process of freeing from foreign or impure matter"[326]
   a. Exercise and sauna
   b. Bowel cleansing, fiber, probiotics, antibiotics, laxatives
   c. Liver and bile stimulators
   d. Cofactors for phase 1 oxidation and phase 2 conjugation
   e. Chelation for heavy metals
   f. Urine alkalinization
3. *Damage control*: managing the consequences of chemical and heavy metal toxicity
   a. Hormone replacement
   b. Antioxidant therapy
   c. Occupational and rehabilitative training
   d. Management of resultant diseases, particularly autoimmune diseases
4. *Political and social action*: Due in large part to corporate influence and government deregulation, environmental contamination with pesticides from American corporations has increased to such an extent over the past few decades that now all Americans show evidence of pesticide accumulation in their bodies. Failure to hold corporations to tight regulatory standards has jeopardized the future of humanity. Voter passivity combined

[323] "The neurobehavioral performance of subjects who consumed tuna fish regularly was significantly worse on color word reaction time, digit symbol reaction time and finger tapping speed (FT)." Carta P, Flore C, Alinovi R, Ibba A, Tocco MG, Aru G, Carta R, Girei E, Mutti A, Lucchini R, Randaccio FS. Sub-clinical neurobehavioral abnormalities associated with low level of mercury exposure through fish consumption. *Neurotoxicology*. 2003 Aug;24(4-5):617-23
[324] "A comprehensive survey of more than 1,300 Americans has found traces of weed- and bug-killers in the bodies of everyone tested, …. The survey, conducted by the U.S. Centers for Disease Control and Prevention, found that the body of the average American contained 13 of these chemicals." Martin Millelstaedt. 13 pesticides in body of average American. *The Globe and Mail*. Friday, May 21, 2004 - Page A17 Available on-line at http://www.theglobeandmail.com/servlet/ArticleNews/TPStory/LAC/20040521/HPEST21/TPEnvironment/ on August 6, 2004
[325] **Vasquez A**. Integrative Rheumatology. IBMRC. http://optimalhealthresearch.com/textbooks/rheumatology.html
[326] Webster's 1913 Dictionary

with collusion between multinational corporations and government officials is the underlying problem. Political action is the solution. The past and recent history on this topic is clear and well documented for those who wish to access the facts.[327,328,329,330,331,332,333, 334,335]

Personal plans for taking responsible action and avoiding political/social passivity that has created the opportunity for regulatory failure and corporate exploitation of the environment that threatens the sustainability of the human species:

_____

_____

_____

_____

_____

_____

_____

_____

_____

_____

_____

_____

[327] Robert Van den Bosch. The pesticide conspiracy. Garden City, NY: Doubleday, 1978. ISBN: 0385133847

[328] "Monsanto Corporation is widely known for its production of the herbicide Roundup and genetically engineered Roundup-ready crops… altered to survive a dousing of the toxic herbicide. …glyphosate, is known to cause eye soreness, headaches, diarrhea, and other flu-like symptoms, and has been linked to non-Hodgkin's lymphoma." Bush Names Former Monsanto Executive as EPA Deputy Administrator. Daily News Archive From March 29, 2001 http://www.beyondpesticides.org/NEWS/daily_news_archive/2001/03_29_01.htm accessed on August 1, 2004

[329] "They pointed to budgets cuts for research and enforcement, to steep declines in the number of cases filed against polluters, to efforts to relax portions of the Clean Air Act, to an acceleration of federal approvals for the spraying of restricted pesticides and more." Patricia Sullivan. Anne Gorsuch Burford, 62, Dies; Reagan EPA Director. *Washington Post.* Thursday, July 22, 2004; Page B06 http://www.washingtonpost.com/wp-dyn/articles/A3418-2004Jul21.html on August 2, 2004

[330] "In fact, amongst the crimes of Reagan and Bush which will go down in history are their emasculation of Federal regulatory apparatus... But in 1988, under the Bush administration, the EPA - illegally, in our view - revoked the Dellaney Law..." Samuel Epstein MD, 1993. Professor of Occupational and Environmental Medicine at the School of Public Health, University of Illinois Medical Center Chicago. http://www.converge.org.nz/pirm/pestican.htm accessed August 1, 2004

[331] "The Environmental Protection Agency will be free to approve pesticides without consulting wildlife agencies to determine if the chemical might harm plants and animals protected by the Endangered Species Act, according to new Bush administration rules.... It also is intended to head off future lawsuits, the officials said." Associated Press. Bush Eases Pesticide Laws http://www.cbsnews.com/stories/2004/07/29/tech/main633009.shtml accessed August 1, 2004

[332] "The new policy also could bolster pesticide makers' contention that federal labeling insulates them from suits alleging that their products cause illness or environmental damage, Olson says. 'It . . . could really be disastrous for public health.'" Bush Exempts Pesticide Companies from Lawsuits. Law on Pesticides Reinterpreted: Government Alters Policy in Effort to Protect Manufacturers. Peter Eisler. *USA TODAY.* October 6, 2003 http://www.organicconsumers.org/foodsafety/bushpesticides100703.cfm Accessed August 1, 2004

[333] WASHINGTON (AP) — "The Environmental Protection Agency will be free to approve pesticides without consulting wildlife agencies to determine if the chemical might harm plants and animals protected by the Endangered Species Act, according to new Bush administration rules." Bush eases pesticide reviews for endangered species. http://www.usatoday.com/news/washington/2004-07-29-epa-pesticides_x.htm?csp=34 Accessed August 2004

[334] "It is simply intolerable that the EPA, instead of providing an example for open scientific discussion, has continuously violated key environmental legislation, stifling legitimate dissent. The failure of EPA to properly encourage and protect whistleblowing has undermined the ability of the EPA and state environmental agencies to enforce environmental laws." Letter to Carol Browner, Administrator U.S. Environmental Protection Agency from Stephen Kohn, Chair National Whistleblower Center Board of Directors dated March 23, 1999. Availble at http://www.whistleblowers.org/statements.htm on October 10, 2004

[335] "The Bush administration has imposed a gag order on the U.S. Environmental Protection Agency from publicly discussing perchlorate pollution, even as two new studies reveal high levels of the rocket-fuel component may be contaminating the nation's lettuce supply." Peter Waldman. Rocket Fuel Residues Found in Lettuce: Bush administration issues gag order on EPA discussions of possible rocket fuel tainted lettuce. *THE WALL STREET JOURNAL.* See http://www.organicconsumers.org/toxic/lettuce042903.cfm http://www.rhinoed.com/epa's_gag_order.htm http://www.peer.org/press/508.html http://yubanet.com/artman/publish/article_13637.shtml

Overview of toxicant exposure and detoxification/depuration

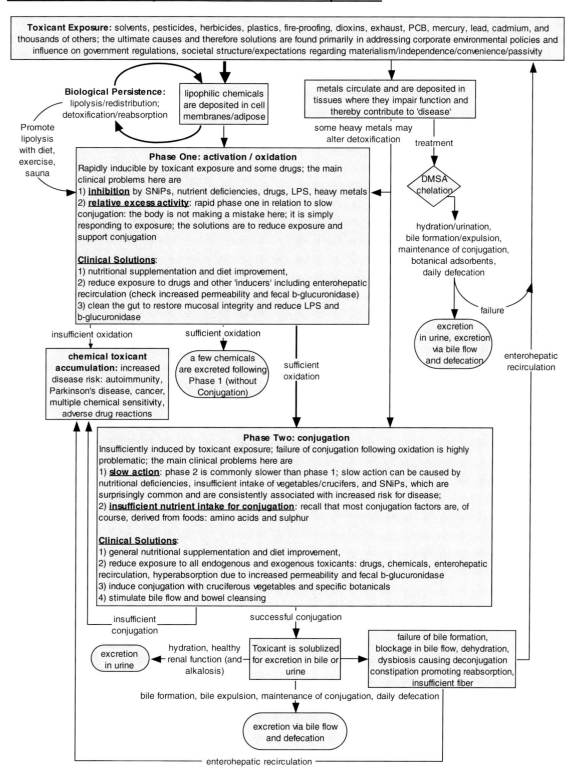

Toxicant Exposure: solvents, pesticides, herbicides, plastics, fire-proofing, dioxins, exhaust, PCB, mercury, lead, cadmium, and thousands of others; the ultimate causes and therefore solutions are found primarily in addressing corporate environmental policies and influence on government regulations, societal structure/expectations regarding materialism/independence/convenience/passivity

Biological Persistence: lipolysis/redistribution; detoxification/reabsorption

Promote lipolysis with diet, exercise, sauna

lipophilic chemicals are deposited in cell membranes/adipose

metals circulate and are deposited in tissues where they impair function and thereby contribute to 'disease'

some heavy metals may alter detoxification

treatment

DMSA chelation

hydration/urination, bile formation/expulsion, maintenance of conjugation, botanical adsorbents, daily defecation

failure

Phase One: activation / oxidation
Rapidly inducible by toxicant exposure and some drugs; the main clinical problems here are
1) **inhibition** by SNiPs, nutrient deficiencies, drugs, LPS, heavy metals
2) **relative excess activity**: rapid phase one in relation to slow conjugation: the body is not making a mistake here; it is simply responding to exposure; the solutions are to reduce exposure and support conjugation

Clinical Solutions:
1) nutritional supplementation and diet improvement,
2) reduce exposure to drugs and other 'inducers' including enterohepatic recirculation (check increased permeability and fecal b-glucuronidase)
3) clean the gut to restore mucosal integrity and reduce LPS and b-glucuronidase

insufficient oxidation

sufficient oxidation

chemical toxicant accumulation: increased disease risk: autoimmunity, Parkinson's disease, cancer, multiple chemical sensitivity, adverse drug reactions

a few chemicals are excreted following Phase 1 (without Conjugation)

sufficient oxidation

excretion in urine, excretion via bile flow and defecation

enterohepatic recirculation

Phase Two: conjugation
Insufficiently induced by toxicant exposure; failure of conjugation following oxidation is highly problematic; the main clinical problems here are
1) **slow action**: phase 2 is commonly slower than phase 1; slow action can be caused by nutritional deficiencies, insufficient intake of vegetables/crucifers, and SNiPs, which are surprisingly common and are consistently associated with increased risk for disease;
2) **insufficient nutrient intake for conjugation**: recall that most conjugation factors are, of course, derived from foods: amino acids and sulphur

Clinical Solutions:
1) general nutritional supplementation and diet improvement,
2) reduce exposure to all endogenous and exogenous toxicants: drugs, chemicals, enterohepatic recirculation, hyperabsorption due to increased permeability and fecal b-glucuronidase
3) induce conjugation with cruciferous vegetables and specific botanicals
4) stimulate bile flow and bowel cleansing

insufficient conjugation

successful conjugation

hydration, healthy renal function (and alkalosis)

excretion in urine

Toxicant is solublized for excretion in bile or urine

failure of bile formation, blockage in bile flow, dehydration, dysbiosis causing deconjugation constipation promoting reabsorption, insufficient fiber

bile formation, bile expulsion, maintenance of conjugation, daily defecation

excretion via bile flow and defecation

enterohepatic recirculation

Integrative/functional healthcare empowers patients with the ability to understand and effectively participate in the course of their life and health

Drug/surgery-based medicine	Paradigm	Holistic natural healthcare
• Doctor as "savior" and indifferent "objective" observer	Role of the doctor	• Doctor as "teacher" and active caring partner and co-participant in the process
• Helpless victim, disempowered, dependent	Role of the patient	• Active participant, empowered, responsible
• Illness is impossibly complex, and treating this with natural means is generally impossible • Treatment is simple: you have this disease, and you need to take one or more drugs for every problem • Diet and lifestyle modifications are generally viewed as secondary to drugs • The disease is more important than the patient	Nature of illness	• Multifactorial: involving many different aspects of lifestyle, diet, exercise, genetic inheritance, psychology, and environment • Many causes allows for many different treatment approaches and different ways of attaining health • Illness can be modified via selective dietary and lifestyle changes and a custom-tailored treatment plan • The patient is more important than the disease
• Disease-centered, drug-centered	Viewpoint	• Patient-centered, wellness-centered
• Drugs, including chemotherapy • Surgery • Radiation • Electroconvulsive treatment • Vaccinations	Treatment and options	• Diet and lifestyle improvement • Relationship/emotional work • Botanical and nutritional medicines • Physical medicine, chiropractic, exercise • Acupuncture • *Selective* rather than *first-line* use of pharmaceuticals and medical procedures
• Symptom suppression • Drug side-effects are a significant cause of death in the US • Only *treats disease*, does not *promote health*; cannot reach optimal health by only reactively treating established health problems • Enormous expense, often subsidized by private or public "insurance"	Long-term outcome	• Improved health • Potential for successful prevention, treatment or eradication of chronic disease • Potential to become optimally healthy • Proven cost-reduction
• Heightened risk, since drugs are foreign chemicals that have action in the body by interfering with the way that the body normally works • Every drug has side-effects, some of which can be life-threatening • Surgery causes irreparable changes to the body, often for the worse. • Radiation and chemotherapy can cause a secondary cancer to develop	Risks	• Reduced risk, since most of the botanical treatments and all of the nutritional medicines have been a major part of the human diet for centuries/millennia and have proven safety • Delayed onset of action: most treatments are not fast-acting enough to be of value in traumatic or acutely life-threatening situations • Patients must be willing to adopt healthier lifestyles
• Allows a doctor to see many patients within a short amount of time, thus increasing profitability • Since drugs do not cure problems, patients must return for lifelong prescription renewals • Therapeutic passivity: minimal action or effort required by patient and doctor • The doctor holds all the power, and the patient is completely dependent on the doctor for treatment	Benefits	• Improved short-term and long-term health • Empowerment • Understanding of body processes as well as healthcare directions and goals • Options

Opposite influences of health promotion vs. disease promotion: Lifestyle concept

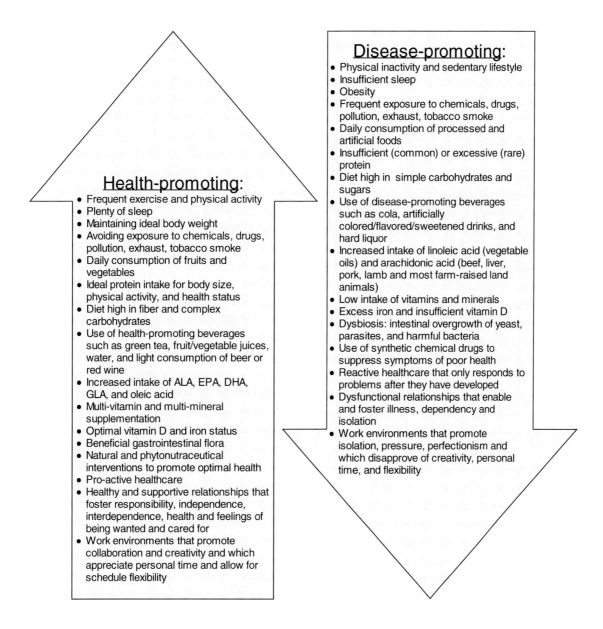

Maximize factors that promote health ◆ Minimize factors that promote disease

Improved clinical outcomes will be attained when doctors and patients attend to both **prescription of health-promoting activities** and **proscription of disease-promoting activities**. Indeed, attention needs to be given to the **ratio** of these disparate and opposing forces, which ultimately influence genetic expression and physiologic function of many organ systems.

Brief Overview of Integrative Primary Healthcare Disciplines

Chiropractic

> "Doctors of Chiropractic are physicians who consider man as an integrated being and give special attention to the physiological and biochemical aspects including structural, spinal, musculoskeletal, neurological, vascular, nutritional, emotional and environmental relationships." *American Chiropractic Association, 2004*[336]

> "The human body represents the actions of three laws—spiritual, mechanical, and chemical—united as one triune. As long as there is perfect union of these three, there is health." *Daniel David Palmer, founder of the modern chiropractic profession*[337]

The basic philosophical model which is taught in many chiropractic colleges is to envision health, disease, and patient care from a conceptual model named the "triad of health" which gives its attention to the three fundamental foundations for well-being: namely, the physical/structural, mental/emotional, and biochemical/nutritional aspects of health. Revolutionary at the time of its inception in the early 1900's, this model now forms the foundation for the increasingly dominant and very popular paradigm of "holistic medicine." It remains a powerful contrast and an attractive alternative to the reductionistic allopathic approach, which generally approaches the human body as if it were simply a conglomerate of independent organ systems that have little or no functional relationship to each other.[338]

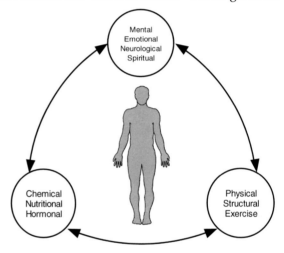

The chiropractic "triad of health"

Using the state of the sciences before the year 1910, chiropractic was founded with a profound appreciation of the integrated nature of health, and the therapeutic focus was on spinal manipulation. In describing the chiropractic model of health, DD Palmer[339] wrote, "The human body represents the actions of three laws—spiritual, mechanical, and chemical—united as one triune. As long as there is perfect union of these three, there is health." While the therapeutic focus of the profession has been spinal manipulation, from its inception the chiropractic profession has emphasized a holistic, integrative model of therapeutic intervention, health, and disease, and chiropractic was the first healthcare profession in America to specifically claim that the optimization of health requires attention to spiritual-emotional-psychological, mechanical-physical-structural, and biochemical-nutritional-hormonal-chemical considerations. Accordingly, these cornerstones are fundamental to the 2005

---

[336] American Chiropractic Association. http://www.amerchiro.org/media/whatis/ Accessed March 13, 2004
[337] Palmer DD. The Science, Art, and Phiosophy, of Chiropractic. Portland, OR; Portland Printing House Company, 1910: 107
[338] Beckman JF, Fernandez CE, Coulter ID. A systems model of health care: a proposal. *J Manipulative Physiol Ther*. 1996 Mar-Apr; 19(3): 208-15
[339] Palmer DD. The Science, Art, and Phiosophy, of Chiropractic. Portland, OR; Portland Printing House Company, 1910: 107

definition of the chiropractic profession articulated by the American Chiropractic Association[340]: "Doctors of Chiropractic are physicians who consider man as an integrated being and give special attention to the physiological and biochemical aspects including structural, spinal, musculoskeletal, neurological, vascular, nutritional, emotional, and environmental relationships."

From its inception, chiropractic was a philosophy of healing that considered the entire health of the patient by addressing the interconnected aspects of our chemical-spiritual-physical being. Later, intraprofessional factions polarized between holistic and vitalistic paradigms; the latter has been presumed to be the philosophy of the entire profession by organizations such as the American Medical Association[341] that have sought to contain and eliminate chiropractic and other forms of natural healthcare[342] by falsifying research[343,344], intentionally misleading the public and manipulating politicians[345,346,347], arriving at illogical conclusions which support the medical paradigm and refute the value of manual therapies[348], and exploiting weaknesses within the profession for its own financial profitability and political advantage.[349] Intentional misrepresentation and defamation of chiropractic continues to occur today, as documented by the 2006 review by Wenban.[350]

Chiropractic Training and Clinical Benefits: In addition to the basic sciences and foundational skills of laboratory and clinical diagnosis, chiropractic physicians receive extensive training in manual physical manipulation, rehabilitation, therapeutic exercise, and clinical nutrition.

An irony exists in the observation that chiropractic education emphasizes anatomy, musculoskeletal therapeutics, and nutrition while these are the very topics that are neglected in allopathic and osteopathic education; the majority medical students and medical physicians who have graduated from allopathic and osteopathic medical schools lack competence in their knowledge of clinical anatomy and musculoskeletal medicine[351,352,353,354,355,356] as well as diet and

[340] American Chiropractic Association. What is Chiropractic? http://amerchiro.org/media/whatis/ Accessed January 9, 2005
[341] American Medical Association. Report 12 of the Council on Scientific Affairs (A-97) Full Text. http://www.ama-assn.org/ama/pub/category/13638.html Accessed September 10, 2005.
[342] Getzendanner S. Permanent injunction order against AMA. *JAMA*. 1988 Jan 1;259(1):81-2
[343] Terrett AG. Misuse of the literature by medical authors in discussing spinal manipulative therapy injury. *J Manipulative Physiol Ther*. 1995 May;18(4):203-10
[344] Morley J, Rosner AL, Redwood D. A case study of misrepresentation of the scientific literature: recent reviews of chiropractic. *J Altern Complement Med*. 2001 Feb;7(1):65-78
[345] Spivak JL. The Medical Trust Unmasked. Louis S. Siegfried Publishers; New York: 1961
[346] Trever W. In the Public Interest. Los Angeles; Scriptures Unlimited; 1972. This is probably the most authoritative documentation of the illegal actions of the AMA up to 1972; contains numerous photocopies of actual AMA documents and minutes of official meetings with overt intentionality of destroying Americans' healthcare options so that the AMA and related organizations would have a monopoly in healthcare.
[347] Wolinsky H, Brune T. The Serpent on the Staff: The Unhealthy Politics of the American Medical Association. GP Putnam and Sons, New York, 1994
[348] Mein EA, Greenman PE, McMillin DL, Richards DG, Nelson CD. Manual medicine diversity: research pitfalls and the emerging medical paradigm. *J Am Osteopath Assoc*. 2001 Aug;101(8):441-4
[349] Wilk CA. Medicine, Monopolies, and Malice: How the Medical Establishment Tried to Destroy Chiropractic. Garden City Park: Avery, 1996
[350] Wenban AB. Inappropriate use of the title 'chiropractor' and term 'chiropractic manipulation' in the peer-reviewed biomedical literature. *Chiropr Osteopat*. 2006;14:16 http://chiroandosteo.com/content/14/1/16
[351] "In summary, seventy (82 per cent) of eighty-five medical school graduates failed a valid musculoskeletal competency examination. We therefore believe that medical school preparation in musculoskeletal medicine is inadequate." Freedman KB, Bernstein J. The adequacy of medical school education in musculoskeletal medicine. *J Bone Joint Surg Am*. 1998;80(10):1421-7
[352] "CONCLUSIONS: According to the standard suggested by the program directors of internal medicine residency departments, a large majority of the examinees once again failed to demonstrate basic competency in musculoskeletal medicine on the examination. It is therefore reasonable to conclude that medical school preparation in musculoskeletal medicine is inadequate." Freedman KB, Bernstein J. Educational deficiencies in musculoskeletal medicine. *J Bone Joint Surg Am*. 2002;84-A(4):604-8
[353] Joy EA, Hala SV. Musculoskeletal Curricula in Medical Education: Filling In the Missing Pieces. *The Physician and Sportsmedicine* 2004; 32: 42-45
[354] "CONCLUSIONS: Seventy-nine percent of the participants failed the basic musculoskeletal cognitive examination. This suggests that training in musculoskeletal medicine is inadequate in both medical school and nonorthopaedic residency training programs." Matzkin E, Smith ME, Freccero CD, Richardson AB. Adequacy of education in musculoskeletal medicine. *J Bone Joint Surg Am*. 2005 Feb;87-A(2):310-4
[355] "Despite generally improved levels of competency with each year at medical school, less than 50% of fourth-year students showed competency. … These results suggested that the curricular approach toward teaching musculoskeletal medicine at this medical school was insufficient and that

nutrition.[357,358,359] In contrast to this replicable data showing that osteopathic and allopathic students and graduates generally fail to demonstrate competence in musculoskeletal medicine and nutrition, one study with 123 chiropractic students and 10 chiropractic doctors showed that chiropractic training in musculoskeletal medicine is significantly superior to allopathic and osteopathic musculoskeletal training.[360]

In accord with the comprehensive chiropractic training in musculoskeletal management, numerous sources of evidence demonstrate that chiropractic management of the most common spinal pain syndromes is safer and less expensive than allopathic medical treatment, particularly for the treatment of low-back pain. In their extensive review of the literature, Manga et al[361] published in 1993 that chiropractic management of low-back pain is superior to allopathic medical management in terms of greater safety, greater effectiveness, and reduced cost; they concluded, "There is an overwhelming body of evidence indicating that chiropractic management of low-back pain is more cost-effective than medical management" and "There would be highly significant cost savings if more management of LBP [low-back pain] was transferred from medical physicians to chiropractors." In a randomized trial involving 741 patients, Meade et al[362] showed, "Chiropractic treatment was more effective than hospital outpatient management, mainly for patients with chronic or severe back pain… The benefit of chiropractic treatment became more evident throughout the follow up period. Secondary outcome measures also showed that chiropractic was more beneficial." A 3-year follow-up study by these same authors[363] in 1995 showed, "At three years the results confirm the findings of an earlier report that when chiropractic or hospital therapists treat patients with low-back pain as they would in day to day practice, those treated by chiropractic derive more benefit and long term satisfaction than those treated by hospitals." More recently, in 2004 Legorreta et al[364] reported that the availability of chiropractic care was associated with significant cost savings among 700,000 patients with chiropractic coverage compared to 1 million patients whose insurance coverage was limited to allopathic medical treatments. Simple extrapolation of the average savings per patient in this study ($208 annual savings associated with chiropractic coverage) to the US population (295 million citizens in 2005[365]) suggests that, if fully implemented in a nation-wide basis, America could save $61,360,000,000 (more than $61 billion per year) in annual healthcare expenses by ensuring chiropractic for all citizens in contrast to failing to provide such coverage; obviously

competency increased when learning was reinforced during the clinical years." Schmale GA. More evidence of educational inadequacies in musculoskeletal medicine. *Clin Orthop Relat Res.* 2005 Aug;(437):251-9

[356] "RESULTS: When the minimum passing level as determined by orthopedic program directors was applied to the results of these examinations, 70.4% of graduating COM students (n=54) and 82% of allopathic graduates (n=85) failed to demonstrate basic competency in musculoskeletal medicine." Stockard AR, Allen TW. Competence levels in musculoskeletal medicine: comparison of osteopathic and allopathic medical graduates. *J Am Osteopath Assoc.* 2006 Jun;106(6):350-5

[357] "CONCLUSIONS: Internal medicine interns' perceive nutrition counseling as a priority, but lack the confidence and knowledge to effectively provide adequate nutrition education." Vetter ML, Herring SJ, Sood M, Shah NR, Kalet AL. What do resident physicians know about nutrition? An evaluation of attitudes, self-perceived proficiency and knowledge. *J Am Coll Nutr.* 2008 Apr;27(2):287-98

[358] "CONCLUSIONS: The amount of nutrition education that medical students receive continues to be inadequate." Adams KM, Kohlmeier M, Zeisel SH. Nutrition education in U.S. medical schools: latest update of a national survey. *Acad Med.* 2010 Sep;85(9):1537-42

[359] CONCLUSIONS: This survey suggests that multiple barriers exist that prevent the primary care practitioner from providing dietary counseling. A multifaceted approach will be needed to change physician counseling behavior." Kushner RF. Barriers to providing nutrition counseling by physicians: a survey of primary care practitioners. *Prev Med.* 1995 Nov;24(6):546-52

[360] Humphreys BK, Sulkowski A, McIntyre K, Kasiban M, Patrick AN. An examination of musculoskeletal cognitive competency in chiropractic interns. *J Manipulative Physiol Ther.* 2007;30(1):44-9

[361] Manga P, Angus D, Papadopoulos C, et al. The Effectiveness and Cost-Effectiveness of Chiropractic Management of Low-Back Pain. Richmond Hill, Ontario: Kenilworth Publishing; 1993

[362] Meade TW, Dyer S, Browne W, Townsend J, Frank AO. Low-back pain of mechanical origin: randomised comparison of chiropractic and hospital outpatient treatment. *BMJ.* 1990;300(6737):1431-7

[363] Meade TW, Dyer S, Browne W, Frank AO. Randomised comparison of chiropractic and hospital outpatient management for low-back pain: results from extended follow up. *BMJ.* 1995;311(7001):349-5

[364] Legorreta AP, Metz RD, Nelson CF, Ray S, Chernicoff HO, Dinubile NA. Comparative analysis of individuals with and without chiropractic coverage: patient characteristics, utilization, and costs. *Arch Intern Med.* 2004;164:1985-92

[365] US Census Bureau http://factfinder.census.gov/home/saff/main.html?_lang=en Accessed January 12, 2005

extrapolations such as this should consider other variables, such as the relatively higher prevalence of injury and death among patients treated with drugs and surgery.[366,367] Furthermore, whether the cost savings associated with chiropractic availability are due to 1) improved overall health and reduced need for pharmacosurgical intervention, 2) greater safety and lower cost of chiropractic treatment versus pharmacosurgical treatment, and/or 3) self-selection by wellness-oriented, perhaps healthier, and higher-income patients, remains to be determined.

A literature review by Dabbs and Lauretti[368] showed that spinal manipulation is safer than the use of NSAIDs in the treatment of neck pain. Contrasting the rates of manipulation-associated cerebrovascular accidents to the dangers of medical and surgical treatments for spinal disorders, Rosner[369] noted, "These rates are 400 times lower than the death rates observed from gastrointestinal bleeding due to the use of nonsteroidal anti-inflammatory drugs and 700 times lower than the overall mortality rate for spinal surgery." Similarly, in his review of the literature comparing the safety of chiropractic manipulation in patients with low-back pain associated with lumbar disc herniation, Oliphant[370] showed that, "The apparent safety of spinal manipulation, especially when compared with other [medically] accepted treatments for [lumbar disk herniation], should stimulate its use in the conservative treatment plan of [lumbar disk herniation]."

The clinical benefits and cost-effectiveness of chiropractic management of musculoskeletal conditions is extensively documented, and that spinal manipulation generally shows superior safety to drug and surgical treatment of back and neck pain is also well established.[371,372,373,374,375,376,377] Adjunctive therapies such as post-isometric relaxation[378] and correction of myofascial dysfunction[379] can lead to tremendous and rapid reductions in musculoskeletal pain without the hazards and expense associated with pharmaceutical drugs. Nonmusculoskeletal benefits of musculoskeletal/spinal manipulation include improved pulmonary function and/or quality of life in patients with asthma[380,381,382,383] and—according to a

---

[366] Rosner AL. Evidence-based clinical guidelines for the management of acute low-back pain: response to the guidelines prepared for the Australian Medical Health and Research Council. *J Manipulative Physiol Ther*. 2001;24(3):214-20

[367] Topol EJ. Failing the public health--rofecoxib, Merck, and the FDA. *N Engl J Med*. 2004 Oct 21;351(17):1707-9

[368] Dabbs V, Lauretti WJ. A risk assessment of cervical manipulation vs. NSAIDs for the treatment of neck pain. *J Manipulative Physiol Ther*. 1995;18:530-6

[369] Rosner AL. Evidence-based clinical guidelines for the management of acute low-back pain: response to the guidelines prepared for the Australian Medical Health and Research Council. *J Manipulative Physiol Ther*. 2001;24(3):214-20

[370] Oliphant D. Safety of spinal manipulation in the treatment of lumbar disk herniations: a systematic review and risk assessment. *J Manipulative Physiol Ther*. 2004;27:197-210

[371] Dabbs V, Lauretti WJ. A risk assessment of cervical manipulation vs. NSAIDs for the treatment of neck pain. *J Manipulative Physiol Ther*. 1995;18:530-6

[372] Rosner AL. Evidence-based clinical guidelines for the management of acute low-back pain: response to the guidelines prepared for the Australian Medical Health and Research Council. *J Manipulative Physiol Ther*. 2001 Mar-Apr;24(3):214-20

[373] Oliphant D. Safety of spinal manipulation in the treatment of lumbar disk herniations: a systematic review and risk assessment. *J Manipulative Physiol Ther*. 2004;27:197-210

[374] Meade TW, Dyer S, Browne W, Townsend J, Frank AO. Low-back pain of mechanical origin: randomised comparison of chiropractic and hospital outpatient treatment. *BMJ*. 1990;300(6737):1431-7

[375] Meade TW, Dyer S, Browne W, Frank AO. Randomised comparison of chiropractic and hospital outpatient management for low-back pain: results from extended follow up. *BMJ*. 1995;311(7001):349-5

[376] Manga P, Angus D, Papadopoulos C, et al. The Effectiveness and Cost-Effectiveness of Chiropractic Management of Low-Back Pain. Richmond Hill, Ontario: Kenilworth Publishing; 1993

[377] Legorreta AP, Metz RD, Nelson CF, Ray S, Chernicoff HO, Dinubile NA. Comparative analysis of individuals with and without chiropractic coverage: patient characteristics, utilization, and costs. *Arch Intern Med*. 2004;164:1985-92

[378] Lewit K, Simons DG. Myofascial pain: relief by post-isometric relaxation. *Arch Phys Med Rehabil*. 1984;65(8):452-6

[379] Ingber RS. Iliopsoas myofascial dysfunction: a treatable cause of "failed" low-back syndrome. *Arch Phys Med Rehabil*. 1989 May;70(5):382-6

[380] Nielson NH, Bronfort G, Bendix T, Madsen F, Wecke B. Chronic asthma and chiropractic spinal manipulation: a randomized clinical trial. *Clin Exp Allergy* 1995;25:80-8

[381] Mein EA, Greenman PE, McMillin DL, Richards DG, Nelson CD. Manual medicine diversity: research pitfalls and the emerging medical paradigm. *J Am Osteopath Assoc*. 2001 Aug;101(8):441-4

[382] "There were small increases (7 to 12 liters per minute) in peak expiratory flow in the morning and the evening in both treatment groups,… Symptoms of asthma and use of beta-agonists decreased and the quality of life increased in both groups, with no significant differences between the groups." Balon

series of cases published by an osteopathic ophthalmologist—improvement or restoration of vision in patients with post-traumatic and acute-onset visual loss.[384,385,386,387,388,389,390,391] More research is required to quantify the potential benefits of spinal manipulation in patients with wide-ranging conditions such as epilepsy[392,393], attention-deficit hyperactivity disorder[394,395], and Parkinson's disease.[396] Given that most pharmaceutical drugs work on single biochemical pathways, spinal manipulation is discordant with the medical/drug paradigm because its effects are numerous (rather than singular) and physical and physiological (rather than biochemical). Thus, when viewed through the allopathic/pharmaceutical lens, spinal manipulation (like acupuncture and other physical modalities) "does not make sense" and will be viewed as "unscientific" simply because it is based in physiology rather than pharmacology. In this case, the fault lies with the viewer and the lens, not with the object.

Research documenting the systemic and "nonmusculoskeletal" benefits of spinal manipulation mandates that our concept of "musculoskeletal" must be expanded to appreciate that **musculoskeletal interventions benefit nonmusculoskeletal body systems and physiologic processes**. This conceptual expansion applies also to soft tissue therapeutics such as massage, which can reduce adolescent aggression[397], improve outcome in preterm infants[398], alleviate premenstrual syndrome[399], and increase serotonin and dopamine levels in patients with low-back pain.[400]

J, Aker PD, Crowther ER, Danielson C, Cox PG, O'Shaughnessy D, Walker C, Goldsmith CH, Duku E, Sears MR. A comparison of active and simulated chiropractic manipulation as adjunctive treatment for childhood asthma. *N Engl J Med*. 1998 Oct 8;339(15):1013-20

[383] Bronfort G, Evans RL, Kubic P, Filkin P. Chronic pediatric asthma and chiropractic spinal manipulation: a prospective clinical series and randomized clinical pilot study. *J Manipulative Physiol Ther*. 2001 Jul-Aug;24(6):369-77

[384] Stephens D, Pollard H, Bilton D, Thomson P, Gorman F. Bilateral simultaneous optic nerve dysfunction after periorbital trauma: recovery of vision in association with chiropractic spinal manipulation therapy. *J Manipulative Physiol Ther*. 1999 Nov-Dec;22(9):615-21

[385] Stephens D, Gorman F, Bilton D. The step phenomenon in the recovery of vision with spinal manipulation: a report on two 13-yr-olds treated together. *J Manipulative Physiol Ther*. 1997;20(9):628-33

[386] Stephens D, Gorman F. The association between visual incompetence and spinal derangement: an instructive case history. *J Manipulative Physiol Ther*. 1997 Jun;20(5):343-50.

[387] Stephens D, Gorman RF. Does 'normal' vision improve with spinal manipulation? *J Manipulative Physiol Ther*. 1996 Jul-Aug;19(6):415-8

[388] Gorman RF. Monocular scotomata and spinal manipulation: the step phenomenon. *J Manipulative Physiol Ther*. 1996 Jun;19(5):344-9

[389] Gorman RF. Monocular visual loss after closed head trauma: immediate resolution associated with spinal manipulation. *J Manipulative Physiol Ther*. 1995 Jun;18(5):308-14

[390] Gorman RF. The treatment of presumptive optic nerve ischemia by spinal manipulation. *J Manipulative Physiol Ther*. 1995;18(3):172-7

[391] Gorman RF. Automated static perimetry in chiropractic. *J Manipulative Physiol Ther*. 1993 Sep;16(7):481-7

[392] Elster EL. Treatment of bipolar, seizure, and sleep disorders and migraine headaches utilizing a chiropractic technique. *J Manipulative Physiol* Ther. 2004 Mar-Apr;27(3):E5

[393] Alcantara J, Heschong R, Plaugher G, Alcantara J. Chiropractic management of a patient with subluxations, low-back pain and epileptic seizures. *J Manipulative Physiol Ther*. 1998;21(6):410-8

[394] Giesen JM, Center DB, Leach RA. An evaluation of chiropractic manipulation as a treatment of hyperactivity in children. *J Manipulative Physiol Ther*. 1989 Oct;12(5):353-63

[395] Bastecki AV, Harrison DE, Haas JW. Cervical kyphosis is a possible link to attention-deficit/hyperactivity disorder. *J Manipulative Physiol Ther*. 2004 Oct;27(8):e14

[396] Elster EL. Upper cervical chiropractic management of a patient with Parkinson's disease: a case report. *J Manipulative Physiol Ther*. 2000 Oct;23(8):573-7

[397] Diego MA, Field T, Hernandez-Reif M, Shaw JA, Rothe EM, Castellanos D, Mesner L. Aggressive adolescents benefit from massage therapy. *Adolescence* 2002 Fall;37(147):597-607

[398] Mainous RO. Infant massage as a component of developmental care: past, present, and future. *Holist Nurs Pract* 2002 Oct;16(5):1-7

[399] Hernandez-Reif M, Martinez A, Field T, Quintero O, Hart S, Burman I. Premenstrual symptoms are relieved by massage therapy. *J Psychosom Obstet Gynaecol* 2000 Mar;21(1):9-15

[400] "RESULTS: By the end of the study, the massage therapy group, as compared to the relaxation group, reported experiencing less pain, depression, anxiety and improved sleep. They also showed improved trunk and pain flexion performance, and their serotonin and dopamine levels were higher." Hernandez-Reif M, Field T, Krasnegor J, Theakston H. Lower back pain is reduced and range of motion increased after massage therapy. *Int J Neurosci* 2001;106(3-4):131-45

Spinal Manipulation: Mechanistic Considerations: Applied to either the spine or peripheral joints, high-velocity low-amplitude (HVLA) joint manipulation appears to have numerous physical and physiological effects, including but not limited to the following:

1. Releasing entrapped intraarticular menisci and synovial folds,
2. Acutely reducing intradiscal pressure, thus promoting replacement of decentralized disc material,
3. Stretching of deep periarticular muscles to break the cycle of chronic autonomous muscle contraction by lengthening the muscles and thereby releasing excessive actin-myosin binding,
4. Promoting restoration of proper kinesthesia and proprioception,
5. Promoting relaxation of paraspinal muscles by stretching facet joint capsules,
6. Promoting relaxation of paraspinal muscles via "postactivation depression", which is the temporary depletion of contractile neurotransmitters,
7. Temporarily elevating plasma beta-endorphin,
8. Temporarily enhancing phagocytic ability of neutrophils and monocytes,
9. Activation of the diffuse descending pain inhibitory system located in the periaqueductal gray matter—this is an important aspect of nociceptive inhibition by intense sensory/mechanoreceptor stimulation, which will be discussed in a following section for its relevance to neurogenic inflammation, and
10. Improving neurotransmitter balance and reducing pain (soft-tissue manipulation).[401]

While the above list of mechanisms-of-action is certainly not complete, for purposes of this paper it is sufficient for the establishment that—indeed—joint manipulation in general and spinal manipulation in particular have objective mechanistic effects that correlate with their clinical benefits. Additional details are provided in numerous published reviews and primary research[402,403,404,405,406,407,408] and by Leach[409], whose extensive description of the mechanisms of action of spinal manipulative therapy is unsurpassed. Given such a wide base of experimental and clinical support published in peer-reviewed journals and widely-available textbooks, denigrations directed toward spinal manipulation on the grounds that it is "unscientific" or "unsupported by research" are unfounded and are indicative of selective ignorance.

---

[401] "RESULTS: By the end of the study, the massage therapy group, as compared to the relaxation group, reported experiencing less pain, depression, anxiety and improved sleep. They also showed improved trunk and pain flexion performance, and their serotonin and dopamine levels were higher." Hernandez-Reif M, Field T, Krasnegor J, Theakston H. Lower back pain is reduced and range of motion increased after massage therapy. *Int J Neurosci* 2001;106(3-4):131-45

[402] Maigne JY, Vautravers P. Mechanism of action of spinal manipulative therapy. *Joint Bone Spine*. 2003;70(5):336-41

[403] Brennan PC, Triano JJ, McGregor M, Kokjohn K, Hondras MA, Brennan DC. Enhanced neutrophil respiratory burst as a biological marker for manipulation forces: duration of the effect and association with substance P and tumor necrosis factor. *J Manipulative Physiol Ther*. 1992 Feb;15(2):83-9

[404] Brennan PC, Kokjohn K, Kaltinger CJ, Lohr GE, Glendening C, Hondras MA, McGregor M, Triano JJ. Enhanced phagocytic cell respiratory burst induced by spinal manipulation: potential role of substance P. *J Manipulative Physiol Ther*. 1991 Sep;14(7):399-408

[405] Heikkila H, Johansson M, Wenngren BI. Effects of acupuncture, cervical manipulation and NSAID therapy on dizziness and impaired head repositioning of suspected cervical origin: a pilot study. *Man Ther*. 2000 Aug;5(3):151-7

[406] Rogers RG. The effects of spinal manipulation on cervical kinesthesia in patients with chronic neck pain: a pilot study. *J Manipulative Physiol Ther*. 1997;20(2):80-5

[407] Bergman, Peterson, Lawrence. Chiropractic Technique. New York: Churchill Livingstone 1993. An updated edition is now availabe from Mosby.

[408] Herzog WH. Mechanical and physiological responses to spinal manipulative treatments. *JNMS: J Neuromusculoskeltal System* 1995; 3: 1-9

[409] Leach RA. (ed). The Chiropractic Theories: A Textbook of Scientific Research, Fourth Edition. Baltimore: Lippincott, Williams & Wilkins, 2004

Mechanoreceptor-Mediated Inhibition of Neurogenic Inflammation: A Possible Mechanism of Action of Spinal Manipulation: Neurogenic inflammation causes catabolism of articular structures and thus promotes joint destruction[410,411], a phenomena that the current author has termed "neurogenic chondrolysis."[412] The biologic and scientific basis for this concept rests on the following sequence of events which ultimately form a self-perpetuating and multisystem cycle:

1. Using joint pain as an example, we know that acute or chronic joint injury results in the release of inflammatory mediators in local tissues as **immunogenic inflammation**.

2. Nociceptive input is received centrally and results in release of inflammatory mediators *from sensory neurons* termed **neurogenic inflammation**[413] and results in a neurologically-mediated catabolic effect in articular cartilage[414,415] termed here as **neurogenic chondrolysis**.

3. As immunogenic and neurogenic inflammation synergize to promote joint destruction, pain from degenerating joints further increases nociceptive afferent transmission to further increase neurogenic and thus immunogenic inflammation. Thus, a *positive feedback* vicious cycle of immunogenic and neurogenic inflammation promotes and perpetuates joint destruction.

4. Further complicating this *regional* cycle of neurogenic-immunogenic inflammation and tissue destruction would be any pain or inflammation *in distant parts of the body*, since pain in one part of the body can exacerbate neurogenic inflammation in another part of the body via **neurogenic switching**[416,417] and immunologic reactivity such as allergy or autoimmunity in one part of the body may be transmitted *via the nervous system* to cause immunogenic inflammation in another part of the body via **immunogenic switching.**[418]

The clinical relevance of neurogenic inflammation and immunogenic switching is that when combined they provide a means *beyond biochemistry* by which to understand how and why inflammation ❶ is *transmitted and perpetuated by the nervous system* and ❷ must be treated with a body-wide *holistic* approach.

      The current author is the first to propose the concept of **mechanoreceptor-mediated inhibition of neurogenic inflammation.**[419] Since neurogenic chondrolysis is inhibited by interference with C-fiber (type IV) mediated afferent transmission[420] and since chiropractic high-velocity low-amplitude (HVLA) manipulation appears to inhibit C-fiber mediated nociception[421,422], then chiropractic-type HVLA manipulation may reduce neurogenic

[410] Gouze-Decaris E, Philippe L, Minn A, Haouzi P, Gillet P, Netter P, Terlain B. Neurophysiological basis for neurogenic-mediated articular cartilage anabolism alteration. *Am J Physiol Regul Integr Comp Physiol*. 2001;280(1):R115-22

[411] Decaris E, Guingamp C, Chat M, Philippe L, Grillasca JP, Abid A, Minn A, Gillet P, Netter P, Terlain B. Evidence for neurogenic transmission inducing degenerative cartilage damage distant from local inflammation. *Arthritis Rheum*. 1999;42(9):1951-60

[412] Vasquez A. *Integrative Orthopedics: Exploring the Structural Aspect of the Matrix*. Applying Functional Medicine in Clinical Practice. Tampa, Florida November 29-December 4, 2004. Hosted by the Institute for Functional Medicine: www.FunctionalMedicine.org

[413] Meggs WJ.Mechanisms of allergy and chemical sensitivity. *Toxicol Ind Health*. 1999 Apr-Jun;15(3-4):331-8

[414] Gouze-Decaris E, Philippe L, Minn A, Haouzi P, Gillet P, Netter P, Terlain B. Neurophysiological basis for neurogenic-mediated articular cartilage anabolism alteration. *Am J Physiol Regul Integr Comp Physiol*. 2001;280(1):R115-22

[415] Decaris E, Guingamp C, Chat M, Philippe L, Grillasca JP, Abid A, Minn A, Gillet P, Netter P, Terlain B. Evidence for neurogenic transmission inducing degenerative cartilage damage distant from local inflammation. *Arthritis Rheum*. 1999;42(9):1951-60

[416] Meggs WJ. Neurogenic Switching: A Hypothesis for a Mechanism for Shifting the Site of Inflammation in Allergy and Chemical Sensitivity. *Environ Health Perspect* 1995; 103:54-56

[417] Meggs WJ. Mechanisms of allergy and chemical sensitivity. *Toxicol Ind Health*. 1999 Apr-Jun;15(3-4):331-8

[418] "...—immunogenic switching—... In this scenario, the afferent stimulation from the cranial vasculature, which is inflamed during a migraine because of neurogenic processes, is rerouted by the CNS to produce immunogenic inflammation at the nose and sinuses." Cady RK, Schreiber CP. Sinus headache or migraine? Considerations in making a differential diagnosis. *Neurology*. 2002;58(9 Suppl 6):S10-4

[419] Vasquez A. *Integrative Orthopedics: Exploring the Structural Aspect of the Matrix*. Applying Functional Medicine in Clinical Practice. Tampa, Florida November 29-December 4, 2004. Hosted by the Institute for Functional Medicine: www.FunctionalMedicine.org

[420] Gouze-Decaris E, Philippe L, Minn A, Haouzi P, Gillet P, Netter P, Terlain B. Neurophysiological basis for neurogenic-mediated articular cartilage anabolism alteration. *Am J Physiol Regul Integr Comp Physiol*. 2001;280(1):R115-22

[421] Gillette R. A speculative argument for the coactivation of diverse somatic receptor populations by forceful chiropractic adjustments. *Man Med* 1987; 3:1-14

[422] Boal RW, Gillette RG. Central neuronal plasticity, low-back pain and spinal manipulative therapy. *J Manipulative Physiol Ther*. 2004;27(5):314-26

inflammation and may promote articular integrity by inhibiting neurogenic chondrolysis. Further, mechanoreceptor-mediated inhibition of neurogenic inflammation would, for example, help explain the benefits of spinal manipulation in the treatment of asthma[423,424,425], since asthma is known to be mediated in large part by neurogenic inflammation.[426,427] Thus, spinal manipulation appears to provide a means—*in addition to the use of other anti-inflammatory interventions such as diet, lifestyle and phytonutritional interventions*—by which pain and inflammation can be treated naturally, without drugs and surgery.

A science-based comprehensive protocol can be implemented against pain and inflammation by using ❶ an anti-inflammatory diet, ❷ frequent exercise, ❸ lifestyle and bodyweight optimization, ❹ nutritional supplementation, ❺ botanical supplementation[428,429], ❻ spinal manipulation (with its kinesthetic, analgesic, *directly* and *indirectly* anti-inflammatory, and *probably* piezoelectric benefits[430]), ❼ stress reduction[431,432], ❽ anti-dysbiosis protocols[433], ❾ hormonal correction ("orthoendocrinology"), and ❿ ancillary treatments such as acupuncture.[434,435] Additional details and citations for these interventions are provided in chapter 3 of *Integrative Orthopedics*[436] and chapter 4 of *Integrative Rheumatology*.[437] Pain and inflammation are self-perpetuating vicious cycles, well suited to intervention with comprehensive and multicomponent treatment plans as profiled above.

Wilk vs American Medical Association

The following two pages provide the transcript of the judgement in 1987 that supposedly ended the American Medical Association's antitrust violations and attempt to destroy the chiropractic profession.

---

[423] Nielson NH, Bronfort G, Bendix T, Madsen F, Wecke B. Chronic asthma and chiropractic spinal manipulation: a randomized clinical trial. *Clin Exp Allergy* 1995;25:80-8

[424] "There were small increases (7 to 12 liters per minute) in peak expiratory flow in the morning and the evening in both treatment groups,… Symptoms of asthma and use of beta-agonists decreased and the quality of life increased in both groups, with no significant differences between the groups." Balon J, Aker PD, Crowther ER, Danielson C, Cox PG, O'Shaughnessy D, Walker C, Goldsmith CH, Duku E, Sears MR. A comparison of active and simulated chiropractic manipulation as adjunctive treatment for childhood asthma. *N Engl J Med*. 1998 Oct 8;339(15):1013-20

[425] Bronfort G, Evans RL, Kubic P, Filkin P. Chronic pediatric asthma and chiropractic spinal manipulation: a prospective clinical series and randomized clinical pilot study. *J Manipulative Physiol Ther*. 2001 Jul-Aug;24(6):369-77

[426] Renz H. Neurotrophins in bronchial asthma. *Respir Res*. 2001;2(5):265-8

[427] Groneberg DA, Quarcoo D, Frossard N, Fischer A. Neurogenic mechanisms in bronchial inflammatory diseases. *Allergy*. 2004 Nov; 59(11): 1139-52

[428] Jancso N, Jancso-Gabor A, Szolcsanyi J. Direct evidence for neurogenic inflammation and its prevention by denervation and by pretreatment with capsaicin. *Br J Pharmacol*. 1967 Sep;31(1):138-51

[429] Miller MJ, Vergnolle N, McKnight W, Musah RA, Davison CA, Trentacosti AM, Thompson JH, Sandoval M, Wallace JL. Inhibition of neurogenic inflammation by the Amazonian herbal medicine sangre de grado. *J Invest Dermatol*. 2001;117(3):725-30

[430] Lipinski B. Biological significance of piezoelectricity in relation to acupuncture, Hatha Yoga, osteopathic medicine and action of air ions. *Med Hypotheses*. 1977;3(1):9-12 See also: Athenstaedt H. Pyroelectric and piezoelectric properties of vertebrates. *Ann N Y Acad Sci*. 1974;238:68-94 See also: Athenstaedt H. "Functional polarity" of the spinal cord caused by its longitudinal electric dipole moment. *Am J Physiol*. 1984;247(3 Pt 2):R482-7

[431] Lutgendorf S, Logan H, Kirchner HL, Rothrock N, Svengalis S, Iverson K, Lubaroff D. Effects of relaxation and stress on the capsaicin-induced local inflammatory response. *Psychosom Med*. 2000;62:524-34

[432] "Couples who demonstrated consistently higher levels of hostile behaviors across both their interactions healed at 60% of the rate of low-hostile couples. High-hostile couples also produced relatively larger increases in plasma IL-6 and tumor necrosis factor alpha…" Kiecolt-Glaser JK, Loving TJ, Stowell JR, Malarkey WB, Lemeshow S, Dickinson SL, Glaser R. Hostile marital interactions, proinflammatory cytokine production, and wound healing. *Arch Gen Psychiatry*. 2005 Dec;62(12):1377-84

[433] Chapter 4 of Integrative Rheumatology and Vasquez A. Reducing Pain and Inflammation Naturally. Part 6: Nutritional and Botanical Treatments Against "Silent Infections" and Gastrointestinal Dysbiosis, Commonly Overlooked Causes of Neuromusculoskeletal Inflammation and Chronic Health Problems. *Nutr Perspect* 2006; Jan http://optimalhealthresearch.com/part6

[434] Joos S, Brinkhaus B, Maluche C, Maupai N, Kohnen R, Kraehmer N, Hahn EG, Schuppan D. Acupuncture and moxibustion in the treatment of active Crohn's disease: a randomized controlled study. *Digestion*. 2004;69(3):131-9

[435] "These results demonstrate an unorthodox new type of neurohumoral regulatory mechanism of sensory fibres and provide a possible mode of action for the anti-inflammatory effect of counter-irritation and acupuncture." Pinter E, Szolcsanyi J. Systemic anti-inflammatory effect induced by antidromic stimulation of the dorsal roots in the rat. *Neurosci Lett*. 1996;212(1):33-6

[436] Vasquez A. Integrative Orthopedics: Second Edition. Fort Worth, Texas; Integrative and Biological Medicine Research and Consulting, 2007 OptimalHealthResearch.com

[437] Vasquez A. Integrative Rheumatology: Second Edition. Fort Worth, Texas; Integrative and Biological Medicine Research and Consulting, 2007 OptimalHealthResearch.com

Special Communication

IN THE UNITED STATES DISTRICT COURT
FOR THE NORTHERN DISTRICT OF ILLINOIS
EASTERN DIVISION

CHESTER A. WILK, et al.,   )
)
            Plaintiffs,)
)
            v.   ) No. 76 C
) 3777
AMERICAN MEDICAL ASSOCIATION,)
et al.,   )
)
            Defendants.)

PERMANENT INJUNCTION ORDER AGAINST AMA

Susan Getzendanner, District Judge

The court conducted a lengthy trial of this case in May and June of 1987 and on August 27, 1987, issued a 101 page opinion finding that the American Medical Association ("AMA") and its members participated in a conspiracy against chiropractors in violation of the nation's antitrust laws. Thereafter an opinion dated September 25, 1987 was substituted for the August 27, 1987 opinion. The question now before the court is the form of injunctive relief that the court will order.

See also p 83.

As part of the injunctive relief to be ordered by the court against the AMA, the AMA shall be required to send a copy of this Permanent Injunction Order to each of its current members. The members of the AMA are bound by the terms of the Permanent Injunction Order if they act in concert with the AMA to violate the terms of the order. Accordingly, it is important that the AMA members understand the order and the reasons why the order has been entered.

The AMA's Boycott and Conspiracy

In the early 1960s, the AMA decided to contain and eliminate chiropractic as a profession. In 1963 the AMA's Committee on Quackery was formed. The committee worked aggressively—both overtly and covertly—to eliminate chiropractic. One of the principal means used by the AMA to achieve its goal was to make it unethical for medical physicians to professionally associate with chiropractors. Under Principle 3 of the AMA's Principles of Medical Ethics, it was unethical for a physician to associate with an "unscientific practitioner," and in 1966 the AMA's House of Delegates passed a resolution calling chiropractic an unscientific cult. To complete the circle, in 1967 the AMA's Judicial Council issued an opinion under Principle 3 holding that it was unethical for a physician to associate professionally with chiropractors.

The AMA's purpose was to prevent medical physicians from referring patients to chiropractors and accepting referrals of patients from chiropractors, to prevent chiropractors from obtaining access to hospital diagnostic services and membership on hospital medical staffs, to prevent medical physicians from teaching at chiropractic colleges or engaging in any joint research, and to prevent any cooperation between the two groups in the delivery of health care services.

Published by order of Susan Getzendanner, US District Judge, Sept 25, 1987.

The AMA believed that the boycott worked—that chiropractic would have achieved greater gains in the absence of the boycott. Since no medical physician would want to be considered unethical by his peers, the success of the boycott is not surprising. However, chiropractic achieved licensing in all 50 states during the existence of the Committee on Quackery.

The Committee on Quackery was disbanded in 1975 and some of the committee's activities became publicly known. Several lawsuits were filed by or on behalf of chiropractors and this case was filed in 1976.

Change in AMA's Position on Chiropractic

In 1977, the AMA began to change its position on chiropractic. The AMA's Judicial Council adopted new opinions under which medical physicians could refer patients to chiropractors, but there was still the proviso that the medical physician should be confident that the services to be provided on referral would be performed in accordance with accepted scientific standards. In 1979, the AMA's House of Delegates adopted Report UU which said that not everything that a chiropractor may do is without therapeutic value, but it stopped short of saying that such things were based on scientific standards. It was not until 1980 that the AMA revised its Principles of Medical Ethics to eliminate Principle 3. Until Principle 3 was formally eliminated, there was considerable ambiguity about the AMA's position. The ethics code adopted in 1980 provided that a medical physician "shall be free to choose whom to serve, with whom to associate, and the environment in which to provide medical services."

The AMA settled three chiropractic lawsuits by stipulating and agreeing that under the current opinions of the Judicial Council a physician may, without fear of discipline or sanction by the AMA, refer a patient to a duly licensed chiropractor when he believes that referral may benefit the patient. The AMA confirmed that a physician may also choose to accept or to decline patients sent to him by a duly licensed chiropractor. Finally, the AMA confirmed that a physician may teach at a chiropractic college or seminar. These settlements were entered into in 1978, 1980, and 1986.

The AMA's present position on chiropractic, as stated to the court, is that it is ethical for a medical physician to professionally associate with chiropractors provided the physician believes that such association is in the best interests of his patient. This position has not previously been communicated by the AMA to its members.

Antitrust Laws

Under the Sherman Act, every combination or conspiracy in restraint of trade is illegal. The court has held that the conduct of the AMA and its members constituted a conspiracy in restraint of trade based on the following facts: the purpose of the boycott was to eliminate chiropractic; chiropractors are in competition with some medical physicians; the boycott had substantial anti-competitive effects; there were no pro-competitive effects of the boycott; and the plaintiffs were injured as a result of the conduct. These facts add up to a violation of the Sherman Act.

In this case, however, the court allowed the defendants the opportunity to establish a "patient care defense" which has the following elements:

(1) that they genuinely entertained a concern for what they perceive as scientific method in the care of each person with whom they have entered into a doctor-patient relationship; (2) that this concern is objectively reasonable; (3) that this concern has been the dominant motivating factor in defendants' promulgation of Principle 3 and in the

conduct intended to implement it; and (4) that this concern for scientific method in patient care could not have been adequately satisfied in a manner less restrictive of competition.

The court concluded that the AMA had a genuine concern for scientific methods in patient care, and that this concern was the dominant factor in motivating the AMA's conduct. However, the AMA failed to establish that throughout the entire period of the boycott, from 1966 to 1980, this concern was objectively reasonable. The court reached that conclusion on the basis of extensive testimony from both witnesses for the plaintiffs and the AMA that some forms of chiropractic treatment are effective and the fact that the AMA recognized that chiropractic began to change in the early 1970s. Since the boycott was not formally over until Principle 3 was eliminated in 1980, the court found that the AMA was unable to establish that during the entire period of the conspiracy its position was objectively reasonable. Finally, the court ruled that the AMA's concern for scientific method in patient care could have been adequately satisfied in a manner less restrictive of competition and that a nationwide conspiracy to eliminate a licensed profession was not justified by the concern for scientific method. On the basis of these findings, the court concluded that the AMA had failed to establish the patient care defense.

None of the court's findings constituted a judicial endorsement of chiropractic. All of the parties to the case, including the plaintiffs and the AMA, agreed that chiropractic treatment of diseases such as diabetes, high blood pressure, cancer, heart disease and infectious disease is not proper, and that the historic theory of chiropractic, that there is a single cause and cure of disease is wrong. There was disagreement between the parties as to whether chiropractors should engage in diagnosis. There was evidence that the chiropractic theory of subluxations was unscientific, and evidence that some chiropractors engaged in unscientific practices. The court did not reach the question of whether chiropractic theory was in fact scientific. However, the evidence in the case was that some forms of chiropractic manipulation of the spine and joints was therapeutic. AMA witnesses, including the present Chairman of the Board of Trustees of the AMA, testified that some forms of treatment by chiropractors, including manipulation, can be therapeutic in the treatment of conditions such as back pain syndrome.

Need for Injunctive Relief

Although the conspiracy ended in 1980, there are lingering effects of the illegal boycott and conspiracy which require an injunction. Some medical physicians' individual decisions on whether or not to professionally associate with chiropractors are still affected by the boycott. The injury to chiropractors' reputations which resulted from the boycott has not been repaired. Chiropractors suffer current economic injury as a result of the boycott. The AMA has never affirmatively acknowledged that there are and should be no collective impediments to professional association and cooperation between chiropractors and medical physicians, except as provided by law. Instead, the AMA has consistently argued that its conduct has not violated the antitrust laws.

Most importantly, the court believes that it is important that the AMA members be made aware of the present AMA position that it is ethical for a medical physician to professionally associate with a chiropractor if the physician believes it is in the best interests of his patient, so that the lingering effects of the illegal group boycott against chiropractors finally can be dissipated.

Under the law, every medical physician, institution, and hospital has the right to make an individual decision as to whether or not that physician, institution, or hospital shall associate professionally with chiropractors. Individual choice by a medical physician voluntarily to associate professionally with chiropractors should be governed only by restrictions under state law, if any, and by the individual medical physician's personal judgment as to what is in the best interest of a patient or patients. Professional association includes referrals, consultations, group practice in partnerships, Health Maintenance Organizations, Preferred Provider Organizations, and other alternative health care delivery systems; the provision of treatment privileges and diagnostic services (including radiological and other laboratory facilities) in or through hospital facilities; association and cooperation in educational programs for students in chiropractic colleges; and cooperation in research, health care seminars, and continuing education programs.

An injunction is necessary to assure that the AMA does not interfere with the right of a physician, hospital, or other institution to make an individual decision on the question of professional association.

Form of Injunction

1. The AMA, its officers, agents and employees, and all persons who act in active concert with any of them and who receive actual notice of this order are hereby permanently enjoined from restricting, regulating or impeding, or aiding and abetting others from restricting, regulating or impeding, the freedom of any AMA member or any institution or hospital to make an individual decision as to whether or not that AMA member, institution, or hospital shall professionally associate with chiropractors, chiropractic students, or chiropractic institutions.

2. This Permanent Injunction does not and shall not be construed to restrict or otherwise interfere with the AMA's right to take positions on any issue, including chiropractic, and to express or publicize those positions, either alone or in conjunction with others. Nor does this Permanent Injunction restrict or otherwise interfere with the AMA's right to petition or testify before any public body on any legislative or regulatory measure or to join or cooperate with any other entity in so petitioning or testifying. The AMA's membership in a recognized accrediting association or society shall not constitute a violation of this Permanent Injunction.

3. The AMA is directed to send a copy of this order to each AMA member and employee, first class mail, postage prepaid, within thirty days of the entry of this order. In the alternative, the AMA shall provide the Clerk of the Court with mailing labels so that the court may send this order to AMA members and employees.

4. The AMA shall cause the publication of this order in JAMA and the indexing of the order under "Chiropractic" so that persons desiring to find the order in the future will be able to do so.

5. The AMA shall prepare a statement of the AMA's present position on chiropractic for inclusion in the current reports and opinions of the Judicial Council with an appropriate heading that refers to professional association between medical physicians and chiropractors, and indexed in the same manner that other reports and opinions are indexed. The court imposes no restrictions on the AMA's statement but only requires that it be consistent with the AMA's statements of its present position to the court.

6. The AMA shall file a report with the court evidencing compliance with this order on or before January 10, 1988.

It is so ordered.

Susan Getzendanner
United States District Judge

Naturopathic Medicine

"The work of the naturopathic physician is to elicit healing by helping patients to create or recreate conditions for health to exist within them. Health will occur where the conditions for health exist. Disease is the product of conditions which allow for it."

Jared Zeff, ND[438]

The diagram to the right is derived from the review by Zeff published in 1997 in *Journal of Naturopathic Medicine* entitled "The process of healing: a unifying theory of naturopathic medicine." By my interpretation, the diagram is important for at least three reasons.

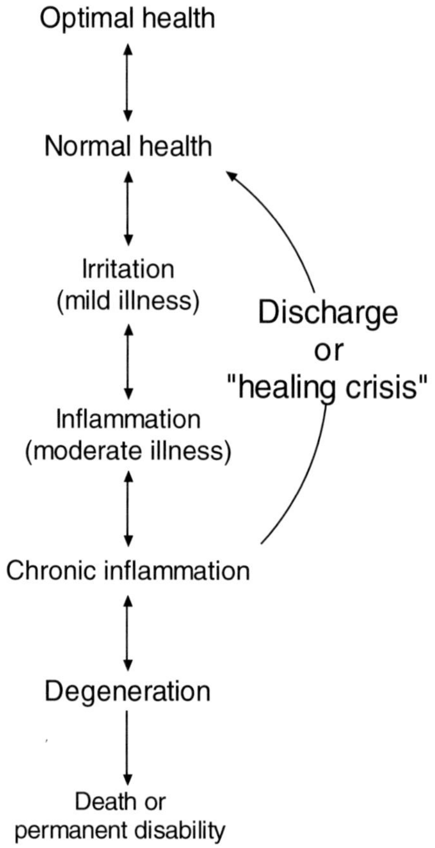

First, whereas the allopathic profession describes the genesis of most diseases as *idiopathic* and therefore [somehow] exclusively serviceable by drugs and surgery, the naturopathic profession describes disease processes as *multifactorial* and *logical* and therefore treatable by the skilled discovery and treatment of the underlying causes. Such underlying causes, which nearly always occur as a plurality, may vary mildly or significantly even within a group of patients with the same diagnosis.

Second, the diagram shows that the development of disease and the restoration of health are both *processes*. The restoration and retention of health requires *intentionality* and *tenacity* in lieu of the simplistic *miracle medicines* and *passive treatments* proffered by the pharmaceutical industry. Generally, disease does not arrive from outside; it is the result of one or more internal imbalances. Chronic illness is generally the result of manifold internal imbalances that culminate in numerous physiologic insults which compromise essential functions to the point that one or more organ systems begin to fail; we as patients and doctors generally label this as some specific "disease" or other, and the general—often erroneous—assumption has been that each *specific disease* (i.e., label, …abstraction, …conceptual entity) requires a *specific treatment* rather than a generalized health-restorative approach. Health is restored through a progressive and stepwise program that addresses as many facets of the illness as possible while vigorously supporting optimal physiologic function.

Third, the fact that Zeff considered the discharge or "healing crisis" so important that it merited inclusion in this diagram shows, indirectly, the naturopathic emphasis on detoxification and the eradication of dysbiosis. Both in the treatment of toxic metal/chemical exposure and in the treatment of chronic infections, patients often go through an acute or subacute phase of feeling ill before experiencing a dramatic alleviation of symptoms; the fact that symptoms may temporarily "get worse before getting better" has been referred to as the "healing crisis." This can

Optimal health

Normal health

Irritation
(mild illness)

Inflammation
(moderate illness)

Discharge
or
"healing crisis"

Chronic inflammation

Degeneration

Death or
permanent disability

---

[438] Zeff JL. The process of healing: a unifying theory of naturopathic medicine. *Journal of Naturopathic Medicine* 1997; 7: 122-5

occur for at least three reasons. First, in the elimination of chemicals and metals from the body, they must first be released from the tissues; the transition from tissues to blood is similar to a subacute re-exposure which triggers symptoms of toxicity until the toxin is excreted via sweat, urine, bile, or breath. Similarly, improvement in nutritional status—a cornerstone of all naturopathic interventions—expedites/facilitates/restores physiologic processes that have been relatively dormant due to lack of enzymatic cofactors such as vitamins and minerals[439]; optimization of nutritional status provides an opportunity for these pathways (such as detoxification of stored xenobiotics) to function again at which time they must "catch up" on work that has not been performed during the time of nutritional deficiency. The activation of these pathways is an essential step toward health restoration but results in an initial upregulation of hepatic phase-1/oxidative biotransformation which often results in the formation of reactive intermediates that temporarily impair physiologic processes and cause an initial exacerbation of symptoms. Third, whether through immunorestoration or the use of botanical/pharmacologic antimicrobial agents, the symptom-exacerbating "die off" reaction—classically called the Jarisch-Herxheimer reaction in the context of treating syphilis—is a result of increased (endo)toxin production/release by bacteria/microbes in response effective antimicrobial processes, whether physiologic or pharmacologic.

Modern naturopathic medicine has grown from deeply rooted European healing traditions reaching back several centuries. Naturopathic physicians have unwaveringly demonstrated respect, love, and appreciation for the healing powers of nature and the process of life itself.[440] Following their coursework in the basic biomedical sciences, naturopathic physicians are trained in urology, oncology, neurology, pediatrics, obstetrics and gynecology, urology, manual physical manipulation (including spinal manipulation), minor surgery, medical procedures, professional ethics, therapeutic diets, clinical and interventional nutrition, botanical medicines, psychological counseling, environmental medicine, and other modalities. Licensed naturopathic physicians commonly practice as generalists and family doctors.[441,442,443,444]

Naturopathic Principles, Concepts, & the *Vis Medicatrix Naturae*

"The healing power of nature is the inherent self-organizing and healing process of living systems… It is the naturopathic physician's role to support, facilitate and augment this process by identifying and removing obstacles to health and recovery, and by supporting the creation of a healthy internal and external environment."[445]

1. **First, Do No Harm (*Primum Non Nocere*)**: Naturopathic physicians use good judgment and compassion to ensure that the treatment does not cause harm to the patient. This

[439] Ames BN. The metabolic tune-up: metabolic harmony and disease prevention. *J Nutr*. 2003 May;133(5 Suppl 1):1544S-8S

[440] Kirchfeld F, Boyle W. Nature Doctors: Pioneers in Naturopathic Medicine. Portland, Oregon; Medicina Biologica (Buckeye Naturopathic Press, East Palestine, Ohio), 1994

[441] Boon HS, Cherkin DC, Erro J, Sherman KJ, Milliman B, Booker J, Cramer EH, Smith MJ, Deyo RA, Eisenberg DM. Practice patterns of naturopathic physicians: results from a random survey of licensed practitioners in two US States. *BMC Complement Altern Med*. 2004;4(1):14

[442] Smith MJ, Logan AC. Naturopathy. *Med Clin North Am*. 2002 Jan;86(1):173-84

[443] Cherkin DC, Deyo RA, Sherman KJ, et al. Characteristics of visits to licensed acupuncturists, chiropractors, massage therapists, and naturopathic physicians. *J Am Board Fam Pract*. 2002 Nov-Dec;15(6):463-72

[444] Cherkin DC, Deyo RA, Sherman KJ, et al. Characteristics of licensed acupuncturists, chiropractors, massage therapists, and naturopathic physicians. *J Am Board Fam Pract*. 2002 Sep-Oct;15(5):378-90

[445] Quoted from the American Association of Naturopathic Physicians website http://aanp.net/Basics/h.naturo.philo.html on February 4, 2001. Other italicized quotes in this section are from the same source. This website has since been replaced by http://naturopathic.org/

contrasts with the effects of allopathic treatment, which collectively kill more than 180,000-220,000 patients per year, at least 493 American patients per day.[446]

2. **Identify and Treat the Causes (Tolle Causam):** *"Illness does not occur without cause."* Naturopathic physicians focus on identifying and addressing the underlying deficiency, toxicity, impairment, or imbalance that is the cause of the health problem or disease.

3. **Treat the Whole Person:** *"The multifactorial nature of health and disease requires a personalized and comprehensive approach to diagnosis and treatment."* On some occasions the illness does take precedence over the person who has it—such in emergency situations like septic arthritis, acute ischemia, and pulmonary edema. In these cases, the situation must be managed appropriately, and these situations are not immediately amenable to long-term lifestyle changes—they require immediate treatment. However, the vast majority of cases in routine outpatient clinical practice will require detailed and bipartite attention to the facets of both **the disease process** and **the person who has the illness**. Our focus as naturopathic physicians on the individual patient is what sets our healing profession apart from others that focus exclusively on the disease and do not consider the manifold intricacies of the individual patient.

4. **The Healing Power of Nature: *Vis Medicatrix Naturae*:** Naturopathic medicine recognizes an inherent self-healing process in the person that is ordered and intelligent. The body has many highly efficient mechanisms for sustaining and regaining health. These mechanisms have their specific and necessary components (e.g., nutrients) and means by which they can be impaired (e.g., xenobiotic immunosuppression). Poor health and disease can result from impairment of these self-healing processes and biologic mechanisms, and thus the body's inherent, natural, self-healing mechanisms—the "healing power of nature"—can be diminished to the state of ineffectiveness or harm (e.g., autoimmunity). Recognizing that the body has this inherent goal of and movement toward self-healing, naturopathic physicians start by identifying and removing "obstacles to cure" rather than ignoring these factors and masking the manifestations of dysfunction with symptom-suppressing drugs.

5. **Prevention:** Healthy lifestyle, proper nutrition, and emotional hygiene go a long way toward preventing (and treating) most conditions. Specific conditions have specific risk factors and causes that have to be considered per patient and condition.

6. **Doctor As Teacher (Docere):** Naturopathic physicians explain the situation and the proposed solution to the patient so that the patient is empowered with understanding and with the comfort of knowing what has happened, what is happening, and the proposed course of upcoming events. Naturopathic physicians strive to let their own lives serve as a models for our patients. This does not mean that naturopathic doctors have to feign perfection; the task is to live the best and most conscious life that we can, to be present with our emotions, qualities, and faults and to treat ourselves with respect and acceptance. We can exemplify health (rather than perfection) to our

> **"Physician, heal thyself.**
> Thus you help your patient, too.
> Let this be his best medicine that he beholds with his eyes: the doctor who heals himself."
>
> Nietzsche FW. Thus Spoke Zarathustra (1892). [Kaufmann W, translator]. Viking Penguin: 1954, page 77

---

[446] "Recent estimates suggest that each year more than 1 million patients are injured while in the hospital and approximately 180,000 die because of these injuries. Furthermore, drug-related morbidity and mortality are common and are estimated to cost more than $136 billion a year." Holland EG, Degruy FV. Drug-induced disorders. *Am Fam Physician*. 1997;56(7):1781-8, 1791-2

patients by being who we authentically are and by so doing we can facilitate their own acceptance of their current health situation, which is a prerequisite to self-initiated change.

7. **Re-Establish the Foundation for Health**: An overview of this important naturopathic concept is provided throughout this chapter.

8. **Removing "obstacles to cure"**: *examples*

Obstacle to the optimization of health	*Example of possible intervention*
o Toxic exposures, medication side-effects	▪ Reduce drug use and dependency
o Toxic relationships, emotional obstacles, past events, unfulfilling occupation,	▪ Improve self-esteem, develop conflict resolution skills, determine life goals and values and a plan for their pursuit
o Social isolation: the typical American has only two friends no-one in whom to confide[447]	▪ Encourage social interaction
o Diet with excess fat, arachidonate, sugar, additives, colorants, and insufficiency of protein, fiber, phytonutrients, and health-promoting fatty acids: ALA, GLA, EPA, DHA, and oleic acid	▪ Diet improvement and nutritional supplementation
o Sedentary lifestyle, lack of exercise	▪ Encourage exercise
o Weight gain/loss as necessary for weight optimization	▪ Encourage self-valuing
o Epidemic exposure to mercury, lead, and xenobiotics	▪ Support detoxification process as a lifestyle

Hierarchy of Therapeutics: This naturopathic concept articulates the importance of addressing *the underlying cause* rather than simply focusing on *the presenting problem*, which is the *symptom of the cause*. Further, interventions are **prioritized**, *for example*:

- Patient-implemented *before* doctor-implemented.
- Removal of harming agent *before* addition of a therapeutic agent: e.g., stop smoking *before* investing in respiratory therapy; implement healthy diet and exercise before higher-risk and higher-cost drugs for hypertension and hypercholesterolemia.
- Low-force interventions *before* high-force interventions.
- Diet *before* nutritional supplements; nutrients *before* botanicals; botanicals *before* drugs; modulatory drugs *before* suppressive/inhibitory drugs; integrative care *before* surgery.
- *See table on following page.*

---

[447] McPherson M, Smith-Lovin L, Brashears ME. Social Isolation in America: Changes in Core Discussion Networks over Two Decades. *American Sociological Review* 2006; 71: 353-75 http://www.asanet.org/galleries/default-file/June06ASRFeature.pdf

Hierarchy of Therapeutics (specifically sequential)	Example of possible intervention
1. Reestablishing the foundation for health	• Mental/emotional/spiritual health • Meditation, freeze-frame, "time out" • Relaxation • Positive visualization, positive expectation, affirmation • Counseling, social contact, group work[448] • Family contact and resolution • Dietary intake and nutritional health which addresses the patient's biochemical individuality[449] and correction of deficiencies or excesses • Identification and elimination of food allergies and food sensitivities • Reduce toxin exposure, promote detoxification • Identification and elimination of exposure to gastrointestinal and inhalant xenobiotics • Remove or reduce specific "obstacles to cure"
2. Stimulation of the "healing power of nature" and the "vital force"	• Constitutional hydrotherapy • Homeopathy • Exercise • Acupuncture, Spinal manipulation • Meditation, rest • Tai Chi, Qigong: "energy-cultivation" • Botanical adaptogens
3. Tonification of weakened systems:	• Botanical medicines and other supplements to help restore normal tissue function • Spinal manipulation to address the primary somatovisceral dysfunction and/or secondary musculoskeletal disorders • Hormonal supplementation • Nutritional supplementation • Exercise • Physiotherapy
4. Correction of structural integrity:	• Spinal manipulation, deep tissue massage, visceral manipulation, lymphatic pump to promote immune surveillance[450] • Stretching, balancing, muscle strengthening, and proprioceptive retraining • Surgery, as a last resort

---

[448] See http://www.mkp.org and www.WomanWithin.org for examples.
[449] Williams RJ. Biochemical Individuality: The Basis for the Genetotrophic Concept. Austin and London: University of Texas Press, 1956
[450] "Lymph flow in the thoracic duct increased from 1.57±0.20 mL·min-1 to a peak TDF of 4.80±1.73 mL·min-1 during abdominal pump, and from 1.20±0.41 mL·min-1 to 3.45±1.61 mL·min-1 during thoracic pump." Knott EM, Tune JD, Stoll ST, Downey HF. Increased lymphatic flow in the thoracic duct during manipulative intervention. *J Am Osteopath Assoc.* 2005 Oct;105(10):447-56 http://www.jaoa.org/cgi/content/full/105/10/447

Osteopathic Medicine

Osteopathic medicine and chiropractic are American-born healthcare professions and paradigms that started at nearly the same time in history and from many of the same foundational principles. Both professions were started in the late 1800's and early 1900's and were founded upon the philosophical premise that the body functioned as a whole and that therefore medicine in general and therapeutic interventions in particular needed to be comprehensive in scope and multifaceted in their application. Further, both professions emphasized the importance of structural integrity as a foundational component of health and thus embraced manual manipulative therapy and spinal manipulation.

From their common origins, subtle differences and chance historic events shaped and further separated these professions from each other. Osteopathy was founded by Andrew Taylor Still, a medical doctor who sought to reform what was then called the "Heroic" paradigm of medicine, which embraced bloodletting and the administration of leeches, purgatives, emetics, and poisons such as mercury as means for "rebalancing" what were perceived to be internal causes of disease, namely the "four humours" of the body which were thought to be blood, phlegm, black bile, and yellow bile. In part because of his training within and identification with the medical profession, Still sought to *reform* rather than *directly oppose* the "mainstream medicine" of his day; in contrast, chiropractic's founder Daniel David Palmer was more strongly opposed to the horrific medicine of his time and thus was more *revolutionary* than *evolutionary* in his approach to forging a new paradigm of health and healthcare. Still's willingness to align with the medical profession and the increasingly powerful and influential pharmaceutical industry unquestionably helped his fledgling profession survive the extinction that otherwise would have been swift at the hands of allopathic groups such as **the American Medical Association (AMA), which labeled osteopathic physicians as "cultists" and systematically restricted inclusion of the osteopathic profession into mainstream healthcare by proclamation in 1953 that "…all voluntary associations with osteopaths are unethical." When osteopathic resistance mounted, the AMA and its co-conspirators, who were later found guilty of violating the nation's antitrust laws by illegally suppressing competition and attempting to build a medical monopoly**[451], acquiesced and accepted osteopaths into its ranks—a strategy which the medical profession believed would eventually destroy the osteopathic profession by forcing it to resign its ideals and identity. In his review of osteopathic history, Gevitz[452] writes, **"…the M.D.'s gradually came to believe that the only way to destroy osteopathy was through the absorption of D.O.'s, much as the homeopaths and eclectics [naturopaths] had been swallowed up early in the century."** Even recently, the AMA has listed osteopathic medicine under "alternative medicine"[453] although several osteopathic medical colleges have consistently provided training that is superior to most "conventional" allopathic medical schools.[454] Today, osteopathic physicians practice in most ways similarly to allopaths—i.e., with unlimited scope of practice in all 50 states, full access to the use of drugs and surgery, and with a very pharmacosurgical paradigm of disease and healthcare. Osteopathic medicine is one of the fastest growing healthcare professions in America.

---

[451] Getzendanner S. Permanent injunction order against AMA. *JAMA*. 1988 Jan 1;259(1):81-2
[452] Gevitz N. The D.O.'s: Osteopathic Medicine in America. Johns Hopkins University Press; 1991; pages 100-103
[453] American Medical Association. Report 12 of the Council on Scientific Affairs (A-97) Full Text http://www.ama-assn.org/ama/pub/category/13638.html Accessed November 23, 2006
[454] Special report. America's best graduate schools. Schools of Medicine. The top schools: primary care. *US News World Rep*. 2004 Apr 12;136(12):74

Osteopathic Manipulative Medicine: Osteopathic manipulative medicine (OMM) is similar to and yet distinct from chiropractic manipulation; the naturopathic profession—true to its eclectic roots—incorporates techniques from all professions. In contrast to chiropractic, OMM terminology and therapeutics focus much more on soft tissues, and the osteopathic lesion—"somatic dysfunction"—is clearly originated from soft tissues in contrast to the chiropractic lesion—the "vertebral subluxation"—which obviously originates from spinal articulations. Whereas the chiropractic intent of correcting or "adjusting" the "subluxation" was historically to improve function of the nervous system, the osteopathic lesion is addressed to more fully improve not only function of the nervous system but also of the vascular, lymphatic, and myofascial systems, too.[455] With regard to the latter, the osteopathic profession has always emphasized the importance of fascia in the genesis of "somatic dysfunction." Indeed, fascia appears to play an important and dynamic (not passive) role in neuromusculoskeletal health, particularly as it is a major contributor to proprioception and may also have a more direct effect through the recently described ability of fascia to actively contract in a smooth-muscle-like manner.[456]

From this author's perspective, an unfortunate consequence of the broadness of osteopathic manipulative conceptualizations/techniques (i.e., vertebral, skeletal, vascular, lymphatic, myofascial,...) is the relative lack (compared to chiropractic) of modernization and sophistication and development of its terminology and training textbooks; two of the most widely used osteopathic texts—*Osteopathic Principles in Practice* (1994) by Kuchera and Kuchera[457], and *Outline of Osteopathic Manipulative Procedures* (2006) by Kimberly[458]—both leave very much to be desired with respect to their clarity, terminology, clinical applicability, and referencing to the scientific literature. *Manipulation of the Spine, Thorax and Pelvis: An Osteopathic Perspective* (2006) by Gibbons and Tehan[459] is much more accessible and clinically applicable; however the text focuses exclusively on high-velocity low-amplitude (HVLA) techniques and therefore does not provide sufficient background and training for students in the very techniques that distinguish osteopathic from chiropractic techniques, namely heightened attention to the myofascial dysfunction that (appropriately) underlies the osteopathic lesion.

> "In contrast to the description of the osteopathic medical profession by the American Osteopathic Association, namely, "doctors of osteopathic medicine, or D.O.s, apply the philosophy of treating the whole person to the prevention, diagnosis and treatment of illness, disease and injury," [the authors of the article in question] essentially reviewed only pharmacologic treatment.
>
> …
>
> It is hoped that future reviews in this journal can include a more balanced survey of the literature, inclusive of non-pharmacologic and "holistic" interventions that are consistent with osteopathic philosophy."
>
> **Vasquez A**. Interventions Need to be Consistent With Osteopathic Philosophy. [Letter] *JAOA: Journal of the American Osteopathic Association* 2006 Sep;106(9):528-9
> http://www.jaoa.org/cgi/content/full/106/9/528

---

[455] Williams N. Managing back pain in general practice--is osteopathy the new paradigm? *Br J Gen Pract*. 1997 Oct;47(423):653-5 http://www.pubmedcentral.nih.gov/articlerender.fcgi?tool=pubmed&pubmedid=9474832
[456] "...the existence of an active fascial contractility could have interesting implications for the understanding of musculoskeletal pathologies with an increased or decreased myofascial tonus. It may also offer new insights and a deeper understanding of treatments directed at fascia, such as manual myofascial release therapies or acupuncture." Schleip R, Klingler W, Lehmann-Horn F. Active fascial contractility: Fascia may be able to contract in a smooth muscle-like manner and thereby influence musculoskeletal dynamics. *Med Hypotheses*. 2005;65(2):273-7
[457] Kuchera WA, Kuchera ML. *Osteopathic Principles In Practice, revised second edition*. Kirksville, MO, KCOM Press; 1994
[458] Kimberly PE. *Outline of Osteopathic Manipulative Procedures. The Kimberly Manual 2006*. Kirksville College of Osteopathic Medicine. Walsworth Publishing Company Marceline, Mo
[459] Gibbons P, Tehan P. *Manipulation of the Spine, Thorax and Pelvis: An Osteopathic Perspective*. Churchill Livingstone; 2006. Isbn: 044310039X

Ironically, the very growth and "allopathicization" of the profession that has threatened the profession's adherence to its holistic tenets has caused a reflexive re-affirmation of these tenets, and the profession has responded with a well-funded and intentional directive to scientifically investigate the mechanisms and efficacy of osteopathic manipulative medicine.[460,461] Recent findings include improved function and reduced pain in patients treated with a comprehensive manipulative technique for the shoulder[462], as well as the significant efficacy of ankle manipulation for patients with recent ankle injuries.[463] Further, OMM treatment of patients medicated for depression was found to triple the effectiveness of drug monotherapy.[464] Other studies have shown benefit of OMM in the treatment of geriatric pneumonia[465], pediatric asthma[466], pediatric dysfunctional voiding[467], carpal tunnel syndrome[468], low-back pain[469], and recovery from cardiac bypass surgery.[470] Replication and validation of these studies—many of which are small or of nonrigorous design (e.g., open clinical trials with no control group)—is important to further define and establish the value of osteopathic manipulation in clinical care.

---

[460] Wisnioski SW 3rd. "Circle Turns Round" to "Allopathic Osteopathy." *J Am Osteopath Assoc* 2006; 106: 423-4 http://www.jaoa.org/cgi/content/full/106/7/423

[461] Teitelbaum HS, Bunn WE 2nd, Brown SA, Burchett AW. Osteopathic medical education: renaissance or rhetoric? *J Am Osteopath Assoc*. 2003 Oct;103(10):489-90 http://www.jaoa.org/cgi/reprint/103/10/489

[462] The "seven stages of Spencer" is an organized technique of range-of-motion exercises and post-isometric stretching to improve functionality of the shoulder. This clinical trial showed improved shoulder function in a group of elderly patients treated with this technique. Knebl JA, Shores JH, Gamber RG, Gray WT, Herron KM. Improving functional ability in the elderly via the Spencer technique, an osteopathic manipulative treatment: a randomized, controlled trial. *J Am Osteopath Assoc*. 2002 Jul;102(7):387-96 http://www.jaoa.org/cgi/reprint/102/7/387 See also "CONCLUSION: Manipulative therapy for the shoulder girdle in addition to usual medical care accelerates recovery of shoulder symptoms." Bergman GJ, Winters JC, Groenier KH, Pool JJ, Meyboom-de Jong B, Postema K, van der Heijden GJ. Manipulative therapy in addition to usual medical care for patients with shoulder dysfunction and pain: a randomized, controlled trial. *Ann Intern Med*. 2004 Sep 21;141(6):432-9 http://www.annals.org/cgi/reprint/141/6/432.pdf

[463] This study shows the rapid onset and benefit of manipulative medicine for the treatment of acute ankle sprains: Eisenhart AW, Gaeta TJ, Yens DP. Osteopathic manipulative treatment in the emergency department for patients with acute ankle injuries. *J Am Osteopath Assoc*. 2003 Sep;103(9):417-21 http://www.jaoa.org/cgi/reprint/103/9/417

[464] This study impressively showed that musculoskeletal manipulation improved treatment effectiveness for depression from 33% to 100%. "After 8 weeks, 100% of the OMT treatment group and 33% of the control group tested normal by psychometric evaluation. ... The findings of this pilot study indicate that OMT may be a useful adjunctive treatment for alleviating depression in women." Plotkin BJ, Rodos JJ, Kappler R, Schrage M, Freydl K, Hasegawa S, Hennegan E, Hilchie-Schmidt C, Hines D, Iwata J, Mok C, Raffaelli D. Adjunctive osteopathic manipulative treatment in women with depression: a pilot study. *J Am Osteopath Assoc*. 2001 Sep;101(9):517-23 http://www.jaoa.org/cgi/reprint/101/9/517

[465] This study showed improved clinical outcomes and reduced antibiotic use in elderly patients with pneumonia when treated with manipulative medicine: "The treatment group had a significantly shorter duration of intravenous antibiotic treatment and a shorter hospital stay." Noll DR, Shores JH, Gamber RG, Herron KM, Swift J Jr. Benefits of osteopathic manipulative treatment for hospitalized elderly patients with pneumonia. *J Am Osteopath Assoc*. 2000 Dec;100(12):776-82 http://www.jaoa.org/cgi/reprint/100/12/776

[466] Osteopathic manipulation improved pulmonary function in pediatric patients with asthma: "With a confidence level of 95%, results for the OMT group showed a statistically significant improvement of 7 L per minute to 9 L per minute for peak expiratory flow rates. These results suggest that OMT has a therapeutic effect among this patient population." Guiney PA, Chou R, Vianna A, Lovenheim J. Effects of osteopathic manipulative treatment on pediatric patients with asthma: a randomized controlled trial. *J Am Osteopath Assoc*. 2005 Jan;105(1):7-12 http://www.jaoa.org/cgi/content/full/105/1/7

[467] "RESULTS: The treatment group exhibited greater improvement in DV symptoms than did the control group (Z=-2.63, p=0.008, Mann-Whitney U-test). Improved or resolution of vesicoureteral reflux and elimination of post-void urine residuals were more prominent in the treatment group." Nemett DR, Fivush BA, Mathews R, Camirand N, Eldridge MA, Finney K, Gerson AC. A randomized controlled trial of the effectiveness of osteopathy-based manual physical therapy in treating pediatric dysfunctional voiding. *J Pediatr Urol*. 2008 Apr;4(2):100-6

[468] Sucher BM, Hinrichs RN, Welcher RL, Quiroz LD, St Laurent BF, Morrison BJ. Manipulative treatment of carpal tunnel syndrome: biomechanical and osteopathic intervention to increase the length of the transverse carpal ligament: part 2. Effect of sex differences and manipulative "priming". *J Am Osteopath Assoc*. 2005 Mar;105(3):135-43. Erratum in: J Am Osteopath Assoc. 2005 May;105(5):238 http://www.jaoa.org/cgi/content/full/105/3/135

[469] "CONCLUSION: OMT significantly reduces low back pain. The level of pain reduction is greater than expected from placebo effects alone and persists for at least three months." Licciardone JC, Brimhall AK, King LN. Osteopathic manipulative treatment for low back pain: a systematic review and meta-analysis of randomized controlled trials. *BMC Musculoskelet Disord*. 2005 Aug 4;6:43 http://www.biomedcentral.com/1471-2474/6/43

[470] This study showed benefit from osteopathic manipulation administered immediately after coronary artery bypass graft surgery: "The observed changes in cardiac function and perfusion indicated that OMT had a beneficial effect on the recovery of patients after CABG surgery. The authors conclude that OMT has immediate, beneficial hemodynamic effects after CABG surgery when administered while the patient is sedated and pharmacologically paralyzed." O-Yurvati AH, Carnes MS, Clearfield MB, Stoll ST, McConathy WJ. Hemodynamic effects of osteopathic manipulative treatment immediately after coronary artery bypass graft surgery. *J Am Osteopath Assoc*. 2005 Oct;105(10):475-81 http://www.jaoa.org/cgi/content/full/105/10/475

Functional Medicine

Note: This section is from the final pre-edited draft which introduces functional medicine in Vasquez A. _Musculoskeletal Pain: Expanded Clinical Strategies_ (2008), published by the Institute for Functional Medicine; used here with permission. Slight modifications were made to this section during revisions in 2011.

Introduction: The purpose of this monograph is to provide healthcare professionals with an overview of the "functional medicine" assessment and management strategies that are applicable to painful neuromusculoskeletal disorders. A comprehensive description of functional medicine from the Institute for Functional Medicine (IFM) is provided later in this section, while a more comprehensive explication is provided in _The Textbook of Functional Medicine_.[471] In recognition of the diversity of this document's readership (inclusive of students, recent graduates, experienced professionals, academicians,

A Functional Medicine Monograph

MUSCULOSKELETAL PAIN:
Expanded Clinical Strategies

Alex Vasquez, DC, ND

THE INSTITUTE FOR FUNCTIONAL MEDICINE

The information in this section on functional medicine is derived from the final pre-edited draft of chapter 1 from Vasquez A. _Musculoskeletal Pain: Expanded Clinical Strategies_, published by the Institute for Functional Medicine in 2008 and available from www.FunctionalMedicine.org

and policymakers) and the pervasive deficiencies in musculoskeletal knowledge among healthcare providers[472,473,474,475,476,477], this monograph on pain will necessarily review some basic concepts; however, this document alone cannot replace professional training in musculoskeletal medicine nor does it include protocols for patient management and differential diagnosis for each of the neuromusculoskeletal problems seen in clinical practice. This text should be used in conjunction with the reader's professional training and other reference texts. Clinicians utilizing a functional medicine approach to patient care must be knowledgeable in the details of integrative physiology and nutritional biochemistry and must also posses the clinical acumen necessary to ensure safe and expedient patient care. These traits and skills are of particular necessity when a serious condition is presented. Life-threatening and limb-threatening neuromusculoskeletal problems are notorious for presenting under the guise of an apparently benign complaint such as fatigue, headache, or simple joint pain.

---

[471] Jones DS (Editor-in-Chief). _Textbook of Functional Medicine_. Institute for Functional Medicine, Gig Harbor, WA 2005

[472] Freedman KB, Bernstein J. The adequacy of medical school education in musculoskeletal medicine. _J Bone Joint Surg Am_. 1998;80(10):1421-7

[473] Freedman KB, Bernstein J. Educational deficiencies in musculoskeletal medicine. _J Bone Joint Surg Am_. 2002;84-A(4):604-8

[474] Joy EA, Hala SV. Musculoskeletal Curricula in Medical Education: Filling In the Missing Pieces. _The Physician and Sportsmedicine_. 2004; 32: 42-45

[475] Matzkin E, Smith ME, Freccero CD, Richardson AB. Adequacy of education in musculoskeletal medicine. _J Bone Joint Surg Am_. 2005 Feb;87-A(2):310-4

[476] Schmale GA. More evidence of educational inadequacies in musculoskeletal medicine. _Clin Orthop Relat Res_. 2005 Aug;(437):251-9

[477] Stockard AR, Allen TW. Competence levels in musculoskeletal medicine: comparison of osteopathic and allopathic medical graduates. _J Am Osteopath Assoc_. 2006 Jun;106(6):350-5

Since approximately 1 of every 7 (14% of total) visits to a primary healthcare provider is for the treatment of musculoskeletal pain or dysfunction[478], every healthcare provider needs to have: 1) knowledge of important concepts related to musculoskeletal medicine, 2) the ability to recognize urgent and emergency conditions, 3) the ability to competently perform orthopedic examination procedures and interpret laboratory assessments, and 4) the knowledge and ability to design and implement effective treatment plans and to coordinate patient management. While this monograph will be thorough in its review of topics discussed, like any other textbook it cannot contain every nuance and examination procedure that clinicians should have in their clinical toolkits. This text should be used in conjunction with the clinician's previous professional training, other textbooks, and best judgment for the delivery of personalized care for each individual patient, including those who present with similar or identical diagnoses. Supportive texts include *Current Medical Diagnosis and Treatment* edited by Tierney et al[479], *Orthopedic Physical Assessment* by Magee[480], and *Integrative Orthopedics* and *Integrative Rheumatology* by Vasquez.[481,482] Further, clinicians can note that this monograph is written primarily for routine outpatient management rather than emergency department management or "playing field" situations.

Musculoskeletal disorders are extremely prevalent and represent a major cause of human suffering, healthcare expenses, and lost productivity. Additionally, many standard medical interventions show high rates of inefficacy and iatrogenesis in addition to their high costs.[483,484,485] The vast majority of painful neuromusculoskeletal disorders can be alleviated and often effectively treated with nutritional interventions, but physicians trained only in standard medicine receive little to no training in nutrition and are therefore generally unable or unwilling to use these science-based interventions to help their patients.[486,487] Further, distain toward nutritional and other nonsurgical and nonpharmacologic interventions is represented in many standard medical textbooks despite proof of efficacy shown in replicable high-quality clinical trials published in top-tier medical journals. For example, despite the more than 800 articles documenting the role of nutritional interventions in the direct or adjunctive treatment of rheumatoid arthritis, the seventeenth edition of *The Merck Manual* published in 1999 wrote that, "Food and diet quackery is common and should be discouraged."[488] Combining these factors with the aforementioned pervasive lack of competence in musculoskeletal knowledge among healthcare providers (exceptions noted[489]), we see that patients with musculoskeletal disorders often face a series of difficult and insurmountable obstacles between their present condition of suffering and the relief that they seek and deserve. Clearly, the field of musculoskeletal medicine

---

[478] American College of Rheumatology Ad Hoc Committee on Clinical Guidelines. Guidelines for the initial evaluation of the adult patient with acute musculoskeletal symptoms. *Arthritis Rheum*. 1996 Jan;39(1):1-8 See also: Vasquez A. Musculoskeletal disorders and iron overload disease: comment on the American College of Rheumatology guidelines. *Arthritis Rheum* 1996;39: 1767-8

[479] Tierney ML. McPhee SJ, Papadakis MA (eds). Current Medical Diagnosis and Treatment. New York: Lange Medical Books. Updated annually

[480] Magee DJ. Orthopedic Physical Assessment. Third edition. Philadelphia: WB Saunders, 1997. Newer editions have been published.

[481] Vasquez A. *Integrative Orthopedics: Second Edition*. Fort Worth, Texas; Integrative and Biological Medicine Research and Consulting, 2007 OptimalHealthResearch.com

[482] Vasquez A. *Integrative Rheumatology: Second Edition*. Fort Worth, Texas; Integrative and Biological Medicine Research and Consulting, 2007 OptimalHealthResearch.com

[483] Moseley JB, O'Malley K, Petersen NJ, Menke TJ, Brody BA, Kuykendall DH, Hollingsworth JC, Ashton CM, Wray NP. A controlled trial of arthroscopic surgery for osteoarthritis of the knee. *N Engl J Med* 2002 Jul 11;347(2):81-8

[484] Kolata G. A Knee Surgery for Arthritis Is Called Sham. *The New York Times*, July 11, 2002

[485] Rosner AL. Evidence-based clinical guidelines for the management of acute low-back pain: response to the guidelines prepared for the Australian Medical Health and Research Council. *J Manipulative Physiol Ther*. 2001;24(3):214-20

[486] Lo C. Integrating nutrition as a theme throughout the medical school curriculum. *Am J Clin Nutr*. 2000 Sep;72(3 Suppl):882S-9S

[487] Adams KM, Lindell KC, Kohlmeier M, Zeisel SH. Status of nutrition education in medical schools. *Am J Clin Nutr*. 2006 Apr;83(4):941S-944S

[488] Beers MH, Berkow R (eds). The Merck Manual. Seventeenth Edition. Whitehouse Station; Merck Research Laboratories: 1999, page 419

[489] Humphreys BK, Sulkowski A, McIntyre K, Kasiban M, Patrick AN. An examination of musculoskeletal cognitive competency in chiropractic interns. *J Manipulative Physiol Ther*. 2007;30(1):44-9

is in need of pervasive paradigm shifts in both physician training and patient management to improve patient care.

Background: Historically, prevailing views of disorders of pain and inflammation were conceptually similar to those of most other diseases and premodern accounts of life in general. Our clinical predecessors did the best they could to understand, describe, and treat the health problems with which their patients presented, and the paradigm from which these clinical entities were viewed and addressed was shaped by the social, religious, and scientific views and limitations of their time. Lacking a molecular and physiologic understanding of disease origination, and restrained by metaphysical and simplistic models of "cause and effect", premodern clinicians devised models for the understanding and treatment of disease that generally appear unsatisfactory today in light of the advances in our understanding in disparate yet interrelated fields such as psychoneuroimmunology, molecular biology, nutrigenomics, environmental medicine and toxicology. Despite these advances, we as a human society and as healthcare providers still carry many of these previous conceptualizations and misconceptualizations with us as we move forward toward a future wherein our views and interventions will be much more precise and "objective" in contrast to the generalized and phenomenalistic approaches that typified premodern medicine and which still permeate certain aspects of clinical care today. For example, we still use the term "stroke" to describe acute cerebrovascular insufficiency, although the term originated from the view that affected patients had been "struck" by the gods or fates perhaps as a form of punishment for some ethical or religious transgression. Even today, patients and clinicians commonly interpret disease as some form of punishment or as an extension of spiritual or intrapersonal shortcoming. Advancing science allows us to disassemble complex events that were previously experienced as *phenomena*, that is, as undecipherable and enigmatic events that overwhelmed comprehension. The **Functional Medicine Matrix** provides an extremely useful tool for helping clinicians grasp a multidimensional decipherable view of disease and its corresponding treatment which facilitates the achievement of higher clinical efficacy, improved patient outcomes, and more favorable safety and cost-effectiveness profiles.

Whereas the advancement of our scientific knowledge often leads us to discard previous models and interventions, occasionally modern science helps us to understand and revisit previous interventions that may have been prematurely or unduly discarded. For example, Hippocrates' admonition to "Let thy food be thy medicine, and thy medicine be thy food" experienced decades of devaluation when dietary, nutritional, and other natural interventions were misbranded as "quackery." On the contrary to these premature and unsubstantiated condemnations, simple natural interventions such as therapeutic fasting and augmentation of vitamin D3 status (via nutritional supplementation or exposure to ultraviolet-B radiation) have shown remarkable safety and efficacy in the mitigation of chronic hypertension, musculoskeletal pain, and autoimmunity.[490,491,492,493,494,495,496,497,498] Furthermore, the appropriate use

---

[490] Goldhamer A, et al. Medically supervised water-only fasting in the treatment of hypertension. *J Manipulative Physiol Ther* 2001 Jun;24(5):335-9

[491] Goldhamer AC, et al. Medically supervised water-only fasting in the treatment of borderline hypertension. *J Altern Complement Med*. 2002 Oct;8(5):643-50

[492] Goldhamer AC. Initial cost of care results in medically supervised water-only fasting for treating high blood pressure and diabetes. *J Altern Complement Med*. 2002 Dec;8(6):696-7

[493] Krause R, Bühring M, Hopfenmüller W, Holick MF, Sharma AM. Ultraviolet B and blood pressure. *Lancet*. 1998 Aug 29;352(9129):709-10

[494] Pfeifer M, Begerow B, Minne HW, Nachtigall D, Hansen C. Effects of a short-term vitamin D(3) and calcium supplementation on blood pressure and parathyroid hormone levels in elderly women. *J Clin Endocrinol Metab*. 2001 Apr;86(4):1633-7

[495] McCarty MF. A preliminary fast may potentiate response to a subsequent low-salt, low-fat vegan diet in the management of hypertension - fasting as a strategy for breaking metabolic vicious cycles. *Med Hypotheses*. 2003 May;60(5):624-33

of vitamin supplements helps prevent chronic disease by numerous mechanisms including modulation of gene transcription, enhancement of DNA repair and stability, and enhancement of metabolic efficiency.[499,500,501] This document will provide a representative survey of current research in the use of dietary, nutritional, and integrative therapeutics commonly utilized in the clinical management of disorders characterized by pain and inflammation.

State of the Evidence: The bulk of information in this monograph is derived from and referenced to peer-reviewed publications indexed in the database known as Medline/Pubmed provided by the U.S. National Library of Medicine and the National Institutes of Health. For the sake of practicality and publishability, not all statements carry citations, but the most important ones do; citations are always provided when referenced to a particular intervention of importance so that clinicians can access the primary source when refining their clinical decisions. A "blanket statement" to cover all the different assessments and interventions described herein would be necessarily inaccurate and therefore each intervention will be considered on the merits of its own rationale, safety, effectiveness, and cost-effectiveness. Again, however, these considerations must ultimately be viewed within the context of the individual patient's condition and the overall cohesion and comprehensiveness of the treatment plan.

      While all clinicians can appreciate the importance of protocols and clinical practice guidelines, we must also perpetually ratify the preeminence of patient individuality and therefore the importance of tailoring treatment to the patient's unique combination of biochemical individuality, comorbid conditions, drug use, personal goals, and willingness to participate in a health-promoting lifestyle. Standardized protocols and practice guidelines are founded on the fallacy of disease homogeneity and the irrelevance of physiologic, psychosocial, and biochemical individuality. As the advancement of biomedical science provides the means for and underscores the importance of customized treatments for each patient, so too has the standard of care begun to shift in the direction of requiring the consideration of these variables before and during the implementation of treatment. Failure to utilize nutritional interventions when such interventions are clinically indicated is inconsistent with the delivery of quality healthcare and may be considered malpractice.[502,503,504,505]

      A clinician who is unaware of the political forces that shape healthcare policy and research is analogous to a captain of an oceangoing ship not knowing how to use a compass, sextant, or coastline map. Medical science and healthcare policy are influenced by a myriad of powerful private interests which are motivated by their own goals, at times different from the stated goals of medicine, which purports to hold paramount the patient's welfare. Scientific objectivity and the guiding ethical principles of informed consent, beneficence, autonomy, and non-malfeasance are subject to different interpretations depending upon the lens through which

---

[496] Hyppönen E, Läärä E, Reunanen A, Järvelin MR, Virtanen SM. Intake of vitamin D and risk of type 1 diabetes: a birth-cohort study. *Lancet*. 2001 Nov 3;358(9292):1500-3

[497] Fuhrman J, Sarter B, Calabro DJ. Brief case reports of medically supervised, water-only fasting associated with remission of autoimmune disease. *Altern Ther Health Med*. 2002 Jul-Aug;8(4):112, 110-1

[498] Holick MF. Vitamin D deficiency: what a pain it is. *Mayo Clin Proc*. 2003 Dec;78(12):1457-9

[499] Fletcher RH, Fairfield KM. Vitamins for chronic disease prevention in adults: clinical applications. *JAMA*. 2002 Jun 19;287(23):3127-9

[500] Heaney RP. Long-latency deficiency disease: insights from calcium and vitamin D. *Am J Clin Nutr*. 2003 Nov;78(5):912-9

[501] Ames BN. The metabolic tune-up: metabolic harmony and disease prevention. *J Nutr*. 2003 May;133(5 Suppl 1):1544S-8S

[502] Heaney RP. Vitamin D, nutritional deficiency, and the medical paradigm. *J Clin Endocrinol Metab*. 2003 Nov;88(11):5107-8

[503] Fletcher RH, Fairfield KM. Vitamins for chronic disease prevention in adults: clinical applications. *JAMA*. 2002 Jun 19;287(23):3127-9

[504] Berg A. Sliding toward nutrition malpractice: time to reconsider and redeploy. *Am J Clin Nutr*. 1993 Jan;57(1):3-7

[505] Cobb DK, Warner D. Avoiding malpractice: the role of proper nutrition and wound management. *J Am Med Dir Assoc*. 2004 Jul-Aug;5(4 Sup):H11-6

a dilemma is viewed. When this "dilemma" is the whole of healthcare, what first appears as order and structure now appears as the disarrayed tug-of-war between factions and private interests, with paradigmatic victory often being awarded to those with the best marketing campaigns and political influence with less importance given to safety, efficacy, and the economic burden to consumers.[506,507,508,509,510,511,512,513,514,515,516,517,518,519,520,521,522,523,524,525,526,527,528,529,530,531,532,533,534,535,536,537] To be ignorant of such considerations is to be blind to the nature of research, policy, and our own biased inclinations for and against particular paradigms, assessments, and interventions.

[506] Editorial. Drug-company influence on medical education in USA. *Lancet.* 2000 Sep 2;356(9232):781

[507] Horton R. Lotronex and the FDA: a fatal erosion of integrity. *Lancet.* 2001 May 19;357(9268):1544-5

[508] Editorial. Politics trumps science at the FDA. *Lancet.* 2005 Nov 26;366(9500):1827

[509] Topol EJ. Failing the public health--rofecoxib, Merck, and the FDA. *N Engl J Med.* 2004 Oct 21;351(17):1707-9

[510] Wolinsky H, Brune T. The Serpent on the Staff: The Unhealthy Politics of the American Medical Association. GP Putnam and Sons, New York, 1994

[511] Wilk CA. Medicine, Monopolies, and Malice: How the Medical Establishment Tried to Destroy Chiropractic. Garden City Park: Avery, 1996

[512] Carter JP. Racketeering in Medicine: The Suppression of Alternatives. Norfolk: Hampton Roads Pub; 1993

[513] National Alliance of Professional Psychology Providers. AMA Seeks To Control and Restrict Psychologist's Scope of Practice. http://www.nappp.org/scope.pdf Accessed November 25, 2006

[514] Daly R, American Psychiatric Association. AMA Forms Coalition to Thwart Non-M.D. Practice Expansion. *Psychiatric News* 2006 March; 41: 17

[515] Angell M. The Truth About the Drug Companies: How They Deceive Us and What to Do About it. Random House; August 2004

[516] Terrett AG. Misuse of the literature by medical authors in discussing spinal manipulative therapy injury. *J Manipulative Physiol Ther.* 1995 May;18(4):203-10

[517] Morley J, Rosner AL, Redwood D. A case study of misrepresentation of the scientific literature: recent reviews of chiropractic. *J Altern Complement Med.* 2001 Feb;7(1):65-78

[518] Wenban AB. Inappropriate use of the title 'chiropractor' and term 'chiropractic manipulation' in the peer-reviewed biomedical literature. *Chiropr Osteopat.* 2006 Aug 22;14:16

[519] Spivak JL. The Medical Trust Unmasked. Louis S. Siegfried Publishers; New York: 1961

[520] Trever W. In the Public Interest. Los Angeles; Scriptures Unlimited; 1972. This is probably the most authoritative documentation of the illegal actions of the AMA up to 1972; contains numerous photocopies of actual AMA documents and minutes of official meetings with overt intentionality of destroying Americans' healthcare options so that the AMA and related organizations would have a monopoly in healthcare.

[521] Getzendanner S. Permanent injunction order against AMA. *JAMA.* 1988 Jan 1;259(1):81-2

[522] "A national study released today reports 20 million American families — or one in seven families — faced hardships paying medical bills last year, which forced many to choose between getting medical attention or paying rent or buying food…" Freeman, Liz. 'Working poor' struggle to afford health care. *Naples Daily News.* Published in Naples, Florida and online at http://www.naplesnews.com/npdn/news/article/0,2071,NPDN_14940_3000546,00.html Accessed July 28, 2004

[523] "The USA's 5.8 million small companies… Health care costs are rising about 15% this year for those with fewer than 200 workers vs. 13.5% for those with 500 or more… But many small employers cite increases of 20% or more. That's made insurance the No. 1 small business problem…" Jim Hopkins. Health care tops taxes as small business cost drain. *USA TODAY.* http://www.usatoday.com/news/health/2003-04-20-small-business-costs_x.htm. Accessed July 28, 2004

[524] "Though the U.S. has slightly fewer doctors per capita than the typical developed nation, we have almost twice as many MRI machines and perform vastly more angioplasties. …at least 31 percent of all the incremental income we'll earn between 1999 and 2010 will go to health care." Pat Regnier, *Money Magazine.* Healthcare myth: We spend too much. October 13, 2003: 11:29 AM EDT http://money.cnn.com/2003/10/08/pf/health_myths_1/ Accessed Monday, July 12, 2004

[525] "Although they spend more on health care than patients in any other industrialized nation, Americans receive the right treatment less than 60 percent of the time, resulting in unnecessary pain, expense and even death…" Ceci Connolly. U.S. Patients Spend More but Don't Get More, Study Finds: Even in Advantaged Areas, Americans Often Receive Inadequate Health Care. *Washington Post*, May 5, 2004; Page A15. On-line at http://www.washingtonpost.com/ac2/wp-dyn/A1875-2004May4 accessed on July 28, 2004

[526] McGlynn EA, Asch SM, Adams J, Keesey J, Hicks J, DeCristofaro A, Kerr EA. The quality of health care delivered to adults in the United States. *N Engl J Med.* 2003 Jun 26;348(26):2635-45

[527] Brennan TA, Leape LL, Laird NM, Hebert L, Localio AR, Lawthers AG, Newhouse JP, Weiler PC, Hiatt HH. Incidence of adverse events and negligence in hospitalized patients: results of the Harvard Medical Practice Study I. 1991. *Qual Saf Health Care.* 2004 Apr;13(2):145-51; discuss 151-2

[528] "Basically, you die earlier and spend more time disabled if you're an American rather than a member of most other advanced countries." Christopher Murray MD PhD, Director of World Health Organization's Global Program on Evidence for Health Policy http://www.who.int/inf-pr-2000/en/pr2000-life.html Accessed July 12, 2004

[529] Shi L. Health care spending, delivery, and outcome in developed countries: a cross-national comparison. *Am J Med Qual* 1997;12(2):83-93

[530] Holland EG, Degruy FV. Drug-induced disorders. *Am Fam Physician.* 1997 Nov 1;56(7):1781-8, 1791-2

[531] Brennan TA, Leape LL, Laird NM, Hebert L, Localio AR, Lawthers AG, Newhouse JP, Weiler PC, Hiatt HH. Incidence of adverse events and negligence in hospitalized patients: results of the Harvard Medical Practice Study I. 1991. *Qual Saf Health Care.* 2004 Apr;13(2):145-51; discuss 151-2

[532] Whitaker R. The case against antipsychotic drugs: a 50-year record of doing more harm than good. *Med Hypotheses.* 2004;62(1):5-13

[533] The relevance of these citations is to show that the misuse of horse estrogens in humans as "hormone replacement therapy" exemplified the application of a strong carcinogen to millions of unsuspecting women: Zhang F, Chen Y, Pisha E, Shen L, Xiong Y, van Breemen RB, Bolton JL. The major metabolite of equilin, 4-hydroxyequilin, autoxidizes to an o-quinone which isomerizes to the potent cytotoxin 4-hydroxyequilenin-o-quinone. *Chem Res Toxicol.* 1999 Feb;12(2):204-13; Pisha E, Lui X, Constantinou AI, Bolton JL. Evidence that a metabolite of equine estrogens, 4-hydroxyequilenin, induces cellular transformation in vitro. *Chem Res Toxicol.* 2001;14(1):82-90; Zhang F, Swanson SM, van Breemen RB, Liu X, Yang Y, Gu C, Bolton JL. Equine estrogen metabolite 4-hydroxyequilenin induces DNA damage in the rat mammary tissues: formation of single-strand breaks, apurinic sites, stable adducts, and oxidized bases. *Chem Res Toxicol.* 2001 Dec;14(12):1654-9

[534] Newman NM, Ling RS. Acetabular bone destruction related to non-steroidal anti-inflammatory drugs. *Lancet.* 1985 Jul 6; 2(8445): 11-4

[535] "In 1983, 2876 people died from medication errors. ... By 1993, this number had risen to 7,391 - a 2.57-fold increase." Phillips DP, Christenfeld N, Glynn LM. Increase in US medication-error deaths between 1983 and 1993. *Lancet.* 1998 Feb 28;351(9103):643-4

[536] Smith R. Medical journals are an extension of the marketing arm of pharmaceutical companies. *PLoS Med.* 2005 May;2(5):e138

[537] van der Steen WJ, Ho VK. Drugs versus diets: disillusions with Dutch health care. *Acta Biotheor.* 2001;49(2):125-40

Research articles and sources of authority must be approached with an artist's delicacy, and with a willingness to receive new information as worthy of preeminence over deeply rooted and well ensconced institutionalized fallacies.

Understanding the Multifaceted Nature of Disease Pathogenesis: The Functional Medicine Matrix as Paradigm and Clinical Tool: At its simplest and most practical level, the Functional Medicine Matrix is a teaching tool and clinical method that facilitates consideration of the different contributions of major intrinsic systems and extrinsic influences that are at play in a given disease process or individual patient. When viewed as a diagram, the web of influences can be appreciated to reveal the interconnected nature of influences and body systems and how imbalance or disruption in one area can lead to problems in another. Once homeostatic reserves and compensatory mechanisms are depleted, the patient experiences progressively worsening health (which may be asymptomatic) and the eventual manifestation of clinical disease.

Over the course of many years and discussions and reconsiderations, the faculty at IFM has elucidated eight preeminent systems or loci ("core clinical imbalances") for clinicians to consider when working with any chronic health disorder. These will be listed and described below with particular consideration of the topic of this monograph, which is neuromusculoskeletal pain and inflammation. Interested readers are directed to IFM's monograph series on topics such as "Depression" and "The Role of Gastrointestinal Inflammation in Systemic Disease" to see how this model is applied to disease states in different organ systems.

2008 rendering of The Functional Medicine Matrix: A concept, model, and clinical tool for evidence-based clinical care. Copyright Institute for Functional Medicine.

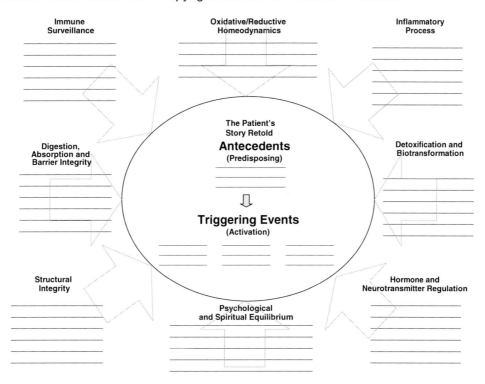

Exploring the Different Aspects of the Functional Medicine Matrix

1. <u>Hormonal and neurotransmitter imbalances</u>: While most clinicians are aware that neurotransmitters can either transmit pain signals or dampen their reception, many clinicians are not aware that neurotransmitter status is somewhat malleable and can be modulated with nutritional supplementation and botanical medicines. The examples that will be considered here are the tryptophan-serotonin-melatonin and the phenylalanine-tyrosine-dopamine-norepinephrine-epinephrine and enkephalin pathways.

   ▪ Tryptophan and 5-hydroxytryptophan (5HTP) are prescription and nonprescription nutritional supplements that are the amino acid precursors for the formation of the neurotransmitter serotonin and, subsequently, the pineal hormone melatonin. Biochemically, these conversions are linear as follows: tryptophan → 5HTP → serotonin → melatonin. Tryptophan depletion and low levels of serotonin are consistently associated with depression, anxiety, exacerbation of eating disorders, and increased sensitivity to acute and chronic pain. Serotonergic pathways are impaired by chronic stress due to increased utilization of serotonin (e.g., serotonin-dependent cortisol release) and increased hepatic degradation of tryptophan by cortisol-stimulated tryptophan pyrrolase.[538] Therapeutically, supplementation with 5HTP augments serotonin and melatonin synthesis and has specific applicability in the alleviation of depression and pain syndromes such as fibromyalgia and headache, including migraine, tension headaches, and juvenile headaches.[539,540] Certainly part of the benefit from 5HTP supplementation is derived from the increased formation of melatonin, as the biological effects of melatonin extend beyond its sleep-promoting role to include powerful antioxidation, anti-infective immunostimulation[541], and preservation of mitochondrial function, a benefit which is of particular relevance to the treatment of fibromyalgia.[542]

   ▪ The conditionally essential fatty acids found in fish oil modulate serotonergic and adrenergic activity in the human brain[543], and given the role of serotonin and norepinephrine in the central processing of pain perception[544], a reasonable hypothesis holds that the pain-relieving activity of fish oil supplementation[545] is partly due to central modulation of pain perception and is not wholly due to modulation of eicosanoid production and inflammatory mediator transcription as previously believed.

   ▪ Vitamin D3 supplementation may also augment serotonergic activity[546], and this mechanism may partly explain the mood-enhancing and pain-relieving benefits of vitamin D3 supplementation. Attentive readers will note that this brief discussion

---

[538] Sandyk R. Tryptophan availability and the susceptibility to stress in multiple sclerosis: a hypothesis. *Int J Neurosci.* 1996 Jul;86(1-2):47-53

[539] Turner EH, Loftis JM, Blackwell AD. Serotonin a la carte: supplementation with the serotonin precursor 5-hydroxytryptophan. *Pharmacol Ther.* 2006 Mar;109(3):325-38

[540] Birdsall TC. 5-Hydroxytryptophan: a clinically-effective serotonin precursor. *Altern Med Rev.* 1998 Aug;3(4):271-80

[541] Gitto E, Karbownik M, Reiter RJ, Tan DX, Cuzzocrea S, Chiurazzi P, Cordaro S, Corona G, Trimarchi G, Barberi I. Effects of melatonin treatment in septic newborns. *Pediatr Res.* 2001 Dec;50(6):756-60

[542] Acuna-Castroviejo D, Escames G, Reiter RJ. Melatonin therapy in fibromyalgia. *J Pineal Res.* 2006 Jan;40(1):98-9

[543] Hibbeln JR, Ferguson TA, Blasbalg TL. Omega-3 fatty acid deficiencies in neurodevelopment, aggression and autonomic dysregulation: opportunities for intervention. *Int Rev Psychiatry.* 2006 Apr;18(2):107-18

[544] Wise TN, Fishbain DA, Holder-Perkins V.Painful physical symptoms in depression: a clinical challenge. *Pain Med.* 2007 Sep;8 Suppl 2:S75-82

[545] Goldberg RJ, Katz J. A meta-analysis of the analgesic effects of omega-3 polyunsaturated fatty acid supplementation for inflammatory joint pain. *Pain.* 2007 May;129(1-2):210-23

[546] Lansdowne AT, Provost SC. Vitamin D3 enhances mood in healthy subjects during winter. *Psychopharmacology* (Berl). 1998 Feb;135(4):319-23

has already begun to bridge the gaps between nutritional status, neurotransmitter synthesis, pain sensitivity, immune function, and mitochondrial bioenergetics.

- Supplementation with DL-phenylalanine (DLPA; racemic mixture of D- and L-forms of the amino acid phenylalanine derived from synthetic production) has long been used in the treatment of pain and depression.[547] The nutritional L-isomer is converted from phenylalanine to tyrosine to L-dopa to dopamine to norepinephrine and epinephrine. Augmentation of this pathway promotes resistance to fatigue, depression, and pain. The synthetic D-isomer augments pain-relieving enkephalin function by inhibiting enkephalin degradation by the enzyme carboxypeptidase A (enkephalinase); the resultant augmentation of enkephalin levels is generally believed to underlie the analgesic and mood-enhancing benefits of DLPA supplementation.
- Therapeutic massage is yet another means to modulate neurotransmitter synthesis for the alleviation of pain. In a study of patients with chronic back pain, massage increased serotonin and dopamine levels (measured in urine).[548]

Hormonal imbalances are particularly relevant to the discussion of chronic pain caused by inflammation characteristic of autoimmune diseases such as rheumatoid arthritis (RA). Often clinically subtle but nonetheless of extreme importance, these hormonal influences on painful inflammation are worthy of their own detailed discussion and thus will be reviewed later in this monograph in the context of the prototypic inflammatory disease RA. Generally speaking and with a few noted exceptions (such as Sjogren's syndrome), the research literature points to a specific pattern of hormonal imbalances among patients with autoimmunity, and this pattern is consistent with the proinflammatory and immunodysregulatory effects of estrogens and prolactin and the anti-inflammatory and immunomodulatory effects of cortisol, dehydroepiandrosterone (DHEA), and testosterone. Patients with autoimmune neuromusculoskeletal inflammation generally display a complete or partial pattern of hormonal disturbances typified by elevated estrogen and prolactin and lowered testosterone, DHEA, and cortisol; appropriate therapeutic correction of these imbalances can safely result in disease amelioration. Rectification of endocrinologic imbalances ("orthoendocrinology") will be discussed in the section on RA and has been detailed with broader clinical applicability elsewhere by this author.[549]

2. <u>Oxidation-reduction imbalances and mitochondropathy</u>: Oxidative stress results from the chronic systemic inflammation seen in painful inflammatory disorders such as RA, and oxidative stress contributes to the perpetuation and exacerbation of inflammatory diseases via expedited tissue destruction and alterations in gene transcription and resultant enhancement of inflammatory mediator production.[550] Immune activation increases production of reactive oxygen species (ROS; "free radicals"), and oxidant stress increases activation of pro-inflammatory transcription factors (such as nuclear factor

---

[547] Russell AL, McCarty MF. DL-phenylalanine markedly potentiates opiate analgesia - an example of nutrient/pharmaceutical up-regulation of the endogenous analgesia system. *Med Hypotheses*. 2000 Oct;55(4):283-8

[548] Hernandez-Reif M, Field T, Krasnegor J, Theakston H. Lower back pain is reduced and range of motion increased after massage therapy. *Int J Neurosci* 2001;106(3-4):131-45

[549] Vasquez A. *Integrative Rheumatology*. Fort Worth, Texas; Integrative & Biological Medicine Research & Consulting, 2007 OptimalHealthResearch.com

[550] Hitchon CA, El-Gabalawy HS. Oxidation in rheumatoid arthritis. *Arthritis Res Ther*. 2004;6(6):265-78

KappaB, NFkB) and also increases spontaneous oxidative modification of endogenous proteins such as cartilage matrix which then undergoes expedited degradation or immunologic attack; thus a vicious cycle of oxidation and inflammation exacerbates and perpetuates various inflammation-associated diseases, resulting in therapeutic recalcitrance and autonomous disease progression.[551,552] A rational clinical approach to breaking this vicious pathogenic cycle can include simultaneous antioxidation and immunomodulation, the former with diet optimization and nutritional supplementation and the latter with allergen avoidance, hormonal correction, xenobiotic detoxification, and specific phytonutritional modulation of pro-inflammatory pathways. Severe and acute inflammation can and often should be suppressed pharmacologically, but sole reliance on pharmacologic immunosuppression leaves the patient vulnerable to iatrogenic immunosuppression and the well-known increased risk for cardiovascular disease, infection, and clinical malignancy while failing to address the underlying biochemical and immunologic imbalances which lie at the bottom of all chronic inflammatory and autoimmune diseases. The contribution of mitochondrial dysfunction to chronic recurrent or persistent pain is most plainly demonstrated in migraine and fibromyalgia (discussed later in this monograph). An important characteristic of migraine is mitochondrial dysfunction, the severity of which correlates positively with the severity of the headache syndrome.[553] In fibromyalgia, numerous abnormalities in cellular bioenergetics are noted, which correlate clinically with the lowered lactate threshold, persistent muscle pain, reduced functional capacity, and the subjective fatigue that characterize the disorder.[554] Nutritional preservation and enhancement of mitochondrial function was termed "mitochondrial resuscitation" by Jeffrey Bland PhD in the 1990s, and clinical implementation of such an approach generally includes, in addition to diet and lifestyle modification, supplementation with coenzyme Q-10, niacin, riboflavin, thiamin, lipoic acid, magnesium, and other nutrients and botanical medicines which enhance production of adenosine triphosphate (ATP).[555]

3. <u>Detoxification and biotransformational imbalances</u>: As our environment becomes increasingly polluted and as researchers and clinicians mature and expand their appreciation and knowledge of the adverse effects of xenobiotics (toxic metals and chemicals), healthcare providers will need to attend to their patients' detoxification capacity and xenobiotic load as a component of the prevention and treatment of disease. By now, senior students and practicing clinicians should be aware of the association of xenobiotics in prototypic diseases such as Parkinson's disease[556,557], adult-onset diabetes mellitus[558,559,560,561], and attention-deficit hyperactivity disorder.[562,563,564] The role of

---

[551] Tak PP, Zvaifler NJ, Green DR, Firestein GS. Rheumatoid arthritis and p53: how oxidative stress might alter the course of inflammatory diseases. *Immunol Today*. 2000 Feb;21(2):78-82

[552] Kurien BT, Hensley K, Bachmann M, Scofield RH. Oxidatively modified autoantigens in autoimmune diseases. *Free Radic Biol Med*. 2006 Aug 15;41(4):549-56

[553] Lodi R, Kemp GJ, Montagna P, Pierangeli G, Cortelli P, Iotti S, Radda GK, Barbiroli B. Quantitative analysis of skeletal muscle bioenergetics and proton efflux in migraine and cluster headache. *J Neurol Sci*. 1997 Feb 27;146(1):73-80

[554] Park JH, Phothimat P, Oates CT, Hernanz-Schulman M, Olsen NJ. Use of P-31 magnetic resonance spectroscopy to detect metabolic abnormalities in muscles of patients with fibromyalgia. *Arthritis Rheum*. 1998 Mar;41(3):406-13

[555] Pieczenik SR, Neustadt J. Mitochondrial dysfunction and molecular pathways of disease. *Exp Mol Pathol*. 2007 Aug;83(1):84-92

[556] Corrigan FM, Wienburg CL, Shore RF, Daniel SE, Mann D. Organochlorine insecticides in substantia nigra in Parkinson's disease. *J Toxicol Environ Health A*. 2000 Feb 25;59(4):229-34

[557] Fleming L, Mann JB, Bean J, Briggle T, Sanchez-Ramos JR. Parkinson's disease and brain levels of organochlorine pesticides. *Ann Neurol*. 1994 Jul;36(1):100-3

[558] Fujiyoshi PT, Michalek JE, Matsumura F. Molecular epidemiologic evidence for diabetogenic effects of dioxin exposure in U.S. Air force veterans of the Vietnam war. *Environ Health Perspect*. 2006 Nov;114(11):1677-83

[559] Lee DH, Lee IK, Song K, Steffes M, Toscano W, Baker BA, Jacobs DR Jr. A strong dose-response relation between serum concentrations of persistent organic pollutants and diabetes: results from the National Health and Examination Survey 1999-2002. *Diabetes Care* 2006 Jul;29(7):1638-44

xenobiotic exposure and impaired detoxification in neuromusculoskeletal pain and inflammatory disorders is more subtle and is generally mediated through the resultant immunotoxicity that manifests as autoimmunity. Occasionally, clinicians will encounter patients with musculoskeletal symptomatology that defies standard diagnosis and treatment but which responds remarkably and permanently to empiric clinical detoxification treatment; such a case will be presented in the Case Reports later in this monograph. The numerous roles of xenobiotic exposure in the genesis and perpetuation of chronic health problems and the role of clinical detoxification in the treatment of such problems has been detailed elsewhere by Crinnion[565,566,567,568,569], Rea[570], Bland[571,572], Vasquez[573,574], and others.[575,576]

4. <u>Immune imbalances</u>: Immune imbalances have an obvious role in musculoskeletal inflammation when discussed in the context of autoimmune diseases such as rheumatoid arthritis, ankylosing spondylitis, and systemic lupus erythematosus. While the standard medical approach to this pathophysiology has focused almost exclusively on the pharmacologic suppression of resultant inflammation and tissue destruction, other disciplines such as naturopathic medicine and functional medicine have emphasized the importance of determining and addressing the underlying causes of such immune imbalance. While clinicians of all disciplines must appreciate the important role of pharmacologic immunosuppression in the treatment of inflammatory exacerbations as seen with giant cell arteritis or neuropsychiatric lupus, they should also appreciate that sole reliance on immunosuppression for long-term management of inflammatory disorders is destined to therapeutic failure insofar as it does not correct the underlying cause of the disease and creates dependency upon perpetual immunosuppression with its attendant costs (not uncommonly in the range of $20,000 - 50,000 per year) and adverse effects including infection and increased risk for cancer. Rather than presuming that immune dysfunction and the resultant inflammation and autoimmunity are results of spontaneous generation, astute clinicians seek to identify and correct the causes of

---

[560] Lee DH, Lee IK, Jin SH, Steffes M, Jacobs DR Jr. Association between serum concentrations of persistent organic pollutants and insulin resistance among nondiabetic adults: results from the National Health and Nutrition Examination Survey 1999-2002. *Diabetes Care*, 2007 Mar;30(3):622-8

[561] Remillard RB, Bunce NJ. Linking dioxins to diabetes: epidemiology and biologic plausibility. *Environ Health Perspect*, 2002 Sep;110(9):853-8

[562] Rauh VA, Garfinkel R, Perera FP, Andrews HF, Hoepner L, Barr DB, Whitehead R, Tang D, Whyatt RW. Impact of prenatal chlorpyrifos exposure on neurodevelopment in the first 3 years of life among inner-city children. *Pediatrics*. 2006 Dec;118(6):e1845-59

[563] Cheuk DK, Wong V. Attention-deficit hyperactivity disorder and blood mercury level: a case-control study in Chinese children. *Neuropediatrics*. 2006 Aug;37(4):234-40

[564] Nigg JT, Knottnerus GM, Martel MM, Nikolas M, Cavanagh K, Karmaus W, Rappley MD. Low blood lead levels associated with clinically diagnosed attention-deficit/hyperactivity disorder and mediated by weak cognitive control. *Biol Psychiatry*. 2008 Feb 1;63(3):325-31

[565] Crinnion W. Results of a Decade of Naturopathic Treatment for Environmental Illnesses: A Review of Clinical Records. *J Naturopathic Medicine* vol. 7; 2, 21-27

[566] Crinnion WJ. Environmental medicine, part 1: the human burden of environmental toxins and their common health effects. *Altern Med Rev*. 2000 Feb;5(1):52-63

[567] Crinnion WJ. Environmental medicine, part 2 - health effects of and protection from ubiquitous airborne solvent exposure. *Altern Med Rev*. 2000 Apr;5(2):133-43

[568] Crinnion WJ. Environmental medicine, part 3: long-term effects of chronic low-dose mercury exposure. *Altern Med Rev*. 2000 Jun;5(3):209-23

[569] Crinnion WJ. Environmental medicine, part 4: pesticides - biologically persistent and ubiquitous toxins. *Altern Med Rev*. 2000 Oct;5(5):432-47

[570] Rea WJ, Pan Y, Johnson AR. Clearing of toxic volatile hydrocarbons from humans. *Bol Asoc Med P R*. 1991 Jul;83(7):321-4

[571] Bland JS, Barrager E, Reedy RG, Bland K. A Medical Food-Supplemented Detoxification Program in the Management of Chronic Health Problems. *Altern Ther Health Med*. 1995 Nov 1;1(5):62-71

[572] Minich DM, Bland JS. Acid-alkaline balance: role in chronic disease and detoxification. *Altern Ther Health Med*. 2007 Jul-Aug;13(4):62-5

[573] Vasquez A. *Integrative Rheumatology: Second Edition*. Fort Worth, Texas; Integrative and Biological Medicine Research and Consulting, 2007 OptimalHealthResearch.com

[574] Vasquez A. Diabetes: Are Toxins to Blame? *Naturopathy Digest* 2007; April

[575] Kilburn KH, Warsaw RH, Shields MG. Neurobehavioral dysfunction in firemen exposed to polycholorinated biphenyls (PCBs): possible improvement after detoxification. *Arch Environ Health*. 1989 Nov-Dec;44(6):345-50

[576] Cecchini M, LoPresti V. Drug residues store in the body following cessation of use: impacts on neuroendocrine balance and behavior--use of the Hubbard sauna regimen to remove toxins and restore health. *Med Hypotheses*. 2007;68(4):868-79

these immune imbalances. By identifying and correcting the underlying causes of immune imbalance (when possible), clinicians can lessen or obviate the need for chronic polypharmaceutical treatment with anti-inflammatory and immunosuppressive agents. Vasquez[577] proposed that secondary immune imbalances (distinguished from primary congenital disorders) generally arise from one or more of five main problems: ❶ habitual consumption of a pro-inflammatory diet, ❷ food allergies and intolerances, ❸ microbial dysbiosis, including multifocal polydysbiosis, ❹ hormonal imbalances, and ❺ xenobiotic exposure and accumulation resulting in immunotoxicity via bystander activation and enhanced processing of autoantigens as well as haptenization and neoantigen formation. These influences may act singularly or when combined may be additive and synergistic. While it is beyond the scope of this monograph to detail each of these here, they will be sufficiently reviewed in later sections dealing with assessment and interventions as well as in the clinical focus subsections, particularly the section on rheumatoid arthritis.

5. Inflammatory imbalances: Inflammatory imbalances may be distinguished from immune imbalances insofar as inflammatory imbalances connote disorders of inflammatory mediator production in the absence of the immunodysfunction that typifies allergy, autoimmunity, or immunosuppression. Here again, long-term consumption of a pro-inflammatory diet[578] is a primary consideration because such a diet typically oversupplies inflammatory precursors such as arachidonate and undersupplies anti-inflammatory phytonutrients such as vitamin D, zinc, selenium, and the numerous phytochemicals that reduce activation of inflammatory pathways.[579,580,581,582] Three of the best examples of correctable inflammatory imbalances are those due to vitamin D deficiency, fatty acid imbalances, and overconsumption of simple sugars and saturated fats. Vitamin D deficiency is a widespread and serious health problem that spans nearly all geographic regions and socioeconomic strata with several important adverse effects. Vitamin D deficiency results in systemic inflammation[583] and chronic musculoskeletal pain[584] which both resolve quickly upon correction of the nutritional deficiency. Similarly and consistent with the Western/American pattern of dietary intake, overconsumption of alpha-linoleic acid and arachidonate along with underconsumption of alpha-linolenic acid (ALA), gamma-linolenic acid (GLA), eicosapentaenoic acid (EPA), docosahexaenoic acid (DHA), and oleic acid subtly yet powerfully shift nutrigenomic tendency and precursor availability in favor of enhanced systemic inflammation. Correction of this imbalance such as with reduced consumption of arachidonate and increased consumption of EPA and DHA has consistently proven to be of significant clinical value in the management of chronic inflammatory disorders.[585,586] Measurable increases in

[577] **Vasquez A**. _Integrative Rheumatology: Second Edition_. Fort Worth, Texas; Integrative and Biological Medicine Research and Consulting, 2007 OptimalHealthResearch.com

[578] Seaman DR. The diet-induced proinflammatory state: a cause of chronic pain and other degenerative diseases? _J Manipulative Physiol Ther_. 2002 Mar-Apr;25(3):168-79

[579] **Vasquez A**. Reducing Pain and Inflammation Naturally. Part 1: New Insights into Fatty Acid Biochemistry and the Influence of Diet. _Nutritional Perspectives_ 2004; October: 5, 7-10, 12, 14

[580] **Vasquez A**. Reducing Pain and Inflammation Naturally. Part 2: New Insights into Fatty Acid Supplementation and Its Effect on Eicosanoid Production and Genetic Expression. _Nutritional Perspectives_ 2005; January: 5-16

[581] **Vasquez A**. Reducing pain and inflammation naturally - Part 3: Improving overall health while safely and effectively treating musculoskeletal pain. _Nutritional Perspectives_ 2005; 28: 34-38, 40-42

[582] **Vasquez A**. Reducing pain and inflammation naturally - Part 4: Nutritional and Botanical Inhibition of NF-kappaB, the Major Intracellular Amplifier of the Inflammatory Cascade. A Practical Clinical Strategy Exemplifying Anti-Inflammatory Nutrigenomics. _Nutritional Perspectives_ 2005;July: 5-12

[583] Timms PM, Mannan N, Hitman GA, Noonan K, Mills PG, Syndercombe-Court D, Aganna E, Price CP, Boucher BJ. Circulating MMP9, vitamin D and variation in the TIMP-1 response with VDR genotype: mechanisms for inflammatory damage in chronic disorders? _QJM_. 2002 Dec;95(12):787-96

[584] Al Faraj S, Al Mutairi K. Vitamin D deficiency and chronic low back pain in Saudi Arabia. _Spine_. 2003 Jan 15;28(2):177-9

[585] James MJ, Gibson RA, Cleland LG. Dietary polyunsaturated fatty acids and inflammatory mediator production. _Am J Clin Nutr_. 2000 Jan;71(1 Suppl):343S-8S

systemic inflammation and oxidative stress follow glucose challenge[587], consumption of saturated fatty acids as found in cream[588], and consumption of a "fast food" breakfast, which triggers the prototypic inflammatory activator NF-kappaB for enhanced production of inflammatory mediators.[589] This triad (vitamin D deficiency, fatty acid imbalance, and overconsumption of sugars and saturated fats) is typical of the Western/American pattern of dietary intake, and the molecular means and clinical consequences of such dietary choices is quite clear, evidenced by burgeoning epidemics of metabolic and inflammatory diseases.

6. <u>Digestive, absorptive, and microbiological imbalances</u>: The grouping of digestive and absorptive considerations suggests that the alimentary tract and its accessory organs of the liver, gall bladder and pancreas will be the focus of these core clinical imbalances, and the addition of microbiological imbalances should remind current clinicians that gastrointestinal dysbiosis is an important and frequent clinical consideration. Impaired digestion begins neither in the stomach nor in the mouth, but it stems rather from any socioeconomic milieu which deprives people of the means to prepare wholesome health-promoting meals and the time to consume those meals in a relaxed parasympathetic-dominant mode, preferably among good company, stimulating conversation, and appropriate ambiance. Poor dentition, xerostomia, hypochlorhydria, cholestasis or cholecystectomy, pancreatic insufficiency, mucosal atrophy, altered gut motility, and bacterial overgrowth of the small bowel are important and common contributors to impaired digestion and absorption; clinicians should consider these frequently and implement treatment with a low threshold for intervention. The relevance of these problems to pain and the musculoskeletal system is generally that of malnutrition and its macro- and micronutrient consequences. Sunlight-deprived individuals must rely on dietary sources of vitamin D, which are hardly adequate for the prevention of overt deficiency; any impairment in digestion, emulsification, or absorption of this fat-soluble vitamin can readily lead to hypovitaminosis D and its resultant musculoskeletal consequences of osteomalacia and unremitting pain.[590] Consumption of foods to which the individual is sensitized ("food allergies") can trigger migraine and other chronic headaches[591,592] as well as generalized musculoskeletal pain and arthritis.[593,594,595] Avoidance of the offending foods often results in amelioration or complete remission of the painful syndrome at low cost and high efficacy without reliance on expensive or potentially harmful or addictive pain-reliving drugs. Occasionally, gluten enteropathy (celiac disease) presents with arthritic pain and chronic synovitis; the pain and

[586] James MJ, Proudman SM, Cleland LG. Dietary n-3 fats as adjunctive therapy in a prototypic inflammatory disease: issues and obstacles for use in rheumatoid arthritis. Prostaglandins *Leukot Essent Fatty Acids*. 2003 Jun;68(6):399-405

[587] Mohanty P, Hamouda W, Garg R, Aljada A, Ghanim H, Dandona P. Glucose challenge stimulates reactive oxygen species (ROS) generation by leucocytes. *J Clin Endocrinol Metab*. 2000 Aug;85(8):2970-3

[588] Mohanty P, Ghanim H, Hamouda W, Aljada A, Garg R, Dandona P. Both lipid and protein intakes stimulate increased generation of reactive oxygen species by polymorphonuclear leukocytes and mononuclear cells. *Am J Clin Nutr*. 2002 Apr;75(4):767-72

[589] Aljada A, Mohanty P, Ghanim H, Abdo T, Tripathy D, Chaudhuri A, Dandona P. Increase in intranuclear nuclear factor kappaB and decrease in inhibitor kappaB in mononuclear cells after a mixed meal: evidence for a proinflammatory effect. *Am J Clin Nutr*. 2004 Apr;79(4):682-90

[590] Basha B, Rao DS, Han ZH, Parfitt AM. Osteomalacia due to vitamin D depletion: a neglected consequence of intestinal malabsorption. *Am J Med*. 2000 Mar;108(4):296-300

[591] Grant EC. Food allergies and migraine. *Lancet*. 1979 May 5;1(8123):966-9

[592] Millichap JG, Yee MM. The diet factor in pediatric and adolescent migraine. *Pediatr Neurol*. 2003 Jan;28(1):9-15

[593] van de Laar MA, Aalbers M, Bruins FG, et al. Food intolerance in rheumatoid arthritis. II. Clinical and histological aspects. *Ann Rheum Dis*. 1992 ;51(3):303-6

[594] Golding DN. Is there an allergic synovitis? *J R Soc Med*. 1990 May;83(5):312-4

[595] Hvatum M, Kanerud L, Hällgren R, Brandtzaeg P. The gut-joint axis: cross reactive food antibodies in rheumatoid arthritis. *Gut*. 2006 Sep;55:1240-7

inflammation remit on a gluten-free diet.[596] Alterations in intestinal microbial balance or an individual's unique response to endogenous bacteria (i.e., dysbiosis) can lead to systemic inflammation, arthritis, vasculitis, and musculoskeletal pain; clinical nuances and molecular mechanisms of gastrointestinal dysbiosis will be surveyed later in this monograph based on a previous review by Vasquez.[597] Clinicians should appreciate that dysbiosis can occur at sites other than the gastrointestinal tract, most importantly the nasopharynx and genitourinary tracts. Eradication of the occult infection or mucosal colonization often results in marked reductions in systemic inflammation and its clinical complications. Interested readers are directed to the excellent review by Noah[598] on the relevance of dysbiosis and its treatment relative to psoriasis; additional citations and clinical applications will be discussed later in this monograph.

7. <u>Structural imbalances from cellular membrane function to the musculoskeletal system</u>: Molecular structural imbalances lie at the heart of the concept of "biochemical individuality" originated by Roger J. Williams[599] in 1956, and this concept was soon thereafter expanded into the theory and practice of "orthomolecular medicine" pioneered by Linus Pauling and colleagues.[600,601] Pauling is considered by many authorities to be the original source of the concept of molecular medicine because he coined the phrase "molecular disease" after his team's discovery in 1949 that sickle cell anemia resulted from a single amino acid substitution that caused physical deformation of the hemoglobin molecule in hypoxic conditions.[602] (One of Pauling's students, Jeffery Bland, continued this legacy with the organization of "functional medicine" which now lives on as the Institute for Functional Medicine.[603]) Single nucleotide polymorphisms (SNP; pronounced "snip") are DNA sequence variations that can result in amino acid substitutions that render the final protein (e.g., structural protein or enzyme) abnormal in structure and therefore function. This aberrancy may or may not cause clinical disease (depending on the severity and importance of the variation), and consequences of the dysfunction may be occult, subtle, or obvious. One of the most powerful and effective means for treating diseases resultant from SNPs that result in enzyme defects is the use of high-dose vitamin supplementation, and this forms the scientific basis for "mega-vitamin therapy" as elegantly and authoritatively reviewed by Bruce Ames, et al.[604] SNP-induced alterations in enzyme structure reduce affinity for vitamin-derived coenzyme binding; this reduced affinity can be "overpowered" by administration of high doses of the required vitamin cofactor to increase tissue concentrations of the nutrient to promote binding of the enzyme with its ligand for the performance of enzymatic function. Thus, the scientific rationale for nutritional therapy is derived in part from the recognition that altered enzymatic function due to altered enzyme structure can often be corrected by administration of supradietary doses of nutrients. Relatedly, the structure and function of

[596] Bourne JT, Kumar P, Huskisson EC, Mageed R, Unsworth DJ, Wojtulewski JA. Arthritis and coeliac disease. *Ann Rheum Dis.* 1985 Sep;44(9):592-8
[597] **Vasquez A**. Reducing Pain and Inflammation Naturally. Part 6: Nutritional and Botanical Treatments Against "Silent Infections" and Gastrointestinal Dysbiosis, Commonly Overlooked Causes of Neuromusculoskeletal Inflammation and Chronic Health Problems. *Nutr Perspect* 2006; Jan: 5-21
[598] Noah PW. The role of microorganisms in psoriasis. *Semin Dermatol.* 1990 Dec;9(4):269-76
[599] Williams RJ. <u>Biochemical Individuality : The Basis for the Genetotrophic Concept</u>. Austin and London: University of Texas Press, 1956. Page x
[600] Pauling L. On the Orthomolecular Environment of the Mind: Orthomolecular Theory. In: Williams RJ, Kalita DK. <u>A Physician's Handbook on Orthomolecular Medicine</u>. New Cannan; Keats Publishing: 1977. Page 76
[601] Pauling L, Robinson AB, Teranishi R, Cary P. Quantitative analysis of urine vapor and breath by gas-liquid partition chromatography. *Proc Natl Acad Sci U S A.* 1971 Oct;68(10):2374-6
[602] Pauling L, Itano HA, Singer SJ, Wells IC. Sickle cell anemia, a molecular disease. *Science.* 1949 Nov 25;110(2865):543-8
[603] Bland JS. Jeffrey S. Bland, PhD, FACN, CNS: functional medicine pioneer. *Altern Ther Health Med.* 2004 Sep-Oct;10(5):74-81
[604] Ames BN, Elson-Schwab I, Silver EA. High-dose vitamin therapy stimulates variant enzymes with decreased coenzyme binding affinity (increased K(m)): relevance to genetic disease and polymorphisms. *Am J Clin Nutr.* 2002 Apr;75(4):616-58

cell membranes is determined by their composition, which is influenced by dietary intake of fatty acids, and which influences production prostaglandins and leukotrienes. This is an important aspect of the scientific rationale for the use of specific fatty acid supplements in the prevention and treatment of painful inflammatory musculoskeletal disease. Cell membrane structure and function can also be altered by systemic oxidative stress; the concomitant alterations in intracellular ions (e.g., calcium) and receptor function along with activation of transcription factors such as NF-kappaB contribute to widespread physiologic impairment which creates a vicious cycle of inflammation, metabolic disturbance, and additional free radical generation.[605,606] Somatic dysfunction, musculoskeletal disorders, and inefficient biomechanics contribute to pain, increased production of inflammatory mediators, and the expedited degeneration of tissues such as collagen and cartilage matrix. Physicians trained in clinical biomechanics and physical medicine appreciate the subtle nuances of musculoskeletal structure-function relationships and address these problems directly with physical and manual means rather than ignoring the physical problem and only treating its biochemical sequelae. While biomechanics, palpatory diagnosis, and manual therapeusis takes years of diligent study for the achievement of proficiency, some of these concepts will be reviewed later in this monograph, particularly in the section on chronic low back pain.

8. Psychological and Spiritual Equilibrium: The connections between physical pain and psychoemotional status and events is worthy of thorough discussion and not merely for the sake of improving upon outdated clinical practices which have typically marginalized these ethereal considerations or considered them only long enough to substantiate psychopharmaceutical intervention. A survey of the literature makes clear the interconnected nature of pain, inflammation, psychoemotional stress, depression, social isolation, and nutritional status; due to space limitations in this monograph, a brief overview must necessarily suffice for the exemplification of representative concepts. Stressful and depressive life events promote the development, persistence, and exacerbation of disorders of pain and inflammation through nutritional, hormonal, immunologic, oxidative, and microbiologic mechanisms. Stated most simply, the perception of stressful events and the resultant neurohormonal cascade results in expedited metabolic utilization and increased urinary excretion of nutrients (e.g., tryptophan , and zinc, magnesium, retinol, respectively) which sum to effect nutritional imbalances and depletion, particularly when the stress response is severe and prolonged.[607,608,609] Specific to the consideration of pain, the depletion of tryptophan (and thus serotonin and melatonin) leaves the patient vulnerable to increased pain from lack of antinociceptive serotonin and to increased inflammation due to impaired endogenous production of anti-inflammatory cortisol, the adrenal release of which requires serotonin-

[605] Evans JL, Maddux BA, Goldfine ID. The molecular basis for oxidative stress-induced insulin resistance. *Antioxid Redox Signal*. 2005 Jul-Aug;7(7-8):1040-52

[606] Joseph JA, Denisova N, Fisher D, Shukitt-Hale B, Bickford P, Prior R, Cao G. Membrane and receptor modifications of oxidative stress vulnerability in aging. Nutritional considerations. *Ann N Y Acad Sci*. 1998 Nov 20;854:268-76

[607] Stephensen CB, Alvarez JO, Kohatsu J, Hardmeier R, Kennedy JI Jr, Gammon RB Jr. Vitamin A is excreted in the urine during acute infection. *Am J Clin Nutr*. 1994 Sep;60(3):388-92

[608] Ingenbleek Y, Bernstein L. The stressful condition as a nutritionally dependent adaptive dichotomy. *Nutrition*. 1999 Apr;15(4):305-20

[609] Henrotte JG, Plouin PF, Lévy-Leboyer C, Moser G, Sidoroff-Girault N, Franck G, Santarromana M, Pineau M. Blood and urinary magnesium, zinc, calcium, free fatty acids, and catecholamines in type A and type B subjects. *J Am Coll Nutr*. 1985;4(2):165-72

dependent stimulation.[610] Severe stress, inflammation, and drugs used to suppress immune-mediated tissue damage (e.g., cyclosporine) increase urinary excretion of magnesium[611], and the eventual magnesium depletion renders the patient more vulnerable to hyperalgesia, depression, and other central nervous system and psychiatric disorders.[612,613] Furthermore, experimental and clinical data have shown that magnesium deficiency leads to a systemic pro-inflammatory state associated with oxidative stress and increased levels of the nociceptive and proinflammatory neurotransmitter substance P.[614] Stress increases secretion of prolactin, a hormone which plays an important pathogenic role in chronic inflammation and autoimmunity.[615,616] An abundance of experimental and clinical research supports the model that chronic psychoemotional stress reduces mucosal immunity, increases intestinal permeability, and allows for increased intestinal colonization by microbes that then stimulate immune responses that cross-react with musculoskeletal tissues and result in the clinical manifestation of autoimmunity and painful rheumatic syndromes which appear clinically as variants of acute and chronic reactive arthritis (formerly Reiter' syndrome[617]) in susceptible patients.[618,619,620,621,622,623,624,625] Very interestingly, certain intestinal bacteria can sense when their human host is stressed, and they take advantage of the situation by becoming more virulent whereas previously these same bacteria may have been incapable of causing disease.[626,627] Psychoemotional stress also reduces mucosal immunity and increases colonization in locations other than the gastrointestinal tract. Microbial colonization of the genitourinary tract ("genitourinary dysbiosis"[628]) appears highly relevant in the genesis and perpetuation of rheumatoid arthritis.[629,630,631,632] Stressful life events also lower

[610] Sandyk R. Tryptophan availability and the susceptibility to stress in multiple sclerosis: a hypothesis. *Int J Neurosci.* 1996 Jul;86(1-2):47-53

[611] DiPalma JR. Magnesium replacement therapy. *Am Fam Physician.* 1990 Jul;42(1):173-6

[612] Murck H. Magnesium and affective disorders. *Nutr Neurosci.* 2002 Dec;5(6):375-89

[613] Hashizume N, Mori M. An analysis of hypermagnesemia and hypomagnesemia. *Jpn J Med.* 1990 Jul-Aug;29(4):368-72

[614] Weglicki W, Quamme G, Tucker K, Haigney M, Resnick L. Potassium, magnesium, and electrolyte imbalance and complications in disease management. *Clin Exp Hypertens.* 2005 Jan;27(1):95-112

[615] Imrich R. The role of neuroendocrine system in the pathogenesis of rheumatic diseases (minireview). *Endocr Regul.* 2002 Jun;36(2):95-106

[616] Orbach H, Shoenfeld Y. Hyperprolactinemia and autoimmune diseases. Autoimmun Rev. 2007 Sep;6(8):537-42

[617] Panush RS, Wallace DJ, Dorff RE, Engleman EP. Retraction of the suggestion to use the term "Reiter's syndrome" sixty-five years later: the legacy of Reiter, a war criminal, should not be eponymic honor but rather condemnation. *Arthritis Rheum.* 2007 Feb;56(2):693-4

[618] Tlaskalová-Hogenová H, Stepánková R, Hudcovic T, Tucková L, Cukrowska B, Lodinová-Zádníková R, Kozáková H, Rossmann P, Bártová J, Sokol D, Funda DP, Borovská D, Reháková Z, Sinkora J, Hofman J, Drastich P, Kokesová A. Commensal bacteria (normal microflora), mucosal immunity and chronic inflammatory and autoimmune diseases. *Immunol Lett.* 2004 May 15;93(2-3):97-108

[619] Collins SM. Stress and the Gastrointestinal Tract IV. Modulation of intestinal inflammation by stress: basic mechanisms and clinical relevance. *Am J Physiol Gastrointest Liver Physiol.* 2001 Mar;280(3):G315-8

[620] Hart A, Kamm MA. Review article: mechanisms of initiation and perpetuation of gut inflammation by stress. *Aliment Pharmacol Ther.* 2002 Dec;16(12):2017-28

[621] Farhadi A, Fields JZ, Keshavarzian A. Mucosal mast cells are pivotal elements in inflammatory bowel disease that connect the dots: stress, intestinal hyperpermeability and inflammation. *World J Gastroenterol.* 2007 Jun 14;13(22):3027-30

[622] Yang PC, Jury J, Söderholm JD, Sherman PM, McKay DM, Perdue MH. Chronic psychological stress in rats induces intestinal sensitization to luminal antigens. *Am J Pathol.* 2006 Jan;168(1):104-14

[623] Rashid T, Ebringer A. Ankylosing spondylitis is linked to Klebsiella--the evidence. *Clin Rheumatol.* 2007 Jun;26(6):858-64

[624] Vasquez A. *Integrative Rheumatology.* Fort Worth, Texas; Integrative and Biological Medicine Research and Consulting, 2007 OptimalHealthResearch.com

[625] Samarkos M, Vaiopoulos G. The role of infections in the pathogenesis of autoimmune diseases. *Curr Drug Targets Inflamm Allergy.* 2005 Feb;4(1):99-103

[626] Alverdy J, Holbrook C, Rocha F, Seiden L, Wu RL, Musch M, Chang E, Ohman D, Suh S. Gut-derived sepsis occurs when the right pathogen with the right virulence genes meets the right host: evidence for in vivo virulence expression in Pseudomonas aeruginosa. *Ann Surg.* 2000 Oct;232(4):480-9

[627] Wu L, Holbrook C, Zaborina O, Ploplys E, Rocha F, Pelham D, Chang E, Musch M, Alverdy J. Pseudomonas aeruginosa expresses a lethal virulence determinant, the PA-I lectin/adhesin, in the intestinal tract of a stressed host: the role of epithelia cell contact and molecules of the Quorum Sensing Signaling System. *Ann Surg.* 2003 Nov;238(5):754-64

[628] **Vasquez A.** *Integrative Rheumatology: Second Edition.* Fort Worth, Texas; Integrative and Biological Medicine Research and Consulting, 2007 OptimalHealthResearch.com

[629] Ebringer A, Rashid T. Rheumatoid arthritis is an autoimmune disease triggered by Proteus urinary tract infection. *Clin Dev Immunol.* 2006 Mar;13(1):41-8

[630] Erlacher L, Wintersberger W, Menschik M, Benke-Studnicka A, Machold K, Stanek G, Söltz-Szöts J, Smolen J, Graninger W. Reactive arthritis: urogenital swab culture is the only useful diagnostic method for the detection of the arthritogenic infection in extra-articularly asymptomatic patients with undifferentiated oligoarthritis. *Br J Rheumatol.* 1995 Sep;34(9):838-42

[631] Rashid T, Ebringer A. Rheumatoid arthritis is linked to Proteus--the evidence. *Clin Rheumatol.* 2007 Jul;26(7):1036-43

testosterone in men and the resultant lack of hormonal immunomodulation can increase the frequency and severity of exacerbations of rheumatoid arthritis[633]; resultant inflammation further suppresses testosterone production and bioavailability[634] leading to a self-perpetuating cycle of hypogonadism and inflammation. Thus, by numerous routes and mechanisms, psychoemotional stress increases the prevalence, persistence, and severity of musculoskeletal inflammation and pain.

Psychiatric codiagnoses are common among patients with painful neuromusculoskeletal disorders, and when the prevailing medical logic cannot solve the musculoskeletal riddle, the disorder is often ascribed to its accompanying mental disorder. The "appropriate" treatment from this perspective is the prescription of psychoactive drugs, generally of the "antidepressant" class. Science-based explanations are needed to expand clinicians' consideration of new possibilities which may someday prevail over commonplace suppositions that leave both clinician and patient trapped within a paradigm of futilely cyclical reasoning and its resultant simplistic symptom-targeting interventions. The following subsections provide alternatives to the "idiopathic pain is caused by its associated depression and both should be treated with antidepressant drugs" hypothesis.

a. <u>Pain, inflammation, and mental depression are final common pathways for nutritional deficiencies and imbalances</u>: As a scientific community we now know that the epidemic problem of vitamin D deficiency leads to both musculoskeletal pain[635] as well as depression[636], and that supplementation with physiologic doses of vitamin D results in an enhanced sense of well-being[637] and high-efficacy alleviation of musculoskeletal pain and depression while providing other major collateral benefits.[638] Since the existence of vitamin D deficiency is more probable than that of antidepressant deficiency, the appropriate intervention for the former is more scientific and rational than that of the latter. Relatedly, research in various fields has shown that Western/American lifestyle and diet patterns diverge radically from human physiologic expectations and human nutritional requirements.[639] With regard to fatty acid intake and the resultant effects on inflammation and neurotransmission, modernized diets are a "set up" for musculoskeletal pain and mental depression, which frequently occur concomitantly and which are both alleviated by corrective fatty acid intervention such as fish oil supplementation as a source of EPA and DHA.[640,641] Correction of

---

[632] Ebringer A, Rashid T, Wilson C. Rheumatoid arthritis: proposal for the use of anti-microbial therapy in early cases. *Scand J Rheumatol.* 2003;32:2-11

[633] James WH. Further evidence that low androgen values are a cause of rheumatoid arthritis: the response of rheumatoid arthritis to seriously stressful life events. *Ann Rheum Dis* 1997;56:566

[634] Karagiannis A, Harsoulis F. Gonadal dysfunction in systemic diseases. *Eur J Endocrinol.* 2005 Apr;152(4):501-13

[635] Plotnikoff GA, Quigley JM. Prevalence of severe hypovitaminosis D in patients with persistent, nonspecific musculoskeletal pain. *Mayo Clin Proc.* 2003 Dec;78(12):1463-70

[636] Wilkins CH, Sheline YI, Roe CM, Birge SJ, Morris JC. Vitamin D deficiency is associated with low mood and worse cognitive performance in older adults. *Am J Geriatr Psychiatry.* 2006 Dec;14(12):1032-40

[637] Vieth R, Kimball S, Hu A, Walfish PG. Randomized comparison of the effects of the vitamin D3 adequate intake versus 100 mcg (4000 IU) per day on biochemical responses and the wellbeing of patients. *Nutr J.* 2004 Jul 19;3:8

[638] **Vasquez A**, Manso G, Cannell J. The clinical importance of vitamin D (cholecalciferol): a paradigm shift with implications for all healthcare providers. *Altern Ther Health Med.* 2004 Sep-Oct;10(5):28-36

[639] O'Keefe JH Jr, Cordain L. Cardiovascular disease resulting from a diet and lifestyle at odds with our Paleolithic genome: how to become a 21st-century hunter-gatherer. *Mayo Clin Proc.* 2004 Jan;79(1):101-8

[640] Kiecolt-Glaser JK, Belury MA, Porter K, Beversdorf DQ, Lemeshow S, Glaser R. Depressive symptoms, omega-6:omega-3 fatty acids, and inflammation in older adults. *Psychosom Med.* 2007 Apr;69(3):217-24

[641] Simopoulos AP. Omega-3 fatty acids in inflammation and autoimmune diseases. *J Am Coll Nutr.* 2002 Dec;21(6):495-505

fatty acid imbalance is therefore more rational in the comanagement of pain and depression than is sole reliance on antidepressant and anti-inflammatory drugs; the latter have their place in treatment but neither addresses the primary cause of the problem and both drug classes have important adverse effects and significant cost in contrast to the safety, affordability, and collateral benefits derived from fatty acid supplementation. Also relevant to this discussion of chronic pain triggered and perpetuated by nutritional imbalances are the pro-inflammatory nature of the Western/American diet[642] and the pain-sensitizing effects of epidemic magnesium deficiency.[643] Therefore, correction of nutritional deficiencies and optimization of nutritional status might supersede the prescription of drugs in patients with concomitant depression and pain.

b. Pain, inflammation, and depression are final common pathways of physical inactivity: Exercising muscle elaborates cytokines ("myokines") with anti-inflammatory activity; a sedentary lifestyle fails to stimulate this endogenous anti-inflammation and is therefore relatively pro-inflammatory.[644] Further, exercise has antidepressant benefits mediated by positive influences on neurotransmission, growth factor elaboration, endocrinologic function, self-image, and social contact.[645] Patients with musculoskeletal pain should be encouraged to exercise to the extent possible given the individual's capacity and type of injury and/or degree of disability. Thus, a prescription for exercise might supersede the prescription of drugs in patients with concomitant depression and pain. Exercise prescriptions must consider frequency, duration, intensity, variety, safety, enjoyment, accountability and objective measures of compliance and progress, as well as appropriate combinations of components which emphasize aerobic fitness, strengthening, flexibility, muscle balancing, and coordination.

c. Pain and depression are final common pathways of inflammation: Several pro-inflammatory cytokines are psychoactive and cause depression, social withdrawal, impaired cognition, and sickness behavior.[646] As an alternative to the use of antidepressant drugs, correction of the underlying inflammatory disorder by natural, pharmacologic, or integrative means may subsequently promote restoration of normal affect and cognitive function.

d. Pain, inflammation, and mental depression are final common pathways for hormonal deficiencies and imbalances: Deficiencies of thyroid hormones, estrogen (insufficiency or excess), testosterone, cortisol, and DHEA can cause depression and impaired neuroemotional status. Hormonal aberrations are common in patients with chronic musculoskeletal pain, particularly of the inflammatory and autoimmune types. Clinical trials have shown that administration of thyroid hormones, testosterone, DHEA, cortisol and suppression prolactin can each provide anti-inflammatory, analgesic, and antidepressant benefits among appropriately selected patients. Thus,

---

[642] Aljada A, Mohanty P, Ghanim H, Abdo T, Tripathy D, Chaudhuri A, Dandona P. Increase in intranuclear nuclear factor kappaB and decrease in inhibitor kappaB in mononuclear cells after a mixed meal: evidence for a proinflammatory effect. *Am J Clin Nutr*. 2004 Apr;79(4):682-90

[643] Park JH, Niermann KJ, Olsen N. Evidence for metabolic abnormalities in the muscles of patients with fibromyalgia. *Curr Rheumatol Rep*. 2000 Apr;2(2):131-40

[644] Petersen AM, Pedersen BK. The anti-inflammatory effect of exercise. *J Appl Physiol*. 2005 Apr;98(4):1154-62

[645] Cotman CW, Berchtold NC, Christie LA. Exercise builds brain health: key roles of growth factor cascades and inflammation. *Trends Neurosci*. 2007 Sep;30(9):464-72

[646] Wilson CJ, Finch CE, Cohen HJ. Cytokines and cognition--the case for a head-to-toe inflammatory paradigm. *J Am Geriatr Soc*. 2002 Dec;50(12):2041-56

identification and correction of hormonal imbalances might supersede the prescription of antidepressant drugs in patients with concomitant depression, inflammation, and pain.

Our cultural and scientific advancements in the knowledge of how the brain and mind function have been paradoxically paralleled by social trends showing increasing depression and social isolation; the typical American has only two friends and no one in whom to confide.[647] In the United States, violent injuries are epidemic, and the level of firearm morbidity and mortality in the US is far higher than anywhere else in the industrialized world.[648] This does to some extent beg the question of the value of "scientific knowledge" of the brain and mind within a social structure that is increasingly violent and fragmented. Further, the mental depression resultant from pandemic social isolation would be better served by physicians' admonition for increased social contact than by the continued overuse of drugs which inhibit neurotransmitter reuptake.

Conclusion: The clinical employment of the functional medicine approach to chronic disease management and health promotion rests upon a foundation of competent patient management and then extends to consider the well documented contributions of the causative *core clinical imbalances* that have allowed the genesis and perpetuation of the problem(s) under consideration. The attainment of wellness, the success of preventive medicine, and the optimization of socioemotional health cannot be attained by pharmacological suppression of the manifestations of dysfunction that result from nutritional and neuroendocrine imbalances, xenobiotic accumulation, sedentary lifestyles, social isolation, and mucosal microbial colonization. Rather, these problems are addressed directly, and these and other causative considerations must remain foremost in the mind of the physician committed to the successful, ethical, and cost-effective long-term prevention and management of chronic health disturbances, particularly those characterized by inflammation and pain.

---

[647] McPherson M, Smith-Lovin L, Brashears ME. Social Isolation in America: Changes in Core Discussion Networks over Two Decades. *American Sociological Review* 2006; 71: 353-75
[648] Preventing firearm violence: a public health imperative. *American College of Physicians. Ann Intern Med.* 1995 Feb 15;122(4):311-3

Functional medicine is a science-based field of health care that is grounded in the following principles:

- **Biochemical individuality** describes the importance of individual variations in metabolic function that derive from genetic and environmental differences among individuals.
- **Patient-centered** medicine emphasizes "patient care" rather than "disease care," following Sir William Osler's admonition that "It is more important to know what patient has the disease than to know what disease the patient has."
- **Dynamic balance** of internal and external factors.
- **Web-like interconnections** of physiological factors – an abundance of research now supports the view that the human body functions as an orchestrated network of interconnected systems, rather than individual systems functioning autonomously and without effect on each other. For example, we now know that immunological dysfunctions can promote cardiovascular disease, that dietary imbalances can cause hormonal disturbances, and that environmental exposures can precipitate neurologic syndromes such as Parkinson's disease.
- **Health as a positive vitality** – not merely the absence of disease.
- **Promotion of organ reserve** as the means to enhance health span.

Functional medicine is anchored by an examination of the core clinical imbalances that underlie various disease conditions. Those imbalances arise as **environmental inputs** such as diet, nutrients (including air and water), exercise, and trauma **are processed** by one's body, mind, and spirit through a unique set of genetic predispositions, attitudes, and beliefs. The **fundamental physiological** processes include communication, both outside and inside the cell; bioenergetics, or the transformation of food into energy; replication, repair, and maintenance of structural integrity, from the cellular to the whole body level; elimination of waste; protection and defense; and transport and circulation. The **core clinical imbalances** that arise from malfunctions within this complex system include:

- **Hormonal and neurotransmitter imbalances**
- **Oxidation-reduction imbalances and mitochondropathy**
- **Detoxification and biotransformational imbalances**
- **Immune imbalances**
- **Inflammatory imbalances**
- **Digestive, absorptive, and microbiological imbalances**
- **Structural imbalances** from cellular membrane function to the musculoskeletal system

Imbalances such as these are the precursors to the signs and symptoms by which we detect and label (diagnose) organ system disease. Improving balance – in the patient's environmental inputs and in the body's fundamental physiological processes – is the precursor to restoring health and it involves much more than treating the symptoms. Functional medicine is dedicated to improving the management of complex, chronic disease by intervening at multiple levels to address these core clinical imbalances and to restore each patient's functionality and health. Functional medicine is not a unique and separate body of knowledge. It is grounded in scientific principles and information widely available in medicine today, combining research from various disciplines into highly detailed yet clinically relevant models of disease pathogenesis and effective clinical management.

Functional medicine emphasizes a definable and teachable **process** of integrating multiple knowledge bases within a pragmatic intellectual matrix that focuses on functionality at many levels, rather than a single treatment for a single diagnosis. Functional medicine uses the patient's story as a key tool for integrating diagnosis, signs and symptoms, and evidence of clinical imbalances into a comprehensive approach to improve both the patient's environmental inputs and his or her physiological function. It is a clinician's discipline, and it directly addresses the need to transform the practice of primary care.

Previously published essays

A Five-Part Nutritional Wellness Protocol That Produces Consistently Positive Results: Brief Review of Scientific Rationale

Alex Vasquez, DC, ND

This article was originally published in *Nutritional Wellness*
http://www.nutritionalwellness.com/archives/2005/sep/09_vasquez.php

When I am lecturing here in the U.S., as well as in Europe, doctors often ask if I will share the details of my protocols with them. Thus, in 2004, I published a 486-page textbook for doctors that includes several protocols and important concepts for the promotion of wellness and treatment of musculoskeletal disorders.[649] In this article, I will share with you what I consider a basic protocol for wellness promotion. I've implemented this protocol as part of the treatment plan for a wide range of clinical problems. In my next column, I will provide several case reports of patients from my office to exemplify the effectiveness of this program and show how it can be the foundation upon which additional treatments can be added as necessary.

Nutrients are required in the proper amounts, forms, and approximate ratios for essential physiologic function; if nutrients are lacking, the body cannot function normally, let alone optimally. Impaired function results in subjective and objective manifestations of what is commonly labeled as "disease." Thus, a powerful and effective alternative to treating diseases with drugs is to re-establish normal/optimal physiologic function by replenishing the body with essential nutrients.

Of course, many diseases are multifactorial and therefore require multicomponent treatment plans, and some diseases actually require the use of drugs. However, while only a relatively small portion of patients actually need drugs for their problems, I am sure we all agree that everyone needs a foundational nutrition plan, as outlined and substantiated below.

1. <u>Health-promoting diet</u>: Following an extensive review of the research literature, I developed what I call the "supplemented Paleo-Mediterranean diet," which I have described in greater detail elsewhere.[650] In essence, this diet plan combines the best of the Mediterranean diet with the best of the Paleolithic diet, the latter of which has been detailed most recently by Dr. Loren Cordain in his book, The Paleo Diet, and his numerous scientific articles.[651] This diet places emphasis on fruits, vegetables, nuts, seeds, and berries that meet the body's needs for fiber, carbohydrates, and most importantly, the 8,000+ phytonutrients that have additive and synergistic health benefits.[652] Preferred protein sources are lean meats such as fish and poultry. In contrast to Cordain's Paleo diet, I also advocate soy and whey for their high-quality protein and anticancer, cardioprotective, and mood-enhancing benefits. Rice and potatoes are discouraged due to their relatively high glycemic indexes and high glycemic loads, and their lack of fiber and phytonutrients (compared to other fruits and vegetables). Generally speaking, grains such as wheat and rye are discouraged due to the high glycemic

---

[649] **Vasquez A**. *Integrative Orthopedics: The Art of Creating Wellness While Managing Acute and Chronic Musculoskeletal Disorders*. 2004, 2007
[650] **Vasquez A**. The Importance of Integrative Chiropractic Health Care in Treating Musculoskeletal Pain and Reducing the Nationwide Burden of Medical Expenses and Iatrogenic Injury and Death: A Concise Review of Current Research and Implications for Clinical Practice and Healthcare Policy. *The Original Internist* 2005; 12(4): 159-182
[651] Cordain L. *The Paleo Diet*. (John Wiley and Sons, 2002). Also: Cordain L. Cereal grains: humanity's double edged sword. *World Rev Nutr Diet* 1999;84:19-73 Access to most of Dr Cordain's articles is available at http://thepaleodiet.com/
[652] Liu RH. Health benefits of fruit and vegetables are from additive and synergistic combinations of phytochemicals. *Am J Clin Nutr* 2003;78(3 Suppl):517S-520S

loads/indexes of most breads and pastries, as well as the allergenicity of gluten, a protein that appears to help trigger disorders such as migraine, celiac disease, psoriasis, epilepsy, and autoimmunity. Sources of simple sugars such as high-fructose corn syrup (e.g., cola, soda) and processed foods (e.g., "TV dinners" and other manufactured snacks and convenience foods) are strictly forbidden. Chemical preservatives, colorants, sweeteners and carrageenan are likewise prohibited. In summary, this diet plan provides plenty of variety, as most dishes comprised of poultry, fish, soy, fruits, vegetables, nuts, berries, and seeds are allowed. The diet also provides plenty of fiber, phytonutrients, carbohydrates, potassium, and protein, while simultaneously being low in fat, sodium, arachidonic acid, and "simple sugars." The diet must be customized with regard to total protein and calorie intake, as determined by the size, status, and activity level of the patient, and individual food allergens should be avoided. Regular consumption of this diet has shown the ability to reduce hypertension, alleviate diabetes, ameliorate migraine headaches, and result in improvement of overall health and a lessening of the severity of many common "diseases." This diet is supplemented with vitamins, minerals, and fatty acids as described below.

2. <u>Multivitamin and multimineral supplementation</u>: Vitamin and mineral supplementation finally received endorsement from "mainstream" medicine when researchers from Harvard Medical School published a review article in Journal of the American Medical Association that concluded, "Most people do not consume an optimal amount of all vitamins by diet alone. ...It appears prudent for all adults to take vitamin supplements."[653] Long-term nutritional insufficiencies experienced by "most people" promote the development of "long-latency deficiency diseases" such as cancer, neuroemotional deterioration, and cardiovascular disease.[654] Impressively, the benefits of multivitamin/multimineral supplementation have been demonstrated in numerous clinical trials. Multivitamin/multimineral supplementation has been shown to improve nutritional status and reduce the risk for chronic diseases[655]. improve mood[656], potentiate antidepressant drug treatment[657], alleviate migraine headaches (when used with diet improvement and fatty acids[658]), improve immune function and infectious disease outcomes in the elderly[659] (especially diabetics[660]), reduce morbidity and mortality in patients with HIV infection[661,662] alleviate premenstrual syndrome[663,664] and bipolar disorder[665], reduce violence and antisocial behavior in children[666] and incarcerated young adults (when used with essential fatty acids[667]), and improve scores of intelligence in children.[668] Vitamin supplementation has anti-inflammatory benefits, as evidenced by significant reduction in C-reactive protein, (CRP) in a double-blind, placebo-controlled trial.[669]

[653] Fletcher RH, Fairfield KM. Vitamins for chronic disease prevention in adults: clinical applications. *JAMA* 2002;287:3127-9

[654] Heaney RP. Long-latency deficiency disease: insights from calcium and vitamin D. *Am J Clin Nutr* 2003;78:912-9

[655] McKay DL, Perrone G, Rasmussen H, Dallal G, Hartman W, Cao G, Prior RL, Roubenoff R, Blumberg JB. The effects of a multivitamin/mineral supplement on micronutrient status, antioxidant capacity and cytokine production in healthy older adults consuming a fortified diet. *J Am Coll Nutr* 2000;19(5):613-21

[656] Benton D, Haller J, Fordy J. Vitamin supplementation for 1 year improves mood. *Neuropsychobiology* 1995;32(2):98-105

[657] Coppen A, Bailey J. Enhancement of the antidepressant action of fluoxetine by folic acid: a randomised, placebo controlled trial. *J Affect Disord* 2000;60:121-30

[658] Wagner W, Nootbaar-Wagner U. Prophylactic treatment of migraine with gamma-linolenic and alpha-linolenic acids. *Cephalalgia* 1997;17:127-30

[659] Langkamp-Henken B, Bender BS, Gardner EM, Herrlinger-Garcia KA, Kelley MJ, Murasko DM, Schaller JP, Stechmiller JK, Thomas DJ, Wood SM. Nutritional formula enhanced immune function and reduced days of symptoms of upper respiratory tract infection in seniors. *J Am Geriatr Soc* 2004;52:3-12

[660] Barringer TA, Kirk JK, Santaniello AC, Foley KL, Michielutte R. Effect of a multivitamin and mineral supplement on infection and quality of life. A randomized, double-blind, placebo-controlled trial. *Ann Intern Med* 2003;138:365-71

[661] Fawzi WW, Msamanga GI, Spiegelman D, et al. A randomized trial of multivitamin supplements and HIV disease progression and mortality. *N Engl J Med* 2004;351:23-32

[662] Burbano X, Miguez-Burbano MJ, McCollister K, Zhang G, Rodriguez A, Ruiz P, Lecusay R, Shor-Posner G. Impact of a selenium chemoprevention clinical trial on hospital admissions of HIV-infected participants. *HIV Clin Trials* 2002;3:483-91

[663] Abraham GE. Nutritional factors in the etiology of the premenstrual tension syndromes. *J Reprod Med* 1983;28(7):446-64

[664] Stewart A. Clinical and biochemical effects of nutritional supplementation on the premenstrual syndrome. *J Reprod Med* 1987;32:435-41

[665] Kaplan BJ, Simpson JS, Ferre RC, Gorman CP, McMullen DM, Crawford SG. Effective mood stabilization with a chelated mineral supplement: an open-label trial in bipolar disorder. *J Clin Psychiatry* 2001;62:936-44

[666] Kaplan BJ, Crawford SG, Gardner B, Farrelly G. Treatment of mood lability and explosive rage with minerals and vitamins: two case studies in children. *J Child Adolesc Psychopharmacol* 2002;12(3):205-19

[667] Gesch CB, Hammond SM, Hampson SE, Eves A, Crowder MJ. Influence of supplementary vitamins, minerals and essential fatty acids on the antisocial behaviour of young adult prisoners. Randomised, placebo-controlled trial. *Br J Psychiatry* 2002;181:22-8

[668] Benton D. Micro-nutrient supplementation and the intelligence of children. *Neurosci Biobehav Rev* 2001;25:297-309

[669] Church TS, Earnest CP, Wood KA, Kampert JB. Reduction of C-reactive protein levels through use of a multivitamin. *Am J Med* 2003;115:702-7

The ability to safely and affordably deliver these benefits makes multimineral-multivitamin supplementation and essential component of any and all health-promoting and disease-prevention strategies. Vitamin A can result in liver damage with chronic consumption of 25,000 IU or more, and intake should generally not exceed 10,000 IU per day in women of childbearing age. Iron should not be supplemented except in patients diagnosed with iron deficiency by a blood test (serum ferritin). Additional vitamin D should be used, as described in the next section.

3. Physiologic doses of vitamin D3: The prevalence of vitamin D deficiency varies from 40 percent (general population) to almost 100 percent (patients with musculoskeletal pain) in the American population. I described the many benefits of vitamin D3 supplementation in the previous issue of *Nutritional Wellness* and in the major monograph published last year.[670] In summary, vitamin D deficiency causes or contributes to depression, hypertension, seizures, migraine, polycystic ovary syndrome, inflammation, autoimmunity, and musculoskeletal pain such as low-back pain. Clinical trials using vitamin D supplementation have proven the cause-and-effect relationship between vitamin D deficiency and these conditions by showing that each of these could be cured or alleviated with vitamin D supplementation. In our review of the literature, we concluded that daily vitamin D doses should be 1,000 IU for infants, 2,000 IU for children, and 4,000 IU for adults. Cautions and contraindications include the use of thiazide diuretics (e.g., hydrochlorothiazide) or any other medications that can promote hypercalcemia, as well as granulomatous diseases such as sarcoidosis, tuberculosis, and certain types of cancer, especially lymphoma. Effectiveness is monitored by measuring serum 25-OH-vitamin D, and safety is monitored by measuring serum calcium.

4. Balanced and complete fatty acid supplementation: A detailed survey of the literature shows there are at least five health-promoting fatty acids commonly found in the human diet.[671] These are alpha-linolenic acid (ALA; omega-3, from flaxseed oil), eicosapentaenoic acid (EPA; omega-3, from fish oil), docosahexaenoic acid (DHA; omega-3, from fish oil and algae), gamma-linolenic acid (GLA; omega-6, most concentrated in borage oil), and oleic acid (omega-9, from olive oil, also flaxseed and borage oils). Each of these fatty acids has health benefits that cannot be fully attained from supplementing a different fatty acid. The benefits of GLA (borage oil) are not attained by consumption of EPA and DHA (fish oil); in fact, consumption of fish oil can actually promote a deficiency of GLA.[672] Likewise, consumption of GLA alone can reduce EPA levels while increasing levels of proinflammatory arachidonic acid; both of these problems are avoided with co-administration of fish oil any time borage oil is used. Using ALA (flaxseed oil) alone only slightly increases EPA but generally leads to no improvement in DHA status and can lead to a reduction of oleic acid; thus, fish oil, olive oil (and borage oil) should be supplemented when flaxseed oil is used.[673] Obviously, the goal here is a balanced intake of all of the health-promoting fatty acids; using only one or two sources of fatty acids is not balanced and results in suboptimal improvement, at best. In clinical practice, I routinely use combination fatty acid therapy comprised of ALA, EPA, DHA, and GLA for essentially all patients. The product also contains a modest amount of oleic acid, and I encourage use of olive oil for salads and cooking. This approach results in complete and balanced fatty acid intake, and the clinical benefits are impressive.

5. Probiotics /gut flora modification: Proper levels of good bacteria promote intestinal health, proper immune function, and support overall health. Excess bacteria or yeast, or the presence of harmful bacteria, yeast, or "parasites" such as amoebas and protozoas, can

[670] **Vasquez A**, Manso G, Cannell J. The clinical importance of vitamin D (cholecalciferol): a paradigm shift with implications for all healthcare providers. *Alternative Therapies in Health and Medicine* 2004;10:28-37 http://optimalhealthresearch.com/cholecalciferol.html

[671] **Vasquez A**. Reducing Pain and Inflammation Naturally. Part 2: New Insights into Fatty Acid Supplementation and Its Effect on Eicosanoid Production and Genetic Expression. *Nutritional Perspectives* 2005; January: 5-16 http://optimalhealthresearch.com/part2

[672] Cleland LG, Gibson RA, Neumann M, French JK. The effect of dietary fish oil supplement upon the content of dihomo-gammalinolenic acid in human plasma phospholipids. *Prostaglandins Leukot Essent Fatty Acids* 1990 May;40(1):9-12

[673] Jantti J, Nikkari T, Solakivi T, Vapaatalo H, Isomaki H. Evening primrose oil in rheumatoid arthritis: changes in serum lipids and fatty acids. *Ann Rheum Dis* 1989;48(2):124-7

cause "leaky gut," systemic inflammation, and a wide range of clinical problems. Intestinal flora can become imbalanced by poor diets, excess stress, immunosuppressive drugs, antibiotics, or exposure to contaminated food or water, all of which are common among American patients. Thus, as a rule, I reinstate the good bacteria by the use of probiotics (good bacteria and yeast), prebiotics (fiber, arabinogalactan, and inulin), and the use of fermented foods such as kefir (in patients not allergic to milk). Harmful yeast, bacteria, and other "parasites" can be eradicated with the combination of dietary change, drugs, and/or herbal extracts. For example, oregano oil in an emulsified, time-released form has proven safe and effective for the elimination of various parasites encountered in clinical practice.[674] Likewise, the herb *Artemisia annua* (sweet wormwood) commonly is used to eradicate specific bacteria and has been used for thousands of years in Asia for the treatment and prevention of infectious diseases, including malaria.[675]

Conclusion:

In this brief review, I have outlined and scientifically substantiated a fundamental protocol that can serve as effective therapy for patients with a wide range of "diseases." Customizing the Paleo-Mediterranean diet to avoid food allergens, using vitamin-mineral supplements along with physiologic doses of vitamin D and broad-spectrum balanced fatty acid supplementation, and ensuring gastrointestinal health with the skillful use of probiotics, prebiotics, and antimicrobial treatments provides an excellent health-promoting and disease-eliminating foundation and lifestyle for many patients. Often, this simple protocol is all that is needed for the effective treatment of a wide range of clinical problems. For other patients with more complex illnesses, of course, additional interventions and laboratory assessments can be used to customize the treatment plan. However, we must always remember that the attainment and preservation of health requires that we meet the body's basic nutritional needs. This five-step protocol begins the process of meeting those needs. In my next article, I'll give you some examples from my clinical practice and additional references to show how safe and effective this protocol can be.

Implementing the Five-Part Nutritional Wellness Protocol for the Treatment of Various Health Problems

Alex Vasquez, DC, ND

This article was originally published in *Nutritional Wellness*
http://www.nutritionalwellness.com/archives/2005/nov/11_vasquez.php

In my last article in *Nutritional Wellness* I described a 5-part nutritional protocol that can be used in the vast majority of patients without adverse effects and with major benefits. For many patients, the basic protocol consisting of 1) the Paleo-Mediterranean diet, 2) multivitamin/multimineral supplementation, 3) additional vitamin D3, 4) combination fatty acid therapy with an optimal balance of ALA, GLA, EPA, DHA, and oleic acid, and 5) probiotics (including the identification and eradication of harmful yeast, bacteria, and other "parasites") is all the treatment that they need. For patients who need additional treatment, this foundational plan still serves as the core of the biochemical aspect of their intervention. Of course, in some cases, we have to use other lifestyle modifications (such as exercise), additional supplements (such as policosanol or antimicrobial herbs), manual treatments (including spinal manipulation) and occasionally select medications (such has hormone modulators) to obtain our goal of maximum improvement.

The following examples show how the 5-part protocol serves to benefit patients with a wide range of conditions. For the sake of saving space, I will use only highly specific citations to the research

---

[674] Force M, Sparks WS, Ronzio RA. Inhibition of enteric parasites by emulsified oil of oregano in vivo. *Phytother Res* 2000;14:213-4
[675] Schuster BG. Demonstrating the validity of natural products as anti-infective drugs. *J Altern Complement Med* 2001;7 Suppl 1:S73-82

literature, since I have provided the other references in the previous issue of *Nutritional Wellness* and elsewhere.[676]

- **A Man with High Cholesterol**: This patient is a 41-year-old slightly overweight man with very high cholesterol. His total cholesterol was 290 (normal < 200), LDL cholesterol was 212 (normal <130), and his triglycerides were 148 (optimal <100). I am quite certain that nearly every medical doctor would have put this man on cholesterol-lowering statin drugs for life. *Treatment*: In contrast, I advised a low-carb Paleo-Mediterranean diet because such diets have been shown to reduce cardiovascular mortality more powerfully that "statin" cholesterol-lowing drugs in older patients.[677] Likewise, fatty acid supplementation is more effective than statin drugs for reducing cardiac and all-cause mortality.[678] We added probiotics, because supplementation with *Lactobacillus* and *Bifidobacterium* has been shown to lower cholesterol levels in humans with high cholesterol.[679] Finally, I also prescribed 20 mg of policosanol for its well-known ability to favorably modify cholesterol levels.[680] *Results*: Within **one month** the patient had lost weight, felt better, and his total cholesterol had dropped to normal at 196 (from 290!), LDL was reduced to 141, and triglycerides were reduced to 80. Basically, this treatment plan was "the protocol + policosanol." Drug treatment of this patient would have been more expensive, more risky, and would not have resulted in global health improvements.

- **A Child with Intractable Seizures**: This is a 4-year-old nonverbal boy with 3-5 seizures per day despite being on two anti-seizure medications and having previously had several other "last resort" medical and surgical procedures. He also had a history of food allergies. *Treatment*: Obviously, there was no room for error in this case. We implemented a moderately low-carb hypoallergenic diet since both carbohydrate restriction[681] and allergy avoidance[682] can reduce the frequency and severity of seizures. Since many "anti-seizure" medications actually cause seizures by causing vitamin D deficiency[683], I added 800 IU per day of emulsified vitamin D3 for its antiseizure benefit.[684] We used 1 tsp per day of a combination fatty acid supplement that provides balanced amounts of ALA, GLA, EPA, and DHA, since fatty acids appear to have potential antiseizure benefits.[685] Vitamin B-6 (250 mg of P5P) and magnesium (bowel tolerance) were also added to reduce brain hyperexcitability.[686] Stool testing showed an absence of *Bifidobacteria* and *Lactobacillus*; probiotics were added for their anti-allergy benefits.[687] *Results*: Within about 2 months seizure frequency reduced from 3-5 per day to one seizure every other day: **an 87% reduction in seizure frequency**. Patient was able to discontinue one of the anti-seizure medications. His parents also noted several global improvements: the boy started making eye contact with people, he was learning again, and intellectually he was "making gains every day." His parents considered this an "amazing difference." Going from 30 seizures per week to 4 seizures per week while reducing medication use by 50% is a major achievement. Notice that we simply used the basic wellness protocol with some additional B6 and magnesium. It is highly unlikely that B6 and magnesium alone would have produced such a favorable response.

---

[676] **Vasquez A**. Integrative Orthopedics. www.OptimalHealthResearch.com and Chiropractic and Naturopathic Medicine for the Promotion of Optimal Health and Alleviation of Pain and Inflammation. http://optimalhealthresearch.com/monograph05
[677] Knoops KT, et al. Mediterranean diet, lifestyle factors, and 10-year mortality in elderly European men and women: the HALE project. *JAMA*. 2004 Sep 22;292(12):1433-9
[678] Studer M, et al. Effect of different antilipidemic agents and diets on mortality: a systematic review. *Arch Intern Med*. 2005;165:725-30
[679] Xiao JZ, et al. Effects of milk products fermented by Bifidobacterium longum on blood lipids in rats and healthy adult male volunteers.*J Dairy Sci*. 2003;86:2452-61
[680] Cholesterol-lowering action of policosanol compares well to that of pravastatin and lovastatin. *Cardiovasc J S Afr*. 2003;14(3):161
[681] Freeman JM, et al. The efficacy of the ketogenic diet-1998: a prospective evaluation of intervention in 150 children. *Pediatrics*. 1998;102:1358-63
[682] Egger J, Carter CM, Soothill JF, Wilson J. Oligoantigenic diet treatment of children with epilepsy and migraine. *J Pediatr*. 1989;114:51-8
[683] Ali FE, Al-Bustan MA, Al-Busairi WA, Al-Mulla FA. Loss of seizure control due to anticonvulsant-induced hypocalcemia. *Ann Pharmacother*. 2004;38:1002-5
[684] Christiansen C, Rodbro P, Sjo O."Anticonvulsant action" of vitamin D in epileptic patients? A controlled pilot study. *Br Med J*. 1974 May 4;2(913):258-9
[685] Yuen AW, et al. Omega-3 fatty acid supplementation in patients with chronic epilepsy: A randomized trial. *Epilepsy Behav*. 2005 Sep;7(2):253-8
[686] Mousain-Bosc M, et al. Magnesium VitB6 intake reduces central nervous system hyperexcitability in children. *J Am Coll Nutr*. 2004;23(5):545S-548S
[687] Majamaa H, Isolauri E.Probiotics: a novel approach in the management of food allergy. *J Allergy Clin Immunol*. 1997 Feb;99(2):179-85

- **A Young Woman with Full-Body Psoriasis Unresponsive to Drug Treatment**: This is a 17-year-old woman with head-to-toe psoriasis since childhood. She wears long pants and long-sleeved shirts year-round, and the psoriasis is a major interference to her social life. Medications have ceased to help. *Treatment*: The Paleo-Mediterranean diet was implemented with an emphasis on food allergy identification.[1] We used a multivitamin-mineral supplement with 200 mcg selenium to compensate for the nutritional insufficiencies and selenium deficiency that are common in patients with psoriasis; likewise 10 mg of folic acid was added to address the relative vitamin deficiencies and elevated homocysteine that are common in these patients.[688] Combination fatty acid therapy with EPA and DHA from fish oil and GLA from borage oil was used for the anti-inflammatory and skin-healing benefits.[689] Vitamin E (1200 IU of mixed tocopherols) and lipoic acid (1,000 mg per day) were added for their anti-inflammatory benefits and to combat the oxidative stress that is characteristic of psoriasis.[690] Of course, probiotics were used to modify gut flora, which is commonly deranged in patients with psoriasis.[691] *Results*: Within a few weeks, this patient's "lifelong psoriasis" was essentially gone. Food allergy identification and avoidance played a major role in the success of this case. When I saw the patient again 9 months later for her second visit, she had no visible evidence of psoriasis. Her "medically untreatable" condition was essentially cured by the use of my basic protocol, with the addition of a few extra nutrients.

- **A Man with Fatigue and Recurrent Numbness in Hands and Feet**. This 40-year-old man had seen numerous neurologists and had spent tens of thousands of dollars on MRIs, CT scans, lumbar punctures, and other diagnostic procedures. No diagnosis had been found, and no effective treatment had been rendered by medical specialists. *Assessments*: We performed a modest battery of lab tests which revealed elevations of fibrinogen and C-reactive protein (CRP), two markers of acute inflammation. Assessment of intestinal permeability with the lactulose-mannitol assay showed major intestinal damage ("leaky gut"). Follow-up parasite testing on different occasions showed dysbiosis caused by *Proteus*, *Enterobacter*, *Klebsiella*, *Citrobacter*, and *Pseudomonas aeruginosa*—of course, these are gram-negative bacteria that can induce immune dysfunction and autoimmunity, as described elsewhere.[1] Specifically, *Pseudomonas aeruginosa* has been linked to the development of nervous system autoimmunity, such as multiple sclerosis.[692] *Treatment*: We implemented a plan of diet modification, vitamins, minerals, fatty acids, and probiotics. The dysbiosis was further addressed with specific antimicrobial herbs (including caprylic acid and emulsified oregano oil[693]) and drugs (such as tetracycline, Bactrim, and augmentin). The antibiotic drugs proved to be ineffective based on repeat stool testing. *Results*: Within one month we witnessed impressive improvements, both subjectively and objectively. Subjectively, the patient reported that the numbness and tingling almost completely resolved. Fatigue was reduced, and energy was improved. Objectively, the patient's elevated CRP plummeted from abnormally high at 11 down to completely normal at 1. Eighteen months later, the patient's CRP had dropped to less than 1 and fatigue and numbness were no longer problematic. Notice that this treatment plan was basically "the protocol" with additional attention to eradicating the dysbiosis we found with specialized stool testing.

- **A 50-year-old Man with Rheumatoid Arthritis**. This patient presented with a 3-year history of rheumatoid arthritis that had been treated unsuccessfully with drugs (methotrexate and intravenous Remicade). The first time I tested his hsCRP level, it was astronomically high at 124 (normal is <3). Because of the severe inflammation and other risk factors for sudden cardiac death, I referred this patient to an osteopathic internist for immune-suppressing drugs;

[688] Vanizor Kural B, et al. Plasma homocysteine and its relationships with atherothrombotic markers in psoriatic patients. *Clin Chim Acta*. 2003 Jun;332(1-2):23-3

[689] **Vasquez A**. Reducing Pain and Inflammation Naturally. Part 2: New Insights into Fatty Acid Supplementation and Its Effect on Eicosanoid Production and Genetic Expression. *Nutritional Perspectives* 2005; January: 5-16 www.OptimalHealthResearch.com/part2

[690] Kokcam I, Naziroglu M. Antioxidants and lipid peroxidation status in the blood of patients with psoriasis. *Clin Chim Acta*. 1999 Nov;289(1-2):23-31

[691] Waldman A, et al. Incidence of Candida in psoriasis--a study on the fungal flora of psoriatic patients. *Mycoses*. 2001 May;44(3-4):77-81

[692] Hughes LE, et al. Antibody responses to Acinetobacter spp. and Pseudomonas aeruginosa in multiple sclerosis: prospects for diagnosis using the myelin-acinetobacter-neurofilament antibody index. *Clin Diagn Lab Immunol*. 2001;8(6):1181-8

[693] Force M, Sparks WS, Ronzio RA. Inhibition of enteric parasites by emulsified oil of oregano in vivo. *Phytother Res*. 2000 May;14(3):213-4

the patient refused, stating that he was no longer willing to rely on immune-suppressing chemical medications. His treatment was entirely up to me. ***Assessments and Treatments***: We implemented the Paleo-Mediterranean diet and a program of vitamins, minerals, optimal combination fatty acid therapy (providing ALA, GLA, EPA, DHA, and oleic acid), and 4000 IU of vitamin D in emulsified form to overcome defects in absorption that are seen in older patients and those with gastrointestinal problems.[694] Hormone testing showed abnormally low DHEA, low testosterone, and slightly elevated estrogen; these problems were corrected with DHEA supplementation and the use of a hormone-modulating drug (Arimidex) that lowers estrogen and raises testosterone. Specialized stool testing showed absence of *Lactobacillus* and *Bifidobacteria* and intestinal overgrowth of *Citrobacter* and *Enterobacter* which was corrected with probiotics and antimicrobial treatments including undecylenic acid and emulsified oregano oil. Importantly, I also decided to inhibit NF-kappaB (the primary transcription factor that upregulates the pro-inflammatory response[695]) by using a combination botanical formula that contains curcumin, piperine, lipoic acid, green tea extract, propolis, rosemary, resveratrol, ginger, and phytolens (an antioxidant extract from lentils that may inhibit autoimmunity[696])—all of these herbs and nutrients have been shown to inhibit NF-kappaB and to thus downregulate inflammatory responses.[697] ***Results***: Within 6 weeks, this patient had happily lost 10 lbs of excess weight and was able to work without pain for the first time in years. Follow-up testing showed that his previously astronomical hsCRP had dropped from 124 to 7—a drop of 114 points in less than one month: better than had ever been achieved even with the use of intravenous immune-suppressing drugs! This patient continues to make significant progress. Obviously this case was complex, and we needed to do more than the basic protocol. Nonetheless, the basic protocol still served as the foundation for the treatment plan. Note that vitamin D has significant anti-inflammatory benefits and can cause major reductions in inflammation measured by CRP.[698] The correction of the hormonal abnormalities and the dysbiosis, and downregulating NF-kappaB with several botanical extracts were also critical components of this successful treatment plan.[1]

Summary and Conclusions

These examples show how the nutritional wellness protocol that I described in the September issue of *Nutritional Wellness* can be used as the foundational treatment for a wide range of health problems. In many cases, implementation of the basic protocol is all that is needed. In more complex situations, we use the basic protocol and then add more specific treatments to address dysbiosis and hormonal problems, and we can add additional nutrients as needed. However, there will never be a substitute for a healthy diet, sufficiencies of vitamin D and all five of the health-promoting fatty acids (i.e., ALA, GLA, EPA, DHA, and oleic acid), and normalization of gastrointestinal flora. Without these basics, survival and the appearance of health are possible, but true health and recovery from "untreatable" illnesses is not possible. In order to attain optimal health, we have to create the conditions that allow for health to be attained[1,] and we start this process by supplying the body with the nutrients that it needs to function optimally. In the words of naturopathic physician Jared Zeff from the *Journal of Naturopathic Medicine*, "*The work of the naturopathic physician is to elicit healing by helping patients to create or recreate the conditions for health to exist within them. Health will occur where the conditions for health exist. Disease is the product of the conditions which allow for it.*"[699] Although the chiropractic profession has

---

[694] **Vasquez A**. Subphysiologic Doses of Vitamin D are Subtherapeutic: Comment on the Study by The Record Trial Group. *TheLancet.com* Accessed June 16, 2005

[695] Tak PP, Firestein GS. NF-kappaB: a key role in inflammatory diseases. *J Clin Invest*. 2001 Jan;107(1):7-11

[696] Sandoval M, et al. Peroxynitrite-induced apoptosis in epithelial (T84) and macrophage (RAW 264.7) cell lines: effect of legume-derived polyphenols (phytolens). *Nitric Oxide*. 1997;1(6):476-83

[697] **Vasquez A**. Reducing pain and inflammation naturally - Part 4: Nutritional and Botanical Inhibition of NF-kappaB, the Major Intracellular Amplifier of the Inflammatory Cascade. A Practical Clinical Strategy Exemplifying Anti-Inflammatory Nutrigenomics. *Nutritional Perspectives* 2005;July: 5-12 www.OptimalHealthResearch.com/part4

[698] Timms PM, et al. Circulating MMP9, vitamin D and variation in the TIMP-1 response with VDR genotype. *QJM*. 2002 Dec;95(12):787-96

[699] Zeff JL. The process of healing: a unifying theory of naturopathic medicine. *Journal of Naturopathic Medicine* 1997; 7: 122-5

emphasized spinal manipulation as its primary therapeutic tool, the profession has always appreciated holistic, integrative models of therapeutic intervention, health and disease.

Chiropractic was the first healthcare profession in America to specifically claim that the optimization of health requires attention to the spiritual (emotional, psychological), mechanical (physical, structural), and chemical (nutritional, hormonal) aspects of our lives.[1] Chiropractic's founder DD Palmer[700] wrote, "The human body represents the actions of three laws—spiritual, mechanical, and chemical—united as one triune. As long as there is perfect union of these three, there is health." Accordingly, these cornerstones are fundamental to the modern definition of the chiropractic profession recently articulated by the American Chiropractic Association[701]: "*Doctors of Chiropractic are physicians who consider man as an integrated being and give special attention to the physiological and biochemical aspects including structural, spinal, musculoskeletal, neurological, vascular, nutritional, emotional and environmental relationships.*" The cases that I have described in this article demonstrate the importance of attending to the nutritional, hormonal, environmental and gastrointestinal aspects of human physiology for helping our patients attain optimal health.

Common Oversights and Shortcomings in the Study and Implementation of Nutritional Supplementation

Alex Vasquez, D.C., N.D.

This article was originally published in *Naturopathy Digest*
http://www.naturopathydigest.com/archives/2007/jun/vasquez.php

Introduction
An impressive discrepancy often exists between the low efficacy of nutritional interventions reported in the research literature and the higher efficacy achieved in the clinical practices of clinicians trained in the use of interventional nutrition (i.e., chiropractic and naturopathic physicians). This discrepancy is dangerous for at least two reasons. First, it results in an undervaluation of the efficacy of nutritional supplementation, which ultimately leaves otherwise treatable patients untreated. Second, such untreated and undertreated patients are often then forced to use dangerous and expensive pharmaceutical drugs and surgical interventions to treat conditions that could have otherwise been easily and safely treated with nutritional supplementation and diet modification. Consequently, the burden of suffering, disease, and healthcare expense in the US is higher than it would be if nutritionally-trained clinicians were more fully integrated into the healthcare system.

Obstacles to Efficacy in the Use of Nutritional Supplementation
Below are listed some of the most common causes for the underachievement of nutritional supplementation in practice and in published research. While this list is not all-inclusive, it will serve as a review for clinicians and an introduction for chiropractic/naturopathic students. In both practice and research, the problems listed below often overlap and function synergistically to reduce the efficacy of nutritional supplementation.

1. **Inadequate dosing (quantity)**: Many clinical trials published in major journals and many doctors in clinical practice have used inadequate doses of vitamins (and other natural therapeutics) and have thus failed to achieve the results that would have easily been obtained had they implemented their protocol with the proper physiologic or supraphysiologic dose of intervention. The best example in my experience centers on vitamin D, where so many of the studies are performed with doses of 400-800 IU per day only to conclude that vitamin supplementation is ineffective for the condition being treated. The problem here is

---

[700] Palmer DD. *The Science, Art, and Phiosophy, of Chiropractic*. Portland, OR; Portland Printing House Company, 1910: 107
[701] American Chiropractic Association. What is Chiropractic? http://amerchiro.org/media/whatis/ Accessed January 9, 2005

that the researchers failed to appreciate that the physiologic requirement for vitamin D3 in adults is approximately 3,000-5,000 IU per day[702] and that therefore their supplemental dose of 400-800 IU is only 10-20% of what is required. Subphysiologic doses are generally subtherapeutic. In this regard, I have had to correct journals such as *The Lancet*[703], *JAMA*[704], and *British Medical Journal*[705] from misleading their readers (many of whom are major policymakers) from concluding that nutritional supplementation is impotent; rather, their researchers and editors were not sufficiently educated in the design and review of studies using nutritional interventions. These journals should hire chiropractic and naturopathic physicians so that they have staff trained in natural treatments and who can thus provide an educated review of studies on these topics.[706]

2. **Inadequate dosing (duration)**: Often the effects of long-term nutritional deficiency are not fully reversible and/or may require a treatment period of months or years to achieve maximal clinical response. For example, full replacement of fatty acids in human brain phospholipids is an ongoing process that occurs over a period of several years; thus studies using fatty acid supplements for a period of weeks or 2-3 months generally underestimate the enhanced effectiveness that can be obtained with administration over many months or several years of treatment. Relatedly, recovery from vitamin D deficiency takes several weeks of high-dose supplementation in order to achieve tissue saturation and subsequent cellular replenishment; studies of short duration are destined to underestimate the results that could have been achieved with supplementation carried out over several months.[707]

3. **Failure to use proper forms of nutrients**: Nutrients are often available in different forms, not the least of which are "active" versus "inactive" and "natural" versus "unnatural." Most vitamin supplements, particularly high-potency B vitamins, are manufactured synthetically and are not from "natural sources" despite the marketing hype promulgated by companies that, for example, mix their synthetic vitamins with a vegetable powder and then call their vitamin supplements "natural." The simple fact is that production of high-potency supplements from purely natural sources would be prohibitively wasteful, inefficient, and expensive. Thus, while it is not necessary for vitamins to be "natural" in order to be useful, it is necessary that the vitamins are useable and preferably not "unnatural." The best example of the use of unnatural supplements is the use of synthetic DL-tocopherol in the so-called "vitamin E" studies; DL-tocopherol is by definition 50% comprised of the L-isomer of tocopherol which is not only unusable by the human body but is actually harmful in that it interferes with normal metabolism and can exacerbate hypertension and cause symptomatic complications (e.g., headaches). Further, tocopherols exist within the body in relationship with the individual forms of the vitamin, such that supplementation with one form (e.g., alpha-tocopherol) can result in a relative deficiency of another form (e.g., gamma-tocopherol). One final example of the failure to use proper forms of nutrients is in the use of pyridoxine HCl as a form of vitamin B6; while this practice itself is not harmful, clinicians need to remember that pyridoxine HCl is ineffective until converted to the more active forms of the vitamin including pyridoxal-5-phosphate. Since this conversion requires co-nutrients such as magnesium and zinc, we can easily see that the reputed failure of B6 supplementation when administered in the form of pyridoxine HCl might actually be due to untreated insufficiencies of required co-nutrients, as discussed in the following section.

[702] Heaney RP, Davies KM, Chen TC, Holick MF, Barger-Lux MJ. Human serum 25-hydroxycholecalciferol response to extended oral dosing with cholecalciferol. *Am J Clin Nutr*. 2003 Jan;77(1):204-10 http://www.ajcn.org/cgi/content/full/77/1/204
[703] **Vasquez A**. Subphysiologic Doses of Vitamin D are Subtherapeutic: Comment on the Study by The Record Trial Group. *The Lancet* 2005 Published on-line May 6 http://OptimalHealthResearch.com/lancet
[704] Muanza DN, **Vasquez A**, Cannell J, Grant WB. Isoflavones and Postmenopausal Women. [letter] *JAMA* 2004; 292: 2337
[705] **Vasquez A**, Cannell J. Calcium and vitamin D in preventing fractures: data are not sufficient to show inefficacy. [letter] *BMJ: British Medical Journal* 2005;331:108-9 http://www.optimalhealthresearch.com/reprints/vasquez-cannell-bmj-reprint.pdf
[706] **Vasquez A**. Allopathic Usurpation of Natural Medicine: The Blind Leading the Sighted. *Naturopathy Digest* 2006 February http://www.naturopathydigest.com/archives/2006/feb/vasquez.php
[707] **Vasquez A**, Manso G, Cannell J. The clinical importance of vitamin D (cholecalciferol): a paradigm shift with implications for all healthcare providers. *Altern Ther Health Med*. 2004 Sep-Oct;10(5):28-36 http://optimalhealthresearch.com/monograph04

4. **Failure to ensure adequacy of co-nutrients**: Vitamins, minerals, amino acids, and fatty acids work together in an intricately choreographed and delicately orchestrated dance that culminates in the successful completion of interconnected physiologic functions. If any of the performers in this event are missing (i.e., nutritional deficiency) or if successive interconversions are impaired due to lack of enzyme function, then the show cannot go on, or—if it does go on—impaired metabolism and defective function will result. So, if we take a patient with "vitamin B6 deficiency" and give him vitamin B6 in the absence of other co-nutrients needed for the proper activation and metabolic utilization of vitamin B6, we cannot honestly expect the "nutritional supplementation" to work in this case; rather, we might see a marginal benefit or perhaps even a negative outcome as an imbalanced system is pushed into a different state of imbalance despite supplementation with the "correct" vitamin. In the case of vitamin B6, necessary co-nutrients include zinc, magnesium, and riboflavin; deficiency of any of these will result in a relative "failure" of B6 supplementation even if a patient has a B6-responsive condition. Notably, overt magnesium deficiency is alarmingly common among patients and citizens in industrialized nations[708,709,710], and this epidemic of magnesium deficiency is due not only to insufficient intake but also to excessive excretion caused by consumption of high-glycemic foods, caffeine, and a diet that promotes chronic metabolic acidosis with resultant urinary acidification.

5. **Failure to achieve urinary alkalinization**: Western/American-style diets typified by overconsumption of grains, dairy, sugar, and salt result in a state of subclinical chronic metabolic acidosis which results in urinary acidification, relative hypercortisolemia, and consequent hyperexcretion of minerals such as calcium and magnesium.[711] [712] Thus, the common conundrum of magnesium replenishment requires not only magnesium supplementation but also dietary interventions to change the internal climate to one that is conducive to bodily retention and cellular uptake of magnesium.[713]

6. **Use of mislabeled supplements**: Even in the professional arena of nutritional supplement manufacturers, some companies habitually underdose their products either in an attempt to spend less in the manufacture of their products or as a consequence of poor quality control. If a product is labeled to contain 1,000 IU of vitamin D but only contains 836 IU of the nutrient, then obviously full clinical efficacy will not be achieved; this was a problem in a recent clinical trial involving vitamin D.[714] The problem for clinicians is in trusting the companies that supply nutritional supplements; some companies do "in house" testing which lacks independent review, while other companies use questionable "independent testing" which is not infrequently performed by a laboratory that is a wholly owned subsidiary of the parent nutritional company. Manufacturing regulations that are sweeping through the industry will cleanse the nutritional supplement world of poorly made products, and these same regulations will sweep some unprepared companies right out the door when they are unable to meet the regulatory requirements.

7. **Assurance of bioavailability and optimal serum/cellular levels**: Clinical trials with nutritional therapies need to monitor serum or cellular levels to ensure absorption, product bioavailability, and the attainment of optimal serum levels. This is particularly relevant in the treatment of chronic disorders such as the autoimmune diseases, wherein so many of these

---

[708] "Altogether 43% of 113 trauma patients had low magnesium levels compared to 30% of noninjured cohorts." Frankel H, Haskell R, Lee SY, Miller D, Rotondo M, Schwab CW. Hypomagnesemia in trauma patients. *World J Surg*. 1999 Sep;23(9):966-9

[709] "There was a 20% overall prevalence of hypomagnesemia among this predominantly female, African American population." Fox CH, Ramsoomair D, Mahoney MC, Carter C, Young B, Graham R. An investigation of hypomagnesemia among ambulatory urban African Americans. *J Fam Pract*. 1999 Aug;48(8):636-9

[710] "Suboptimal levels were detected in 33.7 per cent of the population under study. These data clearly demonstrate that the Mg supply of the German population needs increased attention." Schimatschek HF, Rempis R. Prevalence of hypomagnesemia in an unselected German population of 16,000 individuals. *Magnes Res*. 2001 Dec;14(4):283-90

[711] Cordain L, Eaton SB, Sebastian A, Mann N, Lindeberg S, Watkins BA, O'Keefe JH, Brand-Miller J. Origins and evolution of the Western diet: health implications for the 21st century. *Am J Clin Nutr*. 2005 Feb;81(2):341-54

[712] Maurer M, Riesen W, Muser J, Hulter HN, Krapf R. Neutralization of Western diet inhibits bone resorption independently of K intake and reduces cortisol secretion in humans. *Am J Physiol Renal Physiol*. 2003 Jan;284(1):F32-40

[713] Vormann J,Worlitschek M,Goedecke T,Silver B. Supplementation with alkaline minerals reduces symptoms in patients with chronic low back pain. *J Trace Elem Med Biol*. 2001;15(2-3):179-83

[714] Heaney RP, Davies KM, Chen TC, Holick MF, Barger-Lux MJ. Human serum 25-hydroxycholecalciferol response to extended oral dosing with cholecalciferol. *Am J Clin Nutr*. 2003 Jan;77(1):204-10 http://www.ajcn.org/cgi/content/full/77/1/204

patients have gastrointestinal dysbiosis and often have concomitant nutrient malabsorption.[715] Simply dosing these patients with supplements is not always efficacious; often the gut must be cleared of dysbiosis so that the mucosal lining can be repaired and optimal nutrient absorption can be reestablished.

8. **Coadministration of food with nutritional supplements (sometimes right, sometimes wrong)**: Food can help or hinder the absorption of nutritional supplements. Some supplements, like coenzyme Q10, should be administered with fatty food to enhance absorption. Other supplements, like amino acids, should be administered away from protein-rich foods and are often better administered with simple carbohydrate to enhance cellular uptake; this is especially true with tryptophan.

9. **Correction of gross dietary imbalances enhances supplement effectiveness**: If the diet is grossly imbalanced, then nutritional supplementation is less likely to be effective. The best example of this is in the use of fatty acid supplements, particularly in the treatment of inflammatory disorders. If the diet is laden with dairy, beef, and other sources of arachidonate, then fatty acid supplementation with EPA, DHA, and GLA is much less likely to be effective, or much higher doses of the supplements will need to be used in order to help restore fatty acid balance. Generally speaking, the diet needs to be optimized to enhance the efficacy of nutritional supplementation.

Conclusion

In this brief review, I have listed and discussed some of the most common impediments to the success of nutritional supplementation. I hope that chiropractic and naturopathic students, clinicians, and researchers will find these points helpful in their design of clinical treatment protocols.

Revisiting the Five-Part Nutritional Wellness Protocol: The Supplemented Paleo-Mediterranean Diet

Alex Vasquez, DC, ND, DO

This article was originally published in the January 2011 issue of the American Chiropractic Association's Council on Nutrition's journal *Nutritional Perspectives*

Abstract: This article reviews the five-part nutritional protocol that incorporates a health-promoting nutrient-dense diet and essential supplementation with vitamins/minerals, specific fatty acids, probiotics, and physiologic doses of vitamin D3. This foundational nutritional protocol has proven benefits for disease treatment, disease prevention, and health maintenance and restoration. Additional treatments such as botanical medicines, additional nutritional supplements, and pharmaceutical drugs can be used atop this foundational protocol to further optimize clinical effectiveness. The rationale for this five-part protocol is presented, and consideration is given to adding iodine-iodide as the sixth component of the protocol.

---

[715] **Vasquez A**. Reducing Pain and Inflammation Naturally. Part 6: Nutritional and Botanical Treatments Against "Silent Infections" and Gastrointestinal Dysbiosis, Commonly Overlooked Causes of Neuromusculoskeletal Inflammation and Chronic Health Problems. *Nutritional Perspectives* 2006; January http://www.optimalhealthresearch.com/part6

<u>Introduction</u>: In 2004 and 2005 I first published a "five-part nutrition protocol"[716,717] that provides the foundational treatment plan for a wide range of health disorders. This protocol served and continues to serve as the foundation upon which other treatments are commonly added, and without which those other treatments are likely to fail, or attain suboptimal results at best.[718] Now as then, I will share with you what I consider a basic foundational protocol for wellness promotion and disease treatment. I have used this protocol in my own self-care for many years and have used it in the treatment of a wide range of health-disease conditions in clinical practice.

<u>Review</u>: This nutritional protocol is validated by biochemistry, physiology, experimental research, peer-reviewed human trials, and the clinical application of common sense. It is the most nutrient-dense diet available, satisfying nutritional needs and thereby optimizing metabolic processes while promoting satiety and weight loss/optimization. Nutrients are required in the proper amounts, forms, and approximate ratios for critical and innumerable physiologic functions; if nutrients are lacking, the body cannot function *normally*, let alone *optimally*. Impaired function results in subjective and objective manifestations of what is eventually labeled as "disease." Thus, a powerful and effective alternative to treating diseases with drugs is to re-establish normal/optimal physiologic function by replenishing the body with essential nutrients, reestablishing hormonal balance ("orthoendocrinology"), promoting detoxification of environmental toxins, and by reestablishing the optimal microbial milieu, especially the eradication of (multifocal) dysbiosis; this multifaceted approach can be applied to several diseases, especially those of the inflammatory and autoimmune varieties.[719]

Of course, most diseases are multifactorial and therefore require multicomponent treatment plans, and some diseases actually require the use of drugs in conjunction with assertive interventional nutrition. However, while only a smaller portion of patients actually need drugs for the long-term management their problems, all clinicians should agree that everyone needs a foundational nutrition plan because nutrients—not drugs—are universally required for life and health. This five-part nutrition protocol is briefly outlined below; a much more detailed substantiation of the underlying science and clinical application of this protocol was recently published in a review of more than 650 pages and approximately 3,500 citations.[720]

1. <u>Health-promoting Paleo-Mediterranean diet</u>: Following an extensive review of the research literature, I developed what I call the "supplemented Paleo-Mediterranean diet." In essence, this diet plan combines the best of the Mediterranean diet with the best of the Paleolithic diet, the latter of which has been best distilled by Dr. Loren Cordain in his book "The Paleo Diet"[721] and his numerous scientific articles.[722,723,724] The Paleolithic diet is superior to the Mediterranean diet in nutrient density for promoting satiety, weight loss, and improvements/normalization in overall metabolic function.[725,726] This diet places emphasis on

[716] **Vasquez A**. *Integrative Orthopedics: The Art of Creating Wellness While Managing Acute and Chronic Musculoskeletal Disorders*. 2004, 2007
[717] Vasquez A. A Five-Part Nutritional Protocol that Produces Consistently Positive Results. *Nutritional Wellness* 2005 September Available in the printed version and on-line at http://www.nutritionalwellness.com/archives/2005/sep/09_vasquez.php
[718] **Vasquez A.** Common Oversights and Shortcomings in the Study and Implementation of Nutritional Supplementation. *Naturopathy Digest* 2007 June. http://www.naturopathydigest.com/archives/2007/jun/vasquez.php
[719] **Vasquez A.** Integrative Rheumatology. IBMRC: 2006, 2009. http://optimalhealthresearch.com/rheumatology.html
[720] **Vasquez A.** Chiropractic and Naturopathic Mastery of Common Clinical Disorders. IBMRC: 2009. http://optimalhealthresearch.com/clinical_mastery.html
[721] Cordain L. *The Paleo Diet*. John Wiley and Sons, 2002
[722] O'Keefe JH Jr, Cordain L. Cardiovascular disease resulting from a diet and lifestyle at odds with our Paleolithic genome: how to become a 21st-century hunter-gatherer. *Mayo Clin Proc*. 2004 Jan;79(1):101-8
[723] Cordain L. Cereal grains: humanity's double edged sword. *World Rev Nutr Diet* 1999;84:19-73
[724] Cordain L, Eaton SB, Sebastian A, Mann N, Lindeberg S, Watkins BA, O'Keefe JH, Brand-Miller J. Origins and evolution of the Western diet: health implications for the 21st century. *Am J Clin Nutr*. 2005 Feb;81(2):341-54
[725] "A high micronutrient density diet mitigates the unpleasant aspects of the experience of hunger even though it is lower in calories. Hunger is one of the major impediments to successful weight loss. Our findings suggest that it is not simply the caloric content, but more importantly, the micronutrient density of a diet that influences the experience of hunger. It appears that a high nutrient density diet, after an initial phase of adjustment during which a person experiences "toxic hunger" due to withdrawal from pro-inflammatory foods, can result in a sustainable eating pattern that leads to weight loss and improved health." Fuhrman J, Sarter B, Glaser D, Acocella S. Changing perceptions of hunger on a high nutrient density diet. *Nutr J*. 2010 Nov 7;9:51 http://www.nutritionj.com/content/9/1/51
[726] "The Paleolithic group were as satiated as the Mediterranean group but consumed less energy per day (5.8 MJ/day vs. 7.6 MJ/day, Paleolithic vs. Mediterranean, p=0.04). Consequently, the quotients of mean change in satiety during meal and mean consumed energy from food and drink were higher

fruits, vegetables, nuts, seeds, and berries that meet the body's needs for fiber, carbohydrates, and most importantly, the 8,000+ phytonutrients that have additive and synergistic health effects[727]—including immunomodulating, antioxidant, anti-inflammatory, and anti-cancer benefits. High-quality protein sources such as fish, poultry, eggs, and grass-fed meats are emphasized. Slightly modifying Cordain's paleo diet, I also advocate soy and whey protein isolates for their high-quality protein and their anticancer, cardioprotective, and mood-enhancing (due to the high tryptophan content) benefits. Potatoes and other starchy vegetables, wheat and other grains including rice are discouraged due to their high glycemic indexes and high glycemic loads, and their relative insufficiency of fiber and phytonutrients compared to fruits and vegetables. Grains such as wheat, barley, and rye are discouraged due to the high glycemic loads/indexes of most breads, pastries, and other grain-derived products, as well as due to the immunogenicity of constituents such as gluten, a protein composite (consisting of a prolamin and a glutelin) that can contribute to disorders such as migraine, epilepsy, eczema, arthritis, celiac disease, psoriasis and other types of autoimmunity. Sources of simple sugars and foreign chemicals such as colas/sodas (which contain artificial colors, flavors, and high-fructose corn syrup, which contains mercury[728] and which can cause the hypertensive-diabetic metabolic syndrome[729]) and processed foods (e.g., "TV dinners" and other manufactured snacks and convenience foods) are strictly forbidden. Chemical preservatives, colorants, sweeteners, flavor-enhancers such as monosodium glutamate and carrageenan are likewise avoided. In summary, this diet plan provides plenty of variety, as most dishes comprised of poultry, fish, lean meats, soy, eggs, fruits, vegetables, nuts, berries, and seeds are allowed. The diet provides an abundance of fiber, phytonutrients, carbohydrates, potassium, and protein, while simultaneously being low in fat, sodium, arachidonic acid, and "simple sugars." The diet must be customized with regard to total protein and calorie intake, as determined by the size, status, and activity level of the patient; individual per-patient food allergens should be avoided. Regular consumption of this diet has shown the ability to reduce hypertension, alleviate diabetes, ameliorate migraine headaches, and result in improvement of overall health and a lessening of the severity of many common "diseases", particularly those with an autoimmune or inflammatory component. This Paleo-Mediterranean diet is supplemented with vitamins, minerals, fatty acids, and probiotics—making it the "supplemented Paleo-Mediterranean diet" as described below.

2. <u>Multivitamin and multimineral supplementation</u>: Vitamin and mineral supplementation has been advocated for decades by the chiropractic/naturopathic professions while being scorned by so-called "mainstream medicine." Vitamin and mineral supplementation finally received bipartisan endorsement when researchers from Harvard Medical School published a review article in *Journal of the American Medical Association* that concluded, "Most people do not consume an optimal amount of all vitamins by diet alone. ...it appears prudent for all adults to take vitamin supplements."[730] Long-term nutritional insufficiencies experienced by "most people" promote the development of "long-latency deficiency diseases"[731] such as cancer,

in the Paleolithic group (p=0.03). Also, there was a strong trend for greater Satiety Quotient for energy in the Paleolithic group (p=0.057). Leptin decreased by 31% in the Paleolithic group and by 18% in the Mediterranean group with a trend for greater relative decrease of leptin in the Paleolithic group." Jonsson T, Granfeldt Y, Erlanson-Albertsson C, Ahren B, Lindeberg S. A Paleolithic diet is more satiating per calorie than a Mediterranean-like diet in individuals with ischemic heart disease. *Nutr Metab* (Lond). 2010 Nov 30;7(1):85.
[727] Liu RH. Health benefits of fruit and vegetables are from additive and synergistic combinations of phytochemicals. *Am J Clin Nutr* 2003;78(3 Suppl):517S-520S
[728] "With daily per capita consumption of HFCS in the US averaging about 50 grams and daily mercury intakes from HFCS ranging up to 28 µg, this potential source of mercury may exceed other major sources of mercury especially in high-end consumers of beverages sweetened with HFCS." Dufault R, LeBlanc B, Schnoll R, Cornett C, Schweitzer L, Wallinga D, Hightower J, Patrick L, Lukiw WJ. Mercury from chlor-alkali plants: measured concentrations in food product sugar. *Environ Health*. 2009 Jan 26;8:2 http://www.ehjournal.net/content/8/1/2
[729] **Vasquez A**. Integrative Medicine and Functional Medicine for Chronic Hypertension: An Evidence-based Patient-Centered Monograph for Advanced Clinicians. IBMRC; 2011. http://optimalhealthresearch.com/hypertension_functional_integrative_medicine.html See also: Reungjui S, Roncal CA, Mu W, Srinivas TR, Sirivongs D, Johnson RJ, Nakagawa T. Thiazide diuretics exacerbate fructose-induced metabolic syndrome. *J Am Soc Nephrol*. 2007 Oct;18(10):2724-31 http://jasn.asnjournals.org/content/18/10/2724.full.pdf
[730] Fletcher RH, Fairfield KM. Vitamins for chronic disease prevention in adults: clinical applications. *JAMA* 2002;287:3127-9
[731] Heaney RP. Long-latency deficiency disease: insights from calcium and vitamin D. *Am J Clin Nutr* 2003;78:912-9

neuroemotional deterioration, and cardiovascular disease. Impressively, the benefits of multivitamin/multimineral supplementation have been demonstrated in numerous clinical trials. Multivitamin/multimineral supplementation has been shown to improve nutritional status and reduce the risk for chronic diseases[732], improve mood[733], potentiate antidepressant drug treatment[734], alleviate migraine headaches (when used with diet improvement and fatty acids[735]), improve immune function and infectious disease outcomes in the elderly[736] (especially diabetics[737]), reduce morbidity and mortality in patients with HIV infection[738,739], alleviate premenstrual syndrome[740,741] and bipolar disorder[742], reduce violence and antisocial behavior in children[743] and incarcerated young adults (when used with essential fatty acids[744]), and improve scores of intelligence in children.[745] Multivitamin and multimineral supplementation provides anti-inflammatory benefits, as evidenced by significant reduction in C-reactive protein (CRP) in a double-blind, placebo-controlled trial.[746] The ability to safely and affordably deliver these benefits makes multimineral-multivitamin supplementation an essential component of any and all health-promoting and disease-prevention strategies. A few cautions need to be observed; for example, vitamin A can (rarely) result in liver damage with chronic consumption of 25,000 IU or more, and intake should generally not exceed 10,000 IU per day in women of childbearing age. Also, iron should not be supplemented except in patients diagnosed with iron deficiency by a blood test (serum ferritin).

3. Physiologic doses of vitamin D3: The prevalence of vitamin D deficiency varies from 40-80 percent (general population) to almost 100 percent (patients with musculoskeletal pain) among Americans and Europeans. Vasquez, Manso, and Cannell described the many benefits of vitamin D3 supplementation in an assertive review published in 2004.[747] Our publication showed that vitamin D deficiency causes or contributes to depression, hypertension, seizures, migraine, polycystic ovary syndrome, inflammation, autoimmunity, and musculoskeletal pain, particularly low-back pain. Clinical trials using vitamin D supplementation have proven the cause-and-effect relationship between vitamin D deficiency and most of these conditions by showing that each could be cured or alleviated with vitamin D supplementation. In our review of the literature, we concluded that daily vitamin D doses should be 1,000 IU for infants, 2,000 IU for children, and 4,000 IU for adults, although some adults respond better to higher doses of 10,000 IU per day. Cautions and contraindications include the use of thiazide diuretics (e.g., hydrochlorothiazide) or any other medications that promote hypercalcemia, as well as granulomatous diseases such as sarcoidosis,

[732] McKay DL, Perrone G, Rasmussen H, Dallal G, Hartman W, Cao G, Prior RL, Roubenoff R, Blumberg JB. The effects of a multivitamin/mineral supplement on micronutrient status, antioxidant capacity and cytokine production in healthy older adults consuming a fortified diet. *J Am Coll Nutr* 2000;19(5):613-21

[733] Benton D, Haller J, Fordy J. Vitamin supplementation for 1 year improves mood. *Neuropsychobiology* 1995;32(2):98-105

[734] Coppen A, Bailey J. Enhancement of the antidepressant action of fluoxetine by folic acid: a randomised, placebo controlled trial. *J Affect Disord* 2000;60:121-30

[735] Wagner W, Nootbaar-Wagner U. Prophylactic treatment of migraine with gamma-linolenic and alpha-linolenic acids. *Cephalalgia* 1997;17:127-30

[736] Langkamp-Henken B, Bender BS, Gardner EM, Herrlinger-Garcia KA, Kelley MJ, Murasko DM, Schaller JP, Stechmiller JK, Thomas DJ, Wood SM. Nutritional formula enhanced immune function and reduced days of symptoms of upper respiratory tract infection in seniors. *J Am Geriatr Soc* 2004;52:3-12

[737] Barringer TA, Kirk JK, Santaniello AC, Foley KL, Michielutte R. Effect of a multivitamin and mineral supplement on infection and quality of life. A randomized, double-blind, placebo-controlled trial. *Ann Intern Med* 2003;138:365-71

[738] Fawzi WW, Msamanga GI, Spiegelman D, et al. A randomized trial of multivitamin supplements and HIV disease progression and mortality. *N Engl J Med* 2004;351:23-32

[739] Burbano X, Miguez-Burbano MJ, McCollister K, Zhang G, Rodriguez A, Ruiz P, Lecusay R, Shor-Posner G. Impact of a selenium chemoprevention clinical trial on hospital admissions of HIV-infected participants. *HIV Clin Trials* 2002;3:483-91

[740] Abraham GE. Nutritional factors in the etiology of the premenstrual tension syndromes. *J Reprod Med* 1983;28(7):446-64

[741] Stewart A. Clinical and biochemical effects of nutritional supplementation on the premenstrual syndrome. *J Reprod Med* 1987;32:435-41

[742] Kaplan BJ, Simpson JS, Ferre RC, Gorman CP, McMullen DM, Crawford SG. Effective mood stabilization with a chelated mineral supplement: an open-label trial in bipolar disorder. *J Clin Psychiatry* 2001;62:936-44

[743] Kaplan BJ, Crawford SG, Gardner B, Farrelly G. Treatment of mood lability and explosive rage with minerals and vitamins: two case studies in children. *J Child Adolesc Psychopharmacol* 2002;12(3):205-19

[744] Gesch CB, Hammond SM, Hampson SE, Eves A, Crowder MJ. Influence of supplementary vitamins, minerals and essential fatty acids on the antisocial behaviour of young adult prisoners. Randomised, placebo-controlled trial. *Br J Psychiatry* 2002;181:22-8

[745] Benton D. Micro-nutrient supplementation and the intelligence of children. *Neurosci Biobehav Rev* 2001;25:297-309

[746] Church TS, Earnest CP, Wood KA, Kampert JB. Reduction of C-reactive protein levels through use of a multivitamin. *Am J Med* 2003;115:702-7

[747] **Vasquez A**, Manso G, Cannell J. The clinical importance of vitamin D (cholecalciferol): a paradigm shift with implications for all healthcare providers. *Alternative Therapies in Health and Medicine* 2004;10:28-37 http://optimalhealthresearch.com/cholecalciferol.html

tuberculosis, and certain types of cancer, especially lymphoma. Effectiveness is monitored by measuring serum 25-OH-vitamin D, and safety is monitored by measuring serum calcium. Dosing should be tailored for the attainment of optimal serum levels of 25-hydroxy-vitamin D3, generally 50-100 ng/ml (125-250 nmol/l) as illustrated.

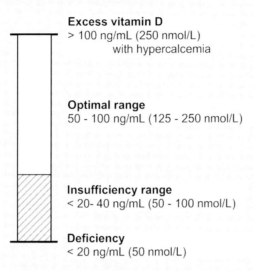

Excess vitamin D
> 100 ng/mL (250 nmol/L)
with hypercalcemia

Optimal range
50 - 100 ng/mL (125 - 250 nmol/L)

Insufficiency range
< 20- 40 ng/mL (50 - 100 nmol/L)

Deficiency
< 20 ng/mL (50 nmol/L)

Interpretation of serum 25(OH) vitamin D levels.
Modified from Vasquez et al, *Alternative Therapies in Health and Medicine* 2004 and Vasquez A. *Musculoskeletal Pain: Expanded Clinical Strategies* (Institute for Functional Medicine) 2008.

4. <u>Balanced and complete fatty acid supplementation</u>: A detailed survey of the literature shows that five fatty acids have major health-promoting disease-preventing benefits and should therefore be incorporated into the daily diet and/or regularly consumed as dietary supplements.[748] These are alpha-linolenic acid (ALA; omega-3, from flaxseed oil), eicosapentaenoic acid (EPA; omega-3, from fish oil), docosahexaenoic acid (DHA; omega-3, from fish oil and algae), gamma-linolenic acid (GLA; omega-6, most concentrated in borage oil but also present in evening primrose oil, hemp seed oil, black currant seed oil), and oleic acid (omega-9, most concentrated in olive oil, which contains in addition to oleic acid many anti-inflammatory, antioxidant, and anticancer phytonutrients). Supplementing with one fatty acid can exacerbate an insufficiency of other fatty acids; hence the importance of balanced combination supplementation. Each of these fatty acids has health benefits that cannot be fully attained from supplementing a different fatty acid; hence, again, the importance of balanced combination supplementation. The benefits of GLA are not attained by consumption of EPA and DHA; in fact, consumption of fish oil can actually promote a deficiency of GLA.[749] Likewise, consumption of GLA alone can reduce EPA levels while increasing levels of proinflammatory arachidonic acid; both of these problems are avoided with co-administration of EPA any time GLA is used because EPA inhibits delta-5-desaturase, which converts dihomo-GLA into arachidonic acid. Using ALA alone only slightly increases EPA but generally leads to no improvement in DHA status and can lead to a reduction of oleic acid; thus, DHA

[748] **Vasquez A**. Reducing Pain and Inflammation Naturally - Part 1: New Insights into Fatty Acid Biochemistry and the Influence of Diet. *Nutritional Perspectives* 2004; October: 5, 7-10, 12, 14 http://optimalhealthresearch.com/reprints/series/
[749] Cleland LG, Gibson RA, Neumann M, French JK. The effect of dietary fish oil supplement upon the content of dihomo-gammalinolenic acid in human plasma phospholipids. *Prostaglandins Leukot Essent Fatty Acids* 1990 May;40(1):9-12

and oleic acid should be supplemented when flaxseed oil is used.[750] Obviously, the goal here is physiologically-optimal (i.e., "balanced") intake of all of the health-promoting fatty acids; using only one or two sources of fatty acids is not balanced and results in suboptimal improvement. In clinical practice, I routinely use combination fatty acid therapy comprised of ALA, EPA, DHA, and GLA for essentially all patients; when one appreciates that the average daily Paleolithic intake of n-3 fatty acids was 7 grams per day contrasted to the average daily American intake of 1 gram per day, we can see that—by using combination fatty acid therapy emphasizing n-3 fatty acids—we are simply meeting physiologic expectations via supplementation, rather than performing an act of recklessness or heroism. The product I use also contains a modest amount of oleic acid that occurs naturally in flax and borage seed oils, and I encourage use of olive oil for salads and cooking. This approach results in complete and balanced fatty acid intake, and the clinical benefits are impressive. Benefits are to be expected in the treatment of premenstrual syndrome, diabetic neuropathy, respiratory distress syndrome, Crohn's disease, lupus, rheumatoid arthritis, cardiovascular disease, hypertension, psoriasis, eczema, migraine headaches, bipolar disorder, borderline personality disorder, mental depression, schizophrenia, osteoporosis, polycystic ovary syndrome, multiple sclerosis, and musculoskeletal pain. The discovery in September 2010 that the G protein-coupled receptor 120 (GPR120) functions as an n-3 fatty acid receptor that, when stimulated with EPA or DHA, exerts broad anti-inflammatory effects (in cell experiments) and enhances systemic insulin sensitivity (in animal study) confirms a new mechanism of action of fatty acid supplementation and shows that we as clinician-researchers are still learning the details of the beneficial effects of commonly used treatments.[751]

5. Probiotics /gut flora modification: Proper levels of good bacteria promote intestinal health, support proper immune function, and encourage overall health. Excess bacteria or yeast, or the presence of harmful bacteria, yeast, or "parasites" such as amoebas and protozoas, can cause "leaky gut," systemic inflammation, and a wide range of clinical problems, especially autoimmunity. Intestinal flora can become imbalanced by poor diets, excess stress, immunosuppressive drugs, and antibiotics, and all of these factors are common among American patients. Thus, as a rule, I reinstate the good bacteria by the use of probiotics (good bacteria and yeast), prebiotics (fiber, arabinogalactan, and inulin), and the use of fermented foods such as kefir and yogurt for patients not allergic to milk. Harmful yeast, bacteria, and other "parasites" can be eradicated with the combination of dietary change, antimicrobial drugs, and/or herbal extracts. For example, oregano oil in an emulsified, time-released form has proven safe and effective for the elimination of various parasites encountered in clinical practice.[752] Likewise, the herb *Artemisia annua* (sweet wormwood) commonly is used to eradicate specific bacteria and has been used for thousands of years in Asia for the treatment and prevention of infectious diseases, including drug-resistant malaria.[753] Restoring microbial balance by providing probiotics, restoring immune function (immunorestoration) and eliminating sources of dysbiosis, especially in the gastrointestinal tract, genitourinary tract, and oropharynx, is a very important component in the treatment plan of autoimmunity and systemic inflammation.[754]

Should combinations of iodine and iodide be the sixth component of the Protocol?: Both iodine and iodide have biological activity in humans. An increasing number of clinicians are using combination iodine-iodide products to provide approximately 12 mg/d; this is consistent with the average daily intake of iodine-iodide in countries such as Japan with a high intake of seafood,

---

[750] Jantti J, Nikkari T, Solakivi T, Vapaatalo H, Isomaki H. Evening primrose oil in rheumatoid arthritis: changes in serum lipids and fatty acids. *Ann Rheum Dis* 1989;48(2):124-7

[751] Oh da Y, Talukdar S, Bae EJ, Imamura T, Morinaga H, Fan W, Li P, Lu WJ, Watkins SM, Olefsky JM. GPR120 is an omega-3 fatty acid receptor mediating potent anti-inflammatory and insulin-sensitizing effects. Cell. 2010 Sep 3;142(5):687-98 http://www.cell.com/abstract/S0092-8674%2810%2900888-3?switch=standard

[752] Force M, Sparks WS, Ronzio RA. Inhibition of enteric parasites by emulsified oil of oregano in vivo. *Phytother Res* 2000;14:213-4

[753] Schuster BG. Demonstrating the validity of natural products as anti-infective drugs. *J Altern Complement Med* 2001;7 Suppl 1:S73-82

[754] **Vasquez A**. Integrative Rheumatology. IBMRC: 2006, 2009. http://optimalhealthresearch.com/rheumatology.html

including fish, shellfish, and seaweed. Collectively, iodine and iodide provide antioxidant, antimicrobial, mucolytic, immunosupportive, antiestrogen, and anticancer benefits that extend far beyond the mere incorporation of iodine into thyroid hormones.[5] Benefits of iodine/iodide in the treatment of asthma[755,756] and systemic fungal infections[757,758] have been documented, and many clinicians use combination iodine/iodide supplementation for the treatment of estrogen-driven conditions such as fibrocystic breast disease.[759] While additional research is needed and already underway to further establish the role of iodine-iodide as a routine component of clinical care, clinicians should begin incorporating this nutrient into their protocols based on the above-mentioned physiologic roles and clinical benefits.

Summary and Conclusions: In this brief review, I have described and substantiated a fundamental protocol that can serve as effective therapy for patients with a wide range of diseases and health disorders. Customizing the Paleo-Mediterranean diet to avoid patient-specific food allergens, using vitamin-mineral supplements along with physiologic doses of vitamin D and broad-spectrum balanced fatty acid supplementation, and ensuring "immunomicrobial" health with the skillful use of probiotics, prebiotics, immunorestoration, and antimicrobial treatments provides an excellent health-promoting and disease-eliminating foundation and lifestyle for many patients. Often, this simple protocol is all that is needed for the effective treatment of a wide range of clinical problems, even those that have been "medical failures" for many years. For other patients with more complex illnesses, of course, additional interventions and laboratory assessments can be used to optimize and further customize the treatment plan. Clinicians should avoid seeking "silver bullet" treatments that ignore overall metabolism, immune function, and inflammatory balance, and we must always remember that the attainment and preservation of health requires that we first meet the body's basic nutritional and physiologic needs. This five-step protocol begins the process of meeting those needs. With it, health can be restored and the need for disease-specific treatment is obviated or reduced; without it, fundamental physiologic needs are not met, and health cannot be obtained and maintained. Addressing core physiologic needs empowers doctors to deliver the most effective healthcare possible, and it allows patients to benefit from such treatment.

---

[755] Tuft L. Iodides in bronchial asthma. *J Allergy Clin Immunol*. 1981 Jun;67(6):497

[756] Falliers CJ, McCann WP, Chai H, Ellis EF, Yazdi N. Controlled study of iodotherapy for childhood asthma. *J Allergy*. 1966 Sep;38(3):183-92

[757] Tripathy S, Vijayashree J, Mishra M, Jena DK, Behera B, Mohapatra A. Rhinofacial zygomycosis successfully treated with oral saturated solution of potassium iodide: a case report. *J Eur Acad Dermatol Venereol*. 2007 Jan;21(1):117-9

[758] Bonifaz A, Saúl A, Paredes-Solis V, Fierro L, Rosales A, Palacios C, Araiza J. Sporotrichosis in childhood: clinical and therapeutic experience in 25 patients. *Pediatr Dermatol*. 2007 Jul-Aug;24(4):369-72

[759] Ghent WR, Eskin BA, Low DA, Hill LP. Iodine replacement in fibrocystic disease of the breast. *Can J Surg*. 1993 Oct;36(5):453-60

Newsletter & Updates

Be alerted to new integrative clinical research and updates to this textbook by registering for the free newsletter, sent 4-6 times per year. Subscribe via www.OptimalHealthResearch.com/newsletter

Self-assessment and challenge questions:

These are sample questions and competencies that can be used as approximate standards of evaluation for students and clinicians. A more extensive sample is published in each new edition of *Integrative Orthopedics, Integrative Rheumatology,* and *Chiropractic and Naturopathic Mastery of Common Clinical Disorders*. To access the most recent complete list of questions and competencies, please go to http://OptimalHealthResearch.com/competencies.

For the following questions specific to the clinical management of hypertension, mark the single best answer for each of the following questions.

1) **A hypertensive patient with end-stage diabetic nephropathy who is treated with an ACE-inhibitor and spironolactone is most likely to suffer which of the following clinical effects as a result of increased intake of fruits and vegetables:**
   A. Hyper-reflexia and clonus
   B. Seizure or paresthesia
   C. Muscle weakness or cardiac arrest
   D. Headaches
   E. Water retention or carpal tunnel syndrome

2) **In a patient experiencing musculoskeletal pain as a result of taking an HMG-CoA reductase (3-hydroxy-3-methyl-glutaryl-CoA reductase) inhibiting drug for cardioprotection, which two nutrients are most likely to be of benefit:**
   A. EPA and DHA
   B. Magnesium and pyridoxine
   C. Ubiquinone and cholecalciferol
   D. Boswellia and Willow extract
   E. Vitamin E and vitamin A

3) **Renal artery stenosis typically occurs in which groups:**
   A. Older women and young children
   B. Young adult women and older men and women
   C. Older men and young adult men
   D. Adolescents and young adult men
   E. Older women and young adult men

4) **Which of the following two patient factors would probably contraindicate the initiation of cholecalciferol replacement with a starting dose of 300,000 IU administered as an intramuscular injection:**
   A. Multiple sclerosis and treatment with prednisone
   B. Fibromyalgia and treatment with Lyrica/ pregabalin
   C. Osteoarthritis and treatment with ibuprofen
   D. Sarcoidosis and treatment with hydrochlorothiazide
   E. Rheumatoid arthritis and treatment with methotrexate and sulfasalazine

5) **Which two antihypertensive nutrients are commonly dosed by determination of bowel tolerance:**
   A. Glutamine and arginine
   B. Vitamin E and selenium
   C. Magnesium and vitamin D
   D. Butyric acid and glutamine
   E. Vitamin C and magnesium

6) **Probenicid and allopurinol might be less necessary or unnecessary for hypertensive patients who avoid which of the following:**
   A. Tortillas baked with unsaturated fatty acids
   B. Wheat bread with a thick crust (resulting from the nonenzymatic glycosylation of lysine residues with a reducing sugar such as lactose or fructose)
   C. Cheese (full fat, from cow's milk)
   D. Aspartame
   E. Corn syrup

7) **Vitamin D3 deficiency causes a specific biochemical-physiologic effect on ion/mineral imbalance within cells due, to a significant degree, to elevated levels of parathyroid hormone. Which of the following drugs most directly offsets this imbalance:**
   A. Furosemide
   B. Amlodipine
   C. Spironolactone
   D. Metoprolol
   E. Lisinopril

8) **As an antihypertensive therapy, fasting lowers blood pressure by which mechanism:**
   A. Increased nocturnal production of melatonin
   B. Increased cortisol sensitivity
   C. Reduced estradiol levels
   D. Reduced insulin levels
   E. Elevated prolactin levels

9) **In a young adult unmedicated hypertensive patient with hyperkalemia and a normal serum creatinine, which of the following tests is required in the next step of the evaluation:**
   A. MRI of the pituitary gland
   B. Serum aldosterone and renin
   C. Serum dehydroepiandrosterone sulfate
   D. Serum reverse triiodothyronine
   E. Serum free thyroxine

10) **Your patient with hypertension is found to have a serum creatinine of 1.8 mg/dl. Which of the following treatments must be discontinued:**
    A. Vitamin D3
    B. Furosemide
    C. L-thyroxine
    D. Metformin
    E. Amlodipine

11) **Which of the following conditions is best known for causing pulmonary hypertension and systemic malignant hypertension as a lethal consequence:**
    A. Systemic sclerosis
    B. Dermatomyositis
    C. Fibromyalgia
    D. Rheumatoid arthritis
    E. Eosinophilic fasciitis

12) **Upper cervical spine subluxation treated with chiropractic manipulation is causally associated with hypertension via which mechanism:**
    1. Sympathetic activation due to pain
    2. Pain causes sympathetic activation and sodium-water retention
    3. Brainstem compression
    4. Basilar invagination
    5. Tentorial herniation
    A. 3,4,5
    B. 2,3,4
    C. 1,2,3
    D. 1,4,5
    E. 2,4,5

13) **Accurate determination of thyroid status includes:**
   A.   Laboratory assessment of TSH is sufficient
   B.   Laboratory assessment of TSH along with monitoring response to therapy with triiodothyronine
   C.   Laboratory assessment of free T4 along with monitoring response to therapy with thyroxine
   D.   Laboratory assessment of free T4 and serum cortisol
   E.   Laboratory assessment of serum testosterone and serum triiodothyronine
   F.   Laboratory assessment of TSH, free T4, antithyroid antibodies, T3:rT3 ratio along with monitoring response to hormone therapy

14) **Which of the following comorbidity patterns suggests vitamin D3 deficiency as a cause of hypertension:**
   A.   Peripheral arthropathy and clonus
   B.   Generalized musculoskeletal pain, migraine, and insulin resistance
   C.   Nonfocal muscle weakness and cardiac arrhythmia
   D.   Diarrhea, tachycardia, and exophthalmos
   E.   Generalized musculoskeletal pain, hyperreflexia, and constipation

15) **Normal body mass index (BMI) is:**
   A.   16-21
   B.   17-22
   C.   18-24
   D.   19-27
   E.   20-28

16) **Per published reviews, the optimal range for serum 25-hydroxy-cholecalciferol is:**
   A.   20-80 ng/ml
   B.   20-80 pg/ml
   C.   50-90 pg/ml
   D.   50-100 ng/ml
   E.   50-100 pg/ml

17) **Which components of the Mediterranean diet are not included in the Paleo diet:**
   A.   Citrus fruit
   B.   Lean meats and fish
   C.   Whole grains
   D.   Leafy green vegetables
   E.   Nuts and seeds

18) **During a water-only fast, if a patient becomes confabulated and does not respond to consumption of a large glass of orange juice, then the problem probably is related to:**
   A.   Magnesium
   B.   Bicarbonate
   C.   Potassium
   D.   Sodium
   E.   Calcium

19) **Intermittent, pulsatile compression of which of the following is most important for the genesis of central neurogenic hypertension?**
   A.   Afferent vagus fibers and nuclei, especially on the right
   B.   Nucleus tractus solitarius
   C.   Efferent vagus fibers and nuclei, especially on the left
   D.   Nucleus accumbens
   E.   Left anterolateral pons

20) **Responding to your newspaper advertisement offering headache treatment, a 75-yo type-2 diabetic new patient in your outpatient office on Thursday afternoon has a blood pressure of 170/120 mm Hg, anisocoria, papilledema, and is alert and oriented x2. Prior-to-visit lab tests performed the previous day show a hemoglobin a1c 10%, serum creatine 1.8 mg/dL, and serum BNP (brain natriuretic peptide) 600 pg/ml. Prior medical and social history reveals widower x6 months, hypothyroidism, and no other prior surgical or medical history. What is the best management strategy:**
   A. Implement the Paleo-Mediterranean diet and appropriate manipulative and mind-body treatments
   B. Implement the Paleo-Mediterranean diet and mind-body treatments, but defer manipulative treatment
   C. Return office visit on Monday to see if the blood pressure is starting to show improvement and if the anisocoria is resolved
   D. Call for an ambulance; admit to hospital urgent care department
   E. Perform appropriate laboratory tests and review with patient (perhaps via phone or brief office visit) the following day (Friday) to ensure patient safety over the weekend
   F. Arrange for nursing care at home
   G. Transfer the patient to a skilled nursing facility

21) **Given that effective nondrug treatment for chronic hypertension can involve lifestyle modification, diet optimization, exercise prescription, nutritional supplementation, manual manipulation of articular structures and soft tissues, and mind-body therapies, which of the following professional groups is LEAST TRAINED to provide nondrug care.**
   A. Allopathic doctors (MD)
   B. Osteopathic doctors (DO)
   C. Chiropractic doctors (DC)
   D. Naturopathic doctors (ND)

22) **Following the use of a specific chiropractic manipulative technique that results in blood pressure reduction, other changes in musculoskeletal structure have been noted. Which pattern of changes follows the cervical spine manipulation and correlates with reduced blood pressure?**
   A. Atlas lateral and rotational positioning (measured by the pre- and post-treatment radiographs), rotational displacement of C-7 through T-5, sagittal-plane pelvic distortion
   B. Lateral displacement of C-7, frontal-plane pelvic distortion, and lateral-plane pelvic distortion, reduction in foot pronation and thus internal rotation of the femur and tibia
   C. Atlas lateral and rotational positioning (measured by the pre- and post-treatment radiographs), lateral displacement of C-7, frontal-plane pelvic distortion, and lateral-plane pelvic distortion
   D. Atlas lateral and rotational positioning (measured by the pre- and post-treatment radiographs), rotational displacement of C-7 through T-5, frontal-plane pelvic distortion, and lateral-plane pelvic distortion

23) **Which manipulative technique has been shown to have a favorable effect on hypertension in a randomized clinical trial of sufficient power to detect statistical and clinical significance?**
   A. Gonstead technique
   B. Diversified technique
   C. Activator technique
   D. Strain and counterstrain (aka: Jones technique)
   E. McKinsey technique
   F. National Upper Cervical Chiropractic Association technique
   G. Active release technique (ART)

24) **Regarding the treatment of hypertension with coenzyme Q-10, which of the following lists the anticipated collateral benefits as supported by clinical research?**
      1. Antioxidant benefits (in addition to inhibition of nuclear transcription factor kappaB)
      2. Improved glucose control and lipid metabolism
      3. Anti-migraine benefit via mitochondrial resuscitation
      4. Renopreservation and renorestoration
  A. 1,3,4
  B. 2,3,4
  C. 1,2,3,4
  D. 1,2

25) **Which of the following antihypertensive drugs provides the secondary benefit of increased renal excretion of uric acid?**
  A. Hydrochlorothiazide
  B. Lisinopril
  C. Clonidine
  D. Amlodipine
  E. Metoprolol
  F. Losartan

26) **Which of the following premanipulative positions most closely resembles the spinal manipulative treatment causally associated with a clinically and statistically significant sustained reduction in blood pressure among hypertensives?**
  A. The premanipulative tension and the therapeutic impulse are established and delivered through the contact hand and the doctor's caudad leg which has compressive contact with the patient's flexed leg.
  B. Body-drop thrust generally superiorly and laterally in the direction of the patient's opposite shoulder; the angle of the thrust changes depending on the spinal-costal level being treated, with more superior segments requiring a more superiorly directed thrust, while lower segments require a progressively laterally-yet-sagittally directed thrust.
  C. Rotational tension is applied and focused at the lumbar spinal segment being treated. Thoracic rotation and lateral flexion are minimized to the extent possible. Modest lumbar lateral flexion toward the table helps to gap the inferior articular process of the superior segment from the superior articular process of the inferior segment.
  D. Lateral flexion at the targeted cervical segment; the slightest amount of contralateral rotation is applied. The doctor establishes an "index" contact on the posterolateral aspect of the cervical vertebrae (i.e., the "paravertebral gutter").

27) **Per the US FDA, antihypertensive efficacy is defined as a placebo-subtracted reduction in diastolic BP of 4-5 mm Hg or more. Which of the following treatments exceeds this criteria according to available clinical data:**
      1. CoQ10 100 mg
      2. Vitamin D3 1000 IU
      3. Ascorbic acid 2000 mg
      4. Milk peptides fermented with *Lactobacillus helveticus*
      5. Extracts from *Theobroma cacao*
      6. Short-term fasting followed by implementation of the Paleo-Mediterranean diet

  A. 1,2,3,4,5 but not 6
  B. 1,3,4,6 but not 2,5
  C. 3,4, but not 1,2,5,6
  D. 2,4,5 but not 1,3,6
  E. 1,2,3,4,6 but not 5

28) **Which of the following would be most appropriate (indicated) and most inappropriate (contraindicated) for a patient with hypertension-induced renal insufficiency with GFR <40:**
1. CoQ10 100 mg
2. Vitamin D3 1000 IU
3. Ascorbic acid 2000 mg
4. Milk peptides fermented with *Lactobacillus helveticus*
5. Extracts from *Theobroma cacao*
6. Short-term fasting followed by implementation of the Paleo-Mediterranean diet

    A. 1 and 2 are indicated; 3 and 6 are contraindicated
    B. 3 and 6 are indicated; 1 and 5 are contraindicated
    C. 4 and 6 are indicated; 3 and 5 are contraindicated
    D. 5 and 6 are indicated; 2 and 4 are contraindicated
    E. 1 and 6 are indicated; 2 and 4 are contraindicated

29) **Which of the following therapeutic interventions is most likely to exacerbate hyperkalemia in a patient treated with lisinopril who also has renal insufficiency?**
1. CoQ10 100 mg
2. Vitamin D3 1000 IU
3. Ascorbic acid 2000 mg
4. Milk peptides fermented with *Lactobacillus helveticus*
5. Extracts from *Theobroma cacao*
6. Short-term fasting followed by implementation of the Paleo-Mediterranean diet

    A. 6 and 1
    B. 6 and 2
    C. 6 and 3
    D. 6 and 4
    E. 6 and 5

30) **What percentage of drug-treated hypertensive patients discontinues treatment by the end of the first year?**
    A. 10%
    B. 25%
    C. 50%
    D. 75%
    E. 90%

31) **Laboratory indicators of which of the following would be expected to increase/decrease following dietary modifications that counteract asymptomatic gastrointestinal dysbiosis?**
    A. NF-kappaB activity would increase; serum lipopolysaccharides will decrease; lactulose:mannitol ratio will decrease
    B. NF-kappaB activity would decrease; serum lipopolysaccharides will decrease; lactulose:mannitol ratio will decrease
    C. NF-kappaB activity would increase; serum lipopolysaccharides will decrease; lactulose:mannitol ratio will increase
    D. NF-kappaB activity would decrease; serum lipopolysaccharides will decrease; lactulose:mannitol ratio will decrease
    E. NF-kappaB activity would increase; serum lipopolysaccharides will increase; lactulose:mannitol ratio will increase

32) **Identify the best indicators of nutritional compliance for the "typical" patient with metabolic syndrome.**
    A. RBC magnesium and urinary calcium
    B. Serum cholesterol and CRP
    C. BMI and serum 25-hydroxy-vitamin D
    D. Weight loss and serum 1,25-dihydroxy-vitamin D3
    E. Serum carotenoids and RBC magnesium

33) **Which of the following medications is most appropriate for an asymptomatic patient with blood pressure of 200/110 mm Hg?**
    A. Oral captopril and oral clonidine
    B. Oral captopril and oral hydrochlorothiazide
    C. Oral captopril and oral furosemide
    D. Oral furosemide and oral hydrochlorothiazide
    E. Intravenous furosemide and Intravenous clonidine

34) **Which of the following medications is most appropriate for an asymptomatic patient with new pulmonary rales, 2+ pitting edema of the lower extremities, and a point-of-care O2 saturation of 89% with blood pressure of 200/110 mm Hg?**
    A. Furosemide
    B. Hydrochlorothiazide
    C. Losartan
    D. Spironolactone
    E. Lisinopril

35) **Which of the following medications and doses is most appropriate for a patient with chest pain and blood pressure of 200/110 mm Hg?**
    A. Intravenous captopril
    B. Intravenous hydrochlorothiazide
    C. Intravenous hydralazine
    D. Intravenous furosemide
    E. Oral losartan

36) **The most common reason for antihypertensive therapeutic inefficacy is:**
    A. Lack of scientific basis
    B. Patient noncompliance
    C. Unreasonable expectations created by exaggerated claims made by drug companies
    D. Lack of physicians' awareness of more comprehensive treatment plans that address the underlying causes of hypertension and that improve therapeutic efficacy in a wide range of patients with varying psychographics, demographics, and comorbidities.
    E. B and D

37) **Discontinuation of which treatment is most likely to cause severe rebound hypertension?**
    A. Magnesium 500 mg bid
    B. Metformin 500 mg bid
    C. Metoprolol 50 mg bid
    D. Mahonia aquifolium (berberine dose 500 mg bid)
    E. Methylcobalamin 500 mcg bid

38) **What percentage of patients with hyperaldosteronemia have normal serum aldosterone levels, thereby requiring testing with the more sensitive aldosterone:renin ratio?**
    A. 0%
    B. 25%
    C. 50%
    D. 75%
    E. 100%

39) **What is the most common documented cause of HTN in children and adolescents?**
    A. Pheochromocytoma
    B. Kidney disease
    C. Adrenal hyperplasia
    D. Stress
    E. Food allergies and intolerances

40) **Consumption of which foods/nutrients are most likely to require more frequent monitoring of a patient's routine INR (international normalized ratio)?**
   A. Gamma-tocopherol and whole-grain breads
   B. Collard greens and ubiquinone
   C. Cholecalciferol and zinc
   D. Dihomo-gamma-linolenic acid and fermented whey peptides
   E. Fermentable oligosacharides and whole-fruit (including the peel) apple juice

41) **Acetyl-L-carnitine increases levels of _____ and thereby results in _____ metabolic/physiologic effects.**
   A. Heat-shock protein; enhanced proteasome
   B. Leptin; vasodilatory
   C. Telomerase; apoptosis
   D. Adiponectin; vasculoprotective
   E. Aldosterone; diuretic

42) **The major source of health education in America is:**
   A. Health and nutrition courses delivered in high school (secondary school).
   B. Medical physicians with training in exercise and nutrition.
   C. Drug companies advertising their products.
   D. Private monthly consultations averaging >2 hours per month (for slightly more than 30 hours per year) with non-allopathic professionals with training in diet, exercise, nutrition, and relationship skills.
   E. Government-employed health counselors.

Index

Now, once more!

"Whoever has really gazed down with an Asiatic and super-Asiatic eye into the most world denying of all possible modes of thought—beyond good and evil—and no longer like Buddha and Schopenhauer under the spell and illusion of morality; perhaps by this very act, without really desiring it, may have opened his eyes to the opposite ideal: the ideal of the most high spirited, energetic, and world affirming man, who has not only learned to come to terms with and assimilate with what it was and is, but who wants to have it again as it was and is to all eternity, insatiably calling out "once more!""

Nietzsche FW. *Beyond Good and Evil*. Essay #56.

Newsletter & Updates

Be alerted to new integrative clinical research and updates to this textbook by signing-up for the free newsletter, sent 6-8 times per year. Contact
newsletter@optimalhealthresearch.com
or
www.OptimalHealthResearch.com/newsletter